SPORTS NUTRITION

Energy Metabolism and Exercise

EDITED BY

IRA WOLINSKY
JUDY A. DRISKELL

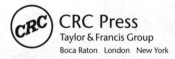

CRC Press
Taylor & Francis Group
Boca Raton   London   New York

CRC Press is an imprint of the
Taylor & Francis Group, an **informa** business

CRC Press
Taylor & Francis Group
6000 Broken Sound Parkway NW, Suite 300
Boca Raton, FL 33487-2742

© 2008 by Taylor & Francis Group, LLC
CRC Press is an imprint of Taylor & Francis Group, an Informa business

No claim to original U.S. Government works
Printed in the United States of America on acid-free paper
10 9 8 7 6 5 4 3 2 1

International Standard Book Number-13: 978-0-8493-7950-5 (Hardcover)

Library of Congress Cataloging-in-Publication Data

Sports nutrition : energy metabolism and exercise / editors, Ira Wolinsky and
  Judy A. Driskell.
       p. ; cm.
  "A CRC title."
  Includes bibliographical references and index.
  ISBN 978-0-8493-7950-5 (alk. paper)
  1. Energy metabolism. 2. Exercise. I. Wolinsky, Ira. II. Driskell, Judy A. (Judy
Anne)
  [DNLM: 1. Energy Metabolism--physiology. 2. Nutrition Physiology. 3. Sports
Medicine. QU 125 S764 2008]
  QP176.S69 2008
  612.3'9--dc22

                                                                              2007017738

Visit the Taylor & Francis Web site at
http://www.taylorandfrancis.com

and the CRC Press Web site at
http://www.crcpress.com

Dedication

We appreciate the opportunity to have worked with the chapter authors, experts all, on this book and on our other books in the area of sports nutrition. We learned from them and dedicate this book to them.

Contents

SECTION 1   Energy-Yielding Nutrients

SECTION 2   Estimation of Energy Requirements

SECTION 3   Physiological Aspects of Energy
Metabolism

Preface

Over recent years, in a close and fruitful collaboration, we have put together a number of books in the area of sports nutrition. During this period we have seen a burgeoning of interest in the area, namely: increased research, new journals, new courses at universities, new professional groups and, of course, new publications such as this one. In this book on energy metabolism and exercise we provide the reader in-depth exploration of important topics that will be of interest to health and nutrition professionals of all walks, as well as the well informed and motivated layman. What is clear from this book and others we have edited is that there must be a range of diets and exercise regimens that will support excellent physical condition and performance. There is not a single diet–exercise treatment that can be the common denominator, and no single formula for health or performance panacea.

Companions to this book are other volumes we edited: Sports Nutrition: Vitamins and Trace Elements, second edition; Nutritional Ergogenic Aids; Nutritional Assessment of Athletes; Nutritional Applications in Exercise and Sport; Energy-Yielding Macronutrients and Energy Metabolism in Sports Nutrition; Macroelements, Water, and Electrolytes in Sports Nutrition. Additionally useful will be the third edition of Nutrition in Exercise and Sport, edited by Ira Wolinsky, and Sports Nutrition, authored by Judy Driskell. Enjoy.

Ira Wolinsky, Ph.D.
Professor Emeritus
University of Houston

Judy A. Driskell, Ph.D., R.D.
Professor
University of Nebraska

The Editors

Ira Wolinsky, Ph.D., is professor emeritus of Nutrition at the University of Houston. He received his B.S. degree in chemistry from the City College of New York and his M.S. and Ph.D. degrees in biochemistry from the University of Kansas. He has served in research and teaching positions at the Hebrew University, the University of Missouri, and The Pennsylvania State University, and has conducted basic research in NASA life sciences facilities and abroad.

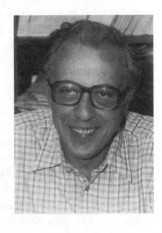

Dr. Wolinsky is a member of the American Society for Nutrition, among other honorary and scientific organizations. He has contributed numerous nutrition research papers in the open literature. His major research interests relate to the nutrition of bone and calcium and trace elements and to sports nutrition. He has been the recipient of research grants from both public and private sources and has been the recipient of several international research fellowships and consultantships to the former Soviet Union, Bulgaria, Hungary, and India. He merited a Fulbright Senior Scholar Fellowship to Greece in 1999.

Dr. Wolinsky has co-authored a book on the history of the science of nutrition, *Nutrition and Nutritional Diseases.* He co-edited *Sports Nutrition: Vitamins and Trace Elements,* first and second editions; *Macroelements, Water, and Electrolytes in Sports Nutrition; Energy-Yielding Macronutrients and Energy Metabolism in Sports Nutrition; Nutritional Applications in Exercise and Sport, Nutritional Assessment of Athletes, Nutritional Ergogenic Aids,* and the current book *Sports Nutrition: Energy Metabolism and Exercise,* all with Judy Driskell. Additionally, he co-edited *Nutritional Concerns of Women,* two editions, with Dorothy Klimis-Zacas; *The Mediterranean Diet: Constituents and Health Promotion* with his Greek colleagues; and *Nutrition in Pharmacy Practice* with Louis Williams. He edited three editions of *Nutrition in Exercise and Sport.* He served also as the editor, or co-editor, for the CRC Series on Nutrition in Exercise and Sport, the CRC Series on Modern Nutrition, the CRC Series on Methods in Nutritional Research, and the CRC Series on Exercise Physiology.

Judy Anne Driskell, Ph.D., R.D. is professor of nutrition and health sciences at the University of Nebraska. She received her B.S. degree in biology from the University of Southern Mississippi in Hattiesburg, and her M.S. and Ph.D. degrees were obtained from Purdue University. She has served in research and teaching positions at Auburn University, Florida State University, Virginia Polytechnic Institute and State University, and the University of Nebraska. She has also served as the nutrition scientist for the U.S. Department of Agriculture/Cooperative State Research Service and as a professor of nutrition and food science at Gadjah Mada and Bogor Universities in Indonesia.

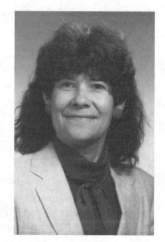

Dr. Driskell is a member of numerous professional organizations including the American Society for Nutrition, the American College of Sports Medicine, the International Society of Sports Nutrition, the Institute of Food Technologists, and the American Dietetic Association. In 1993 she received the Professional Scientist Award of the Food Science and Human Nutrition Section of the Southern Association of Agricultural Scientists. In addition, she was the 1987 recipient of the Borden Award for Research in Applied Fundamental Knowledge of Human Nutrition. She is listed as an expert in B-complex vitamins by the Vitamin Nutrition Information Service.

Dr. Driskell co-edited the CRC books *Sports Nutrition: Minerals and Electrolytes* with Constance V. Kies. In addition, she authored the textbook *Sports Nutrition* and co-authored an advanced nutrition book, *Nutrition: Chemistry and Biology*, both published by CRC. She co-edited *Sports Nutrition: Vitamins and Trace Elements*, first and second editions; *Macroelements; Water, and Electrolytes in Sports Nutrition*; *Energy-Yielding Macronutrients and Energy Metabolism in Sports Nutrition*; *Nutritional Applications in Exercise and Sport*, *Nutritional Assessment of Athletes*, *Nutritional Ergogenic Aids*, and the current book *Sports Nutrition: Energy Metabolism and Exercise*, all with Ira Wolinsky. She has published more than 150 refereed research articles and 13 book chapters as well as several publications intended for lay audiences and has given numerous presentations to professional and lay groups. Her current research interests center around vitamin metabolism and requirements, including the interrelationships between exercise and water-soluble vitamin requirements.

Contributors

Barbara E. Ainsworth,
Ph.D., M.P.H., F.A.C.S.M.
Department of Exercise and Wellness
Arizona State University
Mesa, Arizona

Barry Braun, Ph.D.
Department of Kinesiology
University of Massachusetts
Amherst, Massachusetts

Mauro Di Pasquale, M.D.
CEO, MetabolicDiet.com &
  MDNCC.com
Cobourg, Ontario

J. Andrew Doyle, Ph.D.
Department of Kinesiology and Health
Georgia State University
Atlanta, Georgia

Judy A. Driskell, Ph.D., R.D.
Department of Nutrition and Health
  Sciences
University of Nebraska
Lincoln, Nebraska

J. Larry Durstine, Ph.D., F.A.C.S.M.,
F.A.A.C.V.P.R.
Department of Exercise Science
University of South Carolina
Columbia, South Carolina

Daniel D. Gallaher, Ph.D.
Department of Food Science and
  Nutrition
University of Minnesota
St. Paul, Minnesota

Michael S. Green, M.S.
Department of Kinesiology and Health
Georgia State University
Atlanta, Georgia

Jena G. Hamra, Ph.D.
Department of Biological and
  Environmental Sciences
Texas A&M University–Commerce
Commerce, Texas

G. William Lyerly, M.S., C.S.C.S.,
H.F.I., E.S.
Department of Exercise Science
University of South Carolina
Columbia, South Carolina

Amy C. Maher, M.S.
Department of Medical Science
McMaster University Medical Center
Hamilton, Ontario

Melinda M. Manore, Ph.D., R.D.
Department of Nutrition and Exercise
  Sciences
Oregon State University
Corvallis, Oregon

Robert G. McMurray, Ph.D.
Department of Exercise and Sport
  Science
University of North Carolina at Chapel
  Hill
Chapel Hill, North Carolina

Benjamin F. Miller, Ph.D.
Department of Health and Exercise
  Science
Colorado State University
Fort Collins, Colorado

Jonathan A. Moore, B.S.
Department of Exercise Science
University of South Carolina
Columbia, South Carolina

Kristin S. Ondrak, M.S.
Department of Exercise and Sport
  Science
University of North Carolina
  at Chapel Hill
Chapel Hill, North Carolina

Charilaos Papadopoulos, Ph.D.
Department of Health, Human
  Performance and Nutrition
Central Washington University
Ellensburg, Washington

Kelley K. Pettee, Ph.D.
Department of Exercise and Wellness
Arizona State University
Mesa, Arizona

Mark A. Tarnopolsky, M.D., Ph.D.
Department of Pediatrics and Medicine
McMaster University Medical Centre
Hamilton, Ontario

**Janice L. Thompson, Ph.D.,
F.A.C.S.M.**
Department of Sport, Exercise
  and Health Sciences
University of Bristol
Bristol, U.K.

**Catrine Tudor-Locke, Ph.D.,
F.A.C.S.M**
Department of Exercise and Wellness
Arizona State University
Mesa, Arizona

**Serge P. von Duvillard, Ph.D.,
F.A.C.S.M., F.E.C.S.S.**
Department of Health and Human
  Performance Biological Sciences
Texas A&M University—Commerce
Commerce, Texas

Ira Wolinsky, Ph.D.
Department of Health and Human
  Performance
University of Houston
Houston, Texas

1 Introduction to Sports Nutrition: Energy Metabolism

Barry Braun and Benjamin F. Miller

CONTENTS

I. INTRODUCTION

The interplay between nutrition and physical activity is as frequently misunderstood as the relationship between industrialization and global climate; most people tend to either underemphasize ("as long as I get enough exercise I can eat whatever I want") or overemphasize ("each mouthful of food must conform to rigid requirements") the importance of nutrition to exercise performance. Making sound nutritional choices does not guarantee athletic prowess but consistently making poor choices almost certainly constrains performance. More specifically, sound nutrition is necessary to effectively train and take advantage of training stimuli. From the

1

1920s studies of high carbohydrate versus high fat diets on exercise performance by Krogh and Lindhard[1] through the 1960s glycogen supercompensation studies of Bergstrom and Hultman,[2] to the more recent studies of post-exercise protein feeding on muscle protein synthesis,[3] it is clear that total energy and the macronutrient (i.e., carbohydrate, fat, protein) composition of the diet modulate acute exercise performance and adaptations to training. Understanding how energy is produced and how the demand for energy during exercise drives energy utilization is critical to recommending appropriate dietary choices to replace that energy and refuel for the next exercise bout. The goal of this chapter is to outline these basic principles of energy metabolism and introduce the concepts that will be reviewed in more depth in later chapters.

II. ENERGY TRANSDUCTION

A. GENERAL PRINCIPLES OF BIOENERGETICS

Bioenergetics refers to the Laws of Thermodynamics as applied to biological systems. The first law, that energy cannot be created or destroyed but is transferred between the system and its surroundings, implies that energy flow into the body must balance energy flow out of the body plus or minus energy storage. In the simplest sense, the flow of energy into the body comes from the diet and energy flow out is primarily determined by basal energy requirements and physical activity. Changes in storage are primarily reflected, at least over the long term, by increases or decreases in body fat. Of course, in reality, the flow of energy is a bit more complicated.

The human system, like the systems of most other taxa, has devised mechanisms to store energy. This storage frees the body from the demands of continuously adding energy to the system. Macronutrients in foods contain energy-rich chemical bonds. After digestion and absorption, the energy is stored as chemical bonds in triglyceride (fat), in glycogen (carbohydrate) and, arguably, in skeletal muscle (protein). This stored chemical bond energy is what is used to perform work. In this sense, human energy metabolism is similar to an internal combustion engine wherein energy substrates enter (food or gasoline), are combusted, and heat and work are produced. Metabolic energy is quantified in units of kilocalories (kcal, 1000 calories) and kilojoules (kJ, 1000 joules) or megajoules (MJ, 1000 kJ).

Although the idea of continuously eating without storing energy sounds appealing, it really does not leave much room for anything else in life. Golden-crowned kinglets, tiny (5 grams) birds that inhabit the northeastern United States, eat almost constantly during daylight hours to match their exceptionally high basal metabolic rate and store enough body fat to survive the night. In the winter, kinglets can starve to death after 24 hours without food. The human species is adapted to survive in the face of intermittent food availability, i.e., periods when food is abundant followed by periods of scarcity. Therefore, the efficient storage of food energy in periods of abundance is a metabolic priority. The consequences of maintaining efficient energy storage when food is consistently plentiful has been blamed for the epidemic of obesity and obesity-related diseases in many "Westernized" countries.

B. ENERGY-YIELDING PATHWAYS

The energy-yielding pathways are roughly subdivided into those that require oxygen and those that do not. The ultimate outcome of all the pathways is to convert chemical bond energy in macronutrients to adenosine triphosphate (ATP), the only chemical form of energy the body can use to perform work.

Because ATP storage in the body is severely limited (to provide sufficient energy for an "average" day the supply of ATP is broken down and regenerated around 5000 times a day), there must be storage forms of energy that can be rapidly activated and can respond to changes in energy demand (Figure 1.1). Phosphocreatine (PCr) serves as the most rapidly accessible form of energy "storage." The enzyme creatine kinase (CK) catalyzes a reaction that results in the transfer of a phosphate group from PCr to adenosine diphosphate (ADP) to form ATP. The reaction proceeds quickly in the presence of PCr or ADP and requires no oxygen but is limited by the low availability of PCr. During rapid high-intensity exercise PCr stores are depleted in a few seconds and therefore need to be replenished during a recovery period.

The other non-oxygen-requiring pathway, which is specific to carbohydrate metabolism, is called glycolysis. Glucose molecules freed by breakdown of stored muscle glycogen or entering the muscle cell from the blood via a cellular glucose transport protein (and ultimately derived from breakdown of glycogen stored in the liver) enter the glycolytic pathways. Glycolysis is a series of reactions with an overall favorable free energy change (i.e., there is a net liberation of stored energy) in which the 6-carbon glucose unit is split into 3-carbon units called pyruvate with a net gain of 2 ATP. The pyruvate has several potentials; it can be oxidized within the cell, exported from muscle and taken up by heart or other muscle cells for oxidation, or assembled back into glucose by the liver. Glycolysis has a relatively quick onset compared with aerobic respiration (discussed later). It provides the bulk of energy

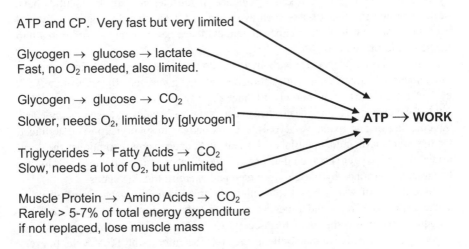

FIGURE 1.1 Schematic drawing showing highlights of the systems used to generate the ATP required to accomplish cellular work.

in the first few minutes of exercise and during sustained exercise at moderate to high intensity (e.g., at greater than about 60% of maximal aerobic capacity).

A very recent hypothesis proposed by Shulman suggests that glycogen breakdown plays an even larger role than previously thought; studies done using magnetic resonance spectroscopy over millisecond time scales suggest that all of the glucose entering the cell, even during exercise, "cycles" through glycogen before entering glycolysis.[4] This theory implies that glycogen breakdown during each muscle contraction is countered by glycogen synthesis between contractions and that the rate of glycogen use is actually the net result of repeating cycles of glycogen breakdown and resynthesis occurring too fast to be seen by more conventional techniques.

Another deviation from the conventional wisdom regarding glycolysis has been the transformation of lactate (a.k.a lactic acid) from metabolic waste product to key energy intermediate.[5] Decades of work by George Brooks and colleagues has generated almost universal acceptance regarding the importance of lactate produced by muscle during exercise as a source of oxidizable energy for neighboring muscle fibers and the heart, and as a key precursor for the synthesis of new glucose by the liver.[5] In addition, biochemistry texts present the pathway of glycolysis as ending with pyruvate; with the pyruvate entering the tricarboxylic acid (TCA) cycle. Although few authors still believe that lactate formation during exercise is caused by lack of oxygen (anaerobiosis), the prevailing viewpoint is that the production of lactate is "initiated" when the rate of glycolysis exceeds the rate of oxidative phosphorylation. This latter view is being re-examined in light of evidence suggesting the existence of an intracellular lactate shuttle.[6,7] In this scheme, lactate is the end product of glycolysis and is moved across the mitochondrial membrane for oxidative phosphorylation. The key components necessary for the cytosolic conversion of pyruvate to lactate, lactate transport into the mitochondria, and the mitochondrial conversion of lactate to pyruvate, have all been identified.[6,8] Although the shuttle hypothesis is gaining experimental evidence in muscle, and similar shuttles have been identified in other tissues such as the brain,[9] it still has not gained universal acceptance and awaits further experimental evidence before being incorporated into the scientific mainstream.[10]

Glycolysis is a gateway for carbohydrate into oxidative phosphorylation in muscle mitochondria. Oxidative phosphorylation refers to the combined processes of the TCA cycle and the electron transport chain. Since glycolysis is more rapidly activated than oxidative phosphorylation and can exceed the oxidative capacity of local mitochondria, the coupling of non-oxidative glycolysis to oxidative phosphorylation is determined by the number of mitochondria in the cell and, under some conditions, the local availability of oxygen. Oxygen delivery and the number of mitochondria will in turn be largely determined by muscle fiber type and exercise training status.

Regardless of whether pyruvate enters the mitochondrial matrix as pyruvate or as lactate, once there, it undergoes oxidative decarboxylation by the pyruvate dehydrogenase enzyme complex to form acetyl-CoA. Acetyl-CoA is an important conversion point in oxidative metabolism since it is the entry to the TCA cycle. In every revolution of the cycle, two carbons enter as acetyl-CoA and two carbons leave as CO_2, and one high-energy phosphate molecule (GTP) is produced. The big payoff, however, is the generation of one molecule of $FADH_2$ and three molecules of NADH that are made in every turn of the cycle. These molecules donate electrons to the electron transport chain, the site where the lion's share of ATP is produced.

The electron transport chain is a microcosm of the complexity and functionality of systems design. In this process electrons given up by the energy-rich electron carriers, NADH and $FADH_2$, are sequentially transferred by a series of four protein complexes (three in the case of $FADH_2$) and two mobile electron carriers. The energetically favorable passage of these electrons through the chain is aided by three of the complexes which are also enzymes; NADH dehydrogenase (Complex I), cytochrome c reductase (Complex III), and cytochrome c oxidase (Complex IV). The final step in the chain is for pairs of electrons to reduce molecular oxygen to water, hence the familiar designation of oxygen as the "terminal electron acceptor". The enzyme complexes also function as pumps which move protons from the mitochondrial matrix to the inter-mitochondrial membrane space. The pumping of these protons creates an electrochemical gradient across the inner mitochondrial membrane (the energy contained in the separation of positive and negative charges is similar to the potential energy contained in a lake being held back by a dam). The potential energy generated by the pumping of protons can be exploited by allowing the protons to fall back across the membrane. In the lake/dam analogy, energy liberated by water spilling out of the dam is harnessed when the flowing water turns a turbine. In the electron transport chain the protons can only fall back across the membrane through an additional complex called ATP synthase. ATP synthase uses the net change in free energy to phosphorylate ADP to ATP. The oxidation of NADH to NAD^+ results in the pumping of six H^+ (two at each enzyme pump), which creates enough energy for the phosphorylation of three ADP to ATP. In the case of $FADH_2$, two ATP are created from the transport chain. The total energy extracted from the complete oxidation of one glucose in the TCA cycle and electron transport chain is 36-37 ATP, depending on whether the glucose was derived from the blood or from muscle glycogen.

As well as being the entry point to the TCA cycle, Acetyl-CoA is the point at which fat and carbohydrate metabolism converge. As opposed to carbohydrate utilization, garnering energy from the utilization of fat can only proceed in the presence of oxygen. Once free fatty acids gain entry to the cell, they are transported to the outer mitochondrial membrane, are activated by the addition of CoA to form fatty acyl-CoA and transported into the mitochondria by the enzymes carnitine palmitoyl transferase I and II. At this point, the fatty acyl-CoA undergoes sequential breakdown to 2-carbon acetyl-CoA units by the process of β-oxidation for entry into the TCA cycle. From here, the pathways leading to ATP production are identical. Because fatty acids usually contain more carbon atoms than does glucose, more ATP are derived from their oxidation. The "typical" fatty acid palmitate contains 16 carbons and generates 129 net ATP when fully oxidized. Although oxidation of fatty acids is a minor component of energy expenditure early in exercise, or during exercise at high intensity (>80% maximal aerobic capacity), sustained exercise at low or moderate intensities would be impossible without a substantial contribution of energy from fat oxidation. The use of intra- and extracellular carbohydrate and lipid energy sources is depicted in Figure 2.

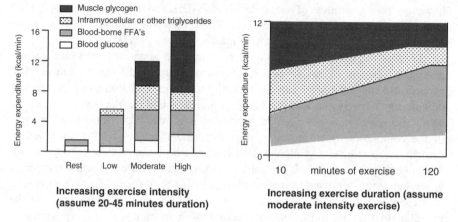

FIGURE 1.2 Opposing effects of exercise intensity and duration on carbohydrate and fat oxidation (FFA = free fatty acids).

Although prevailing wisdom holds that protein, in the form of amino acids, is a relatively minor contributor to exercise energy expenditure, some portion of total energy expenditure (generally 3–6%) is derived from oxidation of amino acids. Amino acids, in particular the branched-chain amino acids leucine, isoleucine and valine, can enter the energy-yielding pathways as pyruvate, acetyl Co-A or at several other points in the TCA cycle. During prolonged exercise, especially when glycogen stores are low, the contribution of amino acids to exercise energy expenditure can exceed 10%. Unlike carbohydrate and fat energy, which are stored in forms that have few structural or functional roles (although even this truism may be revised as a role for glycogen in cell signaling is being elucidated), all body proteins have functions beyond energy storage. The intermittent synthesis and breakdown of skeletal muscle in response to feeding and fasting indicates that skeletal muscle is a storage site for protein. Some would argue, however, that transamination and excretion of excess nitrogen indicate that protein is not stored. The use of protein as an energy source must be repaid by dietary protein or the consequence is a loss of lean tissue.

C. Energy supply

Understanding how stored energy is used to provide energy for exercise gives insight into the probable location, size and accessibility of carbohydrate, fat and protein storage in the body. Each of the storage sites will be considered individually because each is mobilized and utilized quite differently during exercise.

Carbohydrate is stored with water as glycogen in the liver and skeletal muscle. These two stores of glycogen have two distinctly different purposes. Muscle glycogen fuels activity within that muscle or shuttles fuel to other muscle via lactate. Glycogen in the liver maintains blood glucose concentration for tissues, such as central nervous system tissues, that are dependent on glucose. In an average 70 kg male with 15% body fat, the liver contains 0.10 kg of glycogen or 1,600 kJ, whereas skeletal muscle contains 0.40 kg of glycogen or 6,400 kJ.[11] It should be apparent that these stores are finite and limiting. In fact, an overnight fast can be sufficient to deplete most liver glycogen. While the liver can make glucose from 3-carbon precursors such as alanine or lactate via gluconeogenesis when glycogen is in short supply, skeletal muscle does not have that capability. Consequently, skeletal muscle glycogen depletion can be problematic during exercise. Since the pioneering studies of Bergstrom and Hultman,[12] it has been apparent that glycogen depletion correlates with fatigue although the causal mechanism remains unclear. Conversely, increasing stores of glycogen, known as supercompensation, can enhance exercise performance.[2] For these reasons, carbohydrate supplementation has been one of the most intensively studied areas of exercise nutrition.

Fat is stored as triglycerides in skeletal muscle and adipose tissue. In the 70 kg male with 15% body fat example, fat storage would be 10.5 kg or 390,000 kJ (390 MJ).[11] Hence, in even the leanest of athletes, energy stored as fat is, for all practical purposes, considered limitless. The role of the intracellular fat stored within muscle as an energy source during exercise is not clear. When viewed with electron microscopy, skeletal muscle triglycerides and mitochondria are in close proximity.[13] Some experimental results indicate that these triglycerides represent an easily accessible energy source.[14] Other data suggest that working muscle is almost exclusively dependent on the oxidation of carbohydrate, leaving no room for fat use,[15] and that the proximal fat stores are likely used during recovery.[16] The current debate is complicated by methodological issues, which have been reviewed previously in detail.[17] The role of intramyocellular lipid is an active area of research and more answers should be forthcoming.

In a discussion of protein metabolism, it is more accurate to refer to amino acid metabolism since most intermediary metabolism happens as amino acids rather than protein. Our standard male would contain roughly 8.5 kg of protein or about 142,000 kJ (142 MJ).[11] Even given this vast amount of energy, it is incorrect to imply that protein is a significant energy store. The use of branched-chain amino acids does increase during exercise, but the 2-3-fold increase in amino acid oxidation pales in comparison to the 10-20-fold increase in carbohydrate and fat metabolism.[18] In fact, the method most often used to measure substrate oxidation during exercise, the respiratory exchange ratio (RER), ignores the contribution of amino acids. For simplicity then, the dynamic amino acid pool, a product of protein synthesis and breakdown, is usually viewed as being preoccupied with structural metabolism.

D. Energy Demand

Total daily energy expenditure (TDEE) can be roughly divided into three categories: resting metabolic rate (RMR), diet-induced thermogenesis (DIT), and physical activity (PA). Resting metabolism represents the energy demand for maintenance of resting homeostasis and is largely determined by fat-free mass. Skeletal muscle, the largest component of fat-free mass, is a large energy drain because of energy consuming processes such as protein synthesis, ionic regulation, and heat generation. For anyone not performing large amounts of daily PA, RMR is the largest component of energy expenditure. Diet-induced thermogenesis represents the cost of processing, trafficking and storing nutrients and depends mainly on energy intake. Because DIT is difficult to measure reliably in humans, it is usually estimated as representing 10% of total daily energy expenditure. However, this expenditure can vary somewhat with the macronutrient composition of the diet. Physical activity traditionally represents any energy expenditure above doing nothing and is the most variable component of energy expenditure. Physical activity increases energy expenditure because of, among other things, the extra demands of cross-bridge cycling, ion pumping, hormone synthesis, and heat production. Of note is a relatively new concept termed non-exercise activity thermogenesis or NEAT has been coined to include very low intensity activity like fidgeting or simple standing, and is incorporated into measurements of physical activity. For a discussion of energy expenditure, it is useful to consider an American football offensive lineman, a gymnast, and an ultramarathoner.

For an offensive lineman, the requirements for a high absolute power output and to offer considerable resistance to movement by external forces make it advantageous to maintain a large muscle mass. Because of the large muscle mass, this athlete will have a prodigious resting energy expenditure. Given the intermittent nature of their training (practice or weight lifting) and competition, the energy expenditure due to activity will be less significant than resting energy expenditure. This athlete can consume large amounts of energy because it is balanced by their huge resting energy expenditure, and the fact that excess mass will not have negative consequences. For a gymnast, a large muscle mass is advantageous, but excess mass is not. A gymnast will also have a high resting energy expenditure due to their large lean body mass, although not nearly as high as the offensive lineman. Again, given the intermittent nature of a gymnast's activity, energy expenditure due to physical activity will probably not equal resting energy expenditure. This athlete will have to closely monitor energy intake and expenditure since there is a negative consequence for any added mass that is not working skeletal muscle. Finally, an ultra marathoner must maintain a low lean mass since any excess mass, even skeletal muscle, is a clear disadvantage in their sport. In this situation, where prolonged aerobic exercise requires considerable energy output, energy expenditure due to physical activity will likely exceed resting energy expenditure (although the low body fat in the marathon runner causes them to have a higher resting energy expenditure than a comparably-sized sedentary individual).

E. MATCHING SUPPLY TO DEMAND

In meeting the need to match energy supply to energy demand, relevant time spans can range from seconds to years. On the period of seconds, limited stores of ATP and PCr are taxed and must be replenished as other energy producing pathways are activated. Progressing further, exercise bouts of 5 min, 30 min, 1 hr, 4 hr, and 8 hr will all have different supply and demand considerations due to finite energy stores. Finally, over the periods of days, weeks, and years, the matching of supply and demand is dependent on habitual physical activity patterns and dietary habits.

For the time scale of seconds, it is possible to make calculations of the amount of energy needed to perform a bout of work. This can be on a scale as small as the number of ATP needed for twitch activity or the amount of work performed over a 30-second test of maximal bicycling capacity. For longer time periods, the measurement of oxygen consumption (VO_2), known as indirect calorimetry, is a convenient tool for making lab-based measurements of energy demand. These studies are most frequently performed at rest or during steady-state exercise over a defined period of time. Assuming energy is derived from oxidation of carbohydrate and fat in about a 50:50 ratio, for every kJ of aerobic energy production, approximately 50 ml of oxygen is required (or 20.2 kJ/L). Therefore, multiplying VO_2 (L/min) by the energy equivalent of oxygen (20.2 kJ/L) will provide a reasonable estimate of the rate of energy expenditure (kJ/min). By measuring both O_2 consumption and CO_2 production (VCO_2) respiratory exchange ratio ($(RER) = VCO_2/VO_2$) can be calculated. This calculation allows for more accurate measurements of the proportion of carbohydrate and fat (ignores protein) being used as fuels at that time. A ratio near 0.8 indicates primarily fat oxidation, while a ratio near 1.0 indicates primarily carbohydrate oxidation. Obvious limitations of indirect calorimetry are that it can only account for aerobic energy production and ignores non-aerobic energy production, measurements are generally confined to a laboratory environment (although the accuracy of smaller units than can be used in the field is improving), and long-term measurements (anything longer than a few hours) of energy consumption are not practical. Measurements of energy expenditure up to about 24 hours can be made using room calorimeters in the few facilities where they are available.

For longer assessment (days to weeks), the doubly-labeled water technique is the gold standard. The method is expensive but easy to administer. Subjects drink what looks to be an ordinary glass of water, which contains known amounts of a stable isotopic "label" on both the hydrogen and oxygen. The labeled hydrogen equilibrates with the body water pool only, while the labeled oxygen equilibrates with the body water pool and CO_2. Knowing the initial dose of the labels, and measuring the difference in the excretion rates in the body water pool between the two labels, the excretion rate of the unmeasured CO_2 pool can be calculated. Knowing CO_2 production and estimating VCO_2/VO_2 from the composition of the habitual diet, energy expenditure can be calculated. The biggest advantage of this technique is that subjects can be free living, with only a couple of urine samples needed after the initial consumption of the water.

Finally, for truly long-term (weeks to years) changes in energy assessment of dietary intake and body weight can assess energy demand. This measurement is based on the First Law of Thermodynamics. When dietary energy intake exceeds energy expenditure the excess energy will be stored. Over time, energy storage equates to greater body weight. So, by this relatively crude, but reliable and valid, form of energy expenditure assessment, weight gain means that energy intake is exceeding energy demands and weight loss means that energy intake is insufficient for energy demands.

Matching energy supply to energy demand requires several components:

1. A way to assess energy stores and send that information out to the rest of the body;
2. A processing center to integrate information and direct an appropriate response;
3. Systems to change intake and expenditure in the appropriate directions;
4. A signal to the processing center reflecting the new state.

During hard exercise, energy demand can increase by more than 20-fold over the resting metabolism of about 4.2 kj/min (1 kcal/minute), or roughly equivalent to a 100 watt light bulb. Neural, biochemical and hormonal changes that accompany (and even precede) muscle contraction are signals for the change in demand, and energy provision is initiated. For example, the rapid increase in inorganic phosphate (Pi) and ADP in the muscle increases the activity of CK to regenerate ATP from PCr hydrolysis and also accelerates glycolysis. Simultaneously, activation of the sympathetic nervous system and an increase in blood catecholamines (flight or fight response) cause glycogen breakdown in muscle and liver as well as triglyceride breakdown in adipose tissue (and maybe intramuscular triglycerides). So, stored carbohydrate and fat are catabolized to increase the available pool of glucose and fatty acids. A key point is that the matching of supply to demand is almost instantaneous in terms of the magnitude of the response (i.e., there is excellent matching between the kJ required and the kJ provided) but the blend of energy sources is skewed toward the rapidly activated "local" sources in the first few minutes of exercise. Much of the energy early in exercise is derived from PCr and muscle glycogen in order to meet the energetic needs while the other systems are "titrated" into play. As exercise continues, the supply of glucose derived from glycogen, blood glucose, adipose-derived fatty acids, intramyocellular fatty acids and amino acids is continually changing to meet demand. The precise regulation of these interconnected pathways is a topic of much research and certainly has implications for pre-, during, and post-exercise nutritional strategies.

F. Consequences of mismatching supply to demand

Once again, no discussion of the consequences of a mismatch between energy supply and demand is fruitful without considering the appropriate time scale. As previously discussed, PCr can donate its phosphate group for the rapid resynthesis of ATP from ADP. Although PCr stores are about 5 times those of ATP, the supply may be depleted in a couple of seconds during very high intensity exercise. Thereafter, the stores have to recover during rest periods or a transition to less intense aerobic exercise for replenishment. PCr storage has been demonstrated to respond favorably to supplementation and the increase in storage can enhance high-intensity exercise performance,[19,20] which in itself is indirect evidence that PCr stores are limiting in short-duration intense activity. During steady-state exercise, resynthesis of ATP between contractions by PCr, glycolysis and oxidative phosphorylation is usually adequate to keep intracellular ATP concentration from dropping. During very prolonged steady-state exercise, the capacity to completely recycle ATP between contractions can be compromised and ATP concentrations begin to fall. The fall in ATP has been associated with fatigue and inability to maintain exercise performance, however the idea that fatigue is "caused" by a fall in cellular ATP concentration is a dramatic oversimplification of the complex process of fatigue. Nonetheless, it is clear however that an inability to match demand with the appropriate supply will force the individual to reduce exercise intensity to a level that can be sustained with the available energy supply, or even to stop exercise entirely.

The substrates for anaerobic glycolysis are blood glucose and muscle glycogen. Although in most cases blood glucose can be sustained by liver glycogenolysis and gluconeogenesis, muscle glycogen supply is limiting to exercise performance. Like PCr, glycogen satisfies the criteria for being considered limiting in supply; exercise in a glycogen-depleted state will decrease exercise performance, whereas increasing glycogen concentration (supercompensation) will usually enhance exercise performance. Exactly why fatigue is so closely associated with low muscle glycogen is not entirely clear since complete glycogen depletion is not observed even when study subjects fatigue and can no longer maintain exercise.[2] There has been speculation that some minimal concentration of glycogen is "protected" and resistant to use during exercise; perhaps to ensure that some fuel is spared in case of dire necessity (e.g., to keep from becoming dinner). The recent work by Shulman and colleagues suggesting that glucose entering the muscle cell is incorporated into glycogen before being shunted into glycolysis, especially when glycogen stores are low,[4] supports but does not prove that theory. The close connection between glycogen stores and exercise performance have made carbohydrate supplementation before, during and after exercise, one of the most well studied areas of exercise nutrition. In addition, the role of glycogen depletion in exercise performance has crossed into new areas such as energy sensing,[21] cellular signaling,[22] and training-induced adaptations.[23]

As discussed, for all practical purposes fat supply is never limiting to exercise demand. There is an extremely large supply of fat energy stored in the body, and working muscles appear to disdain fat energy during periods of high metabolic flux, i.e., exercise at more than low-moderate intensity. There has been great interest in trying to "train" the athlete to rely more on fat energy by feeding high-fat diets to increase the enzymes required for fat oxidation. While it is possible to induce some of the appropriate metabolic adaptations that increase fat utilization, these interventions do not enhance exercise performance.[24] Thus, as opposed to PCr and glycogen, fat supply does not deplete, it is the capacity to use fat that is limiting, not the supply itself, and supplementation does not improve exercise capacity.

A final point regarding that mismatch of supply and demand during an acute bout of exercise distinguishes between the quantity and quality of fuels. The consequences of mismatching the quantity of energy required results in fatigue, or the inability to maintain the desired force output. On the other hand, the consequences of mismatching the quality of the energy required are more subtle. For example, too much carbohydrate utilization will allow maintenance of a high exercise intensity but will cause rapid glycogen depletion and fatigue. Too little carbohydrate utilization will spare precious glycogen reserves but, by forcing greater reliance of fatty acid oxidation, will constrain exercise to a relatively low intensity. Therefore, the body systems designed to sense, integrate, and deliver the appropriate energy to match demand, must be sensitive to the quality of the energy required as well as the quantity.

Over the long-term (days/weeks/months), energy supply can be mismatched to demand with no acute loss of function, but with potent consequences for body composition and exercise. Caloric restriction or prolonged high energy expenditure will cause energy deficit, whereas prolonged low energy expenditure or excess energy intake results in a surplus. Energy surplus, extended over weeks or months, will result in gain of body mass, which inhibits performance of most exercise tasks.

Decrements in exercise performance will be especially profound if the excess mass is stored as adipose tissue since this tissue does not directly contribute to mechanical work. Chronic energy shortage has profound effects on exercise performance in many different ways. An important advancement in this area is the distinction between inadequate energy intake as opposed to high energy expenditure. Based on pioneering work by Anne Loucks and others,[25,26] the cluster of symptoms (disordered eating, amenorrhea, low bone mineral density) that are often described as the "female athlete triad" is now believed to be more closely related to energy shortage rather than to excess training or low body fat.[25] It has also been observed that chronic energy deficit can alter hormone profiles,[26] cause loss of muscle mass,[27] and change substrate oxidation patterns.[28]

The matching of energy intake and expenditure is especially relevant to performance in an event requiring extremely high energy outputs extended over multiple days or weeks, such as the Tour de France. Researchers from Holland performed the first measurements of energy intake and output during the Tour de France.[29,30] The cyclists in their research group consumed 24.7 MJ/day (5,900 cal/day) with the highest average value for a single day being 32.4 MJ (7,750 kcal). On average, the cyclists expended 29.4–36.0 MJ/day (7020–8600 cal/day). In other words, energy expenditure roughly matched energy intake even though energy expenditure was 3.6–5.3 times the resting metabolic rate. A report by Kirkwood demonstrated that across mammals and birds the maximum possible sustainable energy expenditure was 4–5 times RMR.[31] Therefore, these cyclists at the Tour de France were operating right at the proposed maximum energy expenditure. An intriguing question then emerges as to whether food intake is limiting to exercise performance in an event such as the Tour de France. In other words, it may just be extremely difficult to eat more than 30 MJ/day and therefore, the upper limit to sustainable energy expenditure is 30 MJ/day. Recently there was an effort by another three-week cycling race, the Vuelta a España, to shorten stages to make them more humane and to discourage doping. Rather than take advantage of the "easier" conditions, the riders simply rode faster over the shorter courses.[32] Therefore, even though the stage race was shorter in distance, the athletes were expending the same amount of energy as a longer-distanced stage race. It may be that these athletes are capable of pushing themselves to the physiological limits of energy expenditure no matter how long or short the event is. Further, since the ability to produce energy day after day is dependent on being able to get that energy back into the system, it may be that physiological performance at a tour is limited by how much food can be properly eaten and digested.

G. Factors that Impact Energy Utilization

Intensity and duration of exercise have reciprocal effects on the energy-producing pathways. For example, during both acute exercise and in response to long-term training, as exercise intensity increases the duration that can be sustained decreases. During exercise, glycolytic energy sources increase in concert with increasing exercise intensity. Conversely, as intensity decreases and duration increases, there is a greater contribution from fat sources. A reasonable way to think about this relationship is that exercise intensity determines fuel preference and the fuel preference determines the duration for which a particular bout of exercise can be sustained. Fuel selection during exercise is associated with muscle fiber type so that as exercise intensity increases, muscle fiber recruitment moves from almost purely aerobic type I muscle fibers to incorporate progressively more glycolytic type II fibers; thus changing the capacity for oxidative metabolism. The effect of exercise intensity on fuel preference is well described and is characterized by a point at around 45–50% VO_{2max} where fuel preference "crosses" over from mainly (more than half the energy) fat to mainly carbohydrate sources.[14,33] Since most athletes and other active individuals train and compete at exercise intensities in excess of 50% VO_{2max}, carbohydrate is clearly the preferred energy source. It is important to note, however, that exercise duration has an independent effect by increasing the contribution of fat (and protein) as exercise time elapses and glycogen stores become progressively depleted. The opposing effects of exercise intensity and duration on carbohydrate and lipid metabolism are depicted in Figure 1.3.

The effect of exercise training on fuel preference has been a contentious issue in the past with much of the argument centered on the use of the terms "absolute" and "relative". As one becomes more trained the *relative* contributions of fuels (i.e., proportion of carbohydrate to fat) for a given *relative* exercise intensity (i.e., post-training exercise at the same % of VO_{2max} as pre-training; note that the exercise is now at a higher absolute power output because VO_{2max} increases with training) remains constant. However, after training there is a greater *relative* contribution of fat used for a given *absolute* workload (i.e., post-training exercise at the same power output as pre-training; note that exercise is now at a lower relative intensity because VO_{2max} increases with training). To add complexity, note that at any given *relative* exercise intensity, although the *relative* contribution of fat does not change with training, the total energy demand for the exercise task increases because the absolute

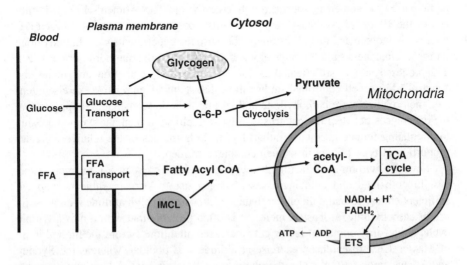

FIGURE 1.3 Schematic of pathways interconnecting carbohydrate and fat utilization (ETS = electron transport system, G-6-P = glucose-6-phospate; IMCL = intramyocellular lipid; TCA = tricarboxylic acid cycle).

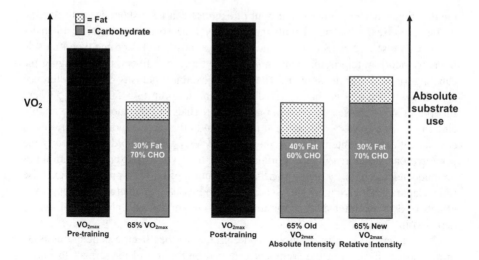

FIGURE 1.4 Absolute and relative workloads and fuel partitioning. Black bars represent VO_{2max} before and after exercise training. Grey and dappled bars represent absolute amounts of carbohydrate and fat, respectively. The relative proportions of the fuels are indicated in the bar.

workload is higher after training. Therefore, the *absolute* amount of fat used does increase. These concepts are represented pictorially in Figure 4.

For many years, all of the examples used in the field of exercise metabolism were based on observations from the standard 70 kg male mentioned above. With increased participation of women in sport through Title IX and The Women's Health Equity Act of the 1990s, physiologists and biochemists began to investigate sex-based differences in women and men. Presumably because the experiments were initially done on men, femaleness (and the physiological effects of the ovarian hormones estrogen and progesterone) is still treated as the "experimental" condition and males the "control". Most well-controlled studies show that at any given relative exercise intensity, men oxidize more carbohydrate and less fat than do women.[34,35] It appears that the differences between the patterns of relative fuel use in men and women are due to circulating female hormones rather than male hormones or the relatively greater proportion of type I fibers in women compared to men.[35-37]

Several environmental factors also change fuel preferences. For example, exercise in both heat and cold increases glycogen use.[38] Also, in subjects who eat sufficient energy to maintain energy balance, exposure to high altitude increases the use of carbohydrate, at least in men.[39] It is often the case that with a new Olympic cycle, a new environmental factor gets increased attention. Before the high altitude of Mexico City, research on exercise at altitude was popular, whereas the Sydney and Athens games stimulated research on exercise in the heat. A legitimate concern for the 2008 Olympics in Beijing is air quality. Although it is not clear whether air pollutants alter substrate use, it is possible that medications used to treat asthma, such as Clenbuterol, do change fuel preference.[40]

III. HOW DOES DIET INFLUENCE ENERGY UTILIZATION?

A. GROSS ENERGY INTAKE

Energy deficit is induced by decreased caloric intake or increased energy expenditure. Caloric restriction lowers RMR, energy expended via PA, and DIT. Therefore all three components of TDEE respond to caloric restriction in a direction that conserves expended energy and minimizes accumulated weight loss:

$$\text{Caloric Restriction Energy Deficit:} \quad \begin{array}{cccc} \text{RMR} + \text{DIT} + \text{PA} = \text{TDEE} \\ \downarrow \quad \downarrow \quad \downarrow \quad \downarrow\downarrow \end{array}$$

Instead of caloric restriction, energy deficit can also be induced by maintaining caloric intake and increasing energy expended by PA (exercise). Since exercise helps preserve lean tissue mass, RMR may not decline, and may even increase if there is a significant change in body composition. Since DIT is primarily determined by caloric intake, energy expended by DIT should not decrease if energy intake is not restricted. Therefore, a weight management program based on increasing energy expenditure by PA could result in a strikingly different pattern of changes to TDEE that are more likely to promote continued weight loss:

$$\text{Exercise Energy Deficit:} \quad \begin{array}{cccc} \text{RMR} + \text{DIT} + \text{PA} = \text{TDEE} \\ \leftrightarrow \quad \leftrightarrow \quad \uparrow \quad \uparrow \end{array}$$

The response to exercise-induced energy deficit may be mediated by a different endocrine response from that observed with caloric restriction. How exercise-induced energy deficit impacts endocrine signals has not been systematically studied. In addition, sex differences in the neuroendocrine response to exercise training have been noted in rodents.[35] Data from human and animal studies indeed suggest that increased physical activity, with ad libitum feeding, causes loss of body weight in males but not in females.[41] Whether this is a true sex difference or an artifact of experimental design (to maintain the same relative exercise energy expenditure, women expend fewer absolute kJ in the training intervention because they tend to have lower baseline daily energy expenditure) remains to be decided.

B. MACRONUTRIENT COMPOSITION

In recent years there has been considerable discussion about the effect of macronutrient intake on energy expenditure. At rest, substitution of one macronutrient for another could change energy expenditure because of a difference in the thermic effect of the different macronutrients. A recent review summarized the effect of substituting one macronutrient for another on total energy expenditure.[42] According to these authors, there is little effect when fat is substituted for carbohydrate. However, increasing protein to 30–35% of energy intake increases energy expenditure.

The magnitude of the increased energy expenditure is small, 2.7% for an average caloric intake in the short-term,[42] but may have some implications for long-term weight management as small consistent changes integrated over long time frames can add up to physiologically relevant effects.

Macronutrient composition of the diet also changes energy utilization by mediating the proportion of fuels used for energy production. The relative economy of storage of the primary energy-producing macronutrients (carbohydrate and fat) is useful for illustrating how macronutrient intake effects energy utilization. Digestible carbohydrates contain, on average, 17.6 kJ/gram (4.2 kcal/gram), two moles of ATP are used to store one mole of glucose as glycogen, and 2.7 grams of water are also stored per gram of glycogen. Lipids (triglycerides) contain 39.3 kJ/gram (9.4 kcal/gram), there is no ATP cost for storage, and triglycerides are hydrophobic so that body fat is almost 90% pure lipid. In total, the energy value of stored glycogen is about 4.2 kJ/gram (1 kcal/gram) while stored fat has an energy content of approximately 33.6 kJ/gram (8 kcal/gram).[43] Storing energy as triglycerides in adipose tissue is therefore extremely efficient; the same quantity of energy can be stored with considerably less weight. Storage of the 390,000 kJ mentioned earlier as carbohydrate (glycogen) instead of fat would increase body weight by more than 36 kg. Therefore, while this huge increase in weight would not be a problem for an oak tree (which may explain why plants generally store a great majority of their energy as carbohydrate in the form of starch), it would clearly be a huge disadvantage for animals that need to move to catch dinner (or avoid becoming dinner). In summary, carbohydrate is not stored efficiently, is continually required for specific tissue functions (e.g., central nervous system), and is a more oxygen efficient fuel compared to fat. Therefore, dietary fat is preferentially stored while dietary carbohydrate is preferentially oxidized.

Despite the fact that dietary carbohydrate can be converted to fat in the liver,[44] the rate at which this process (*de novo* lipogenesis) occurs is negligible under most conditions. Instead, carbohydrate intake is rapidly matched by an increase in carbohydrate use and RER approaches 1.0 (all carbohydrate). Even after the consumption of a mixed meal, RER rises toward 1.0 indicating an increased contribution of carbohydrate to energy expenditure. Carbohydrate intake is well matched by carbohydrate use during both rest and exercise. During exercise, exogenous carbohydrate provision (e.g., consuming a sports drink) can be matched by oxidation of the ingested glucose up until glucose transporters in the gut become saturated.[45]

IV. HOW DOES EXERCISE INFLUENCE DIETARY REQUIREMENTS?

A. ENERGY NEEDS

Exercise increases total energy needs due to a rise in the PA component of TDEE. As discussed above, competitive events like the Tour de France put huge demands on energy intake. Insight regarding the energy demands in a variety of sports was obtained by using four to seven-day diet records in Dutch athletes.[46] Average dietary intake varied from 110 kJ/kg/day (26 kcal/kg/day) in female body builders and 157 kJ/kg/day (38 kcal/kg/day) in female top-level gymnasts to 272 kJ/kg/day (65 kcal/kg/day) in male triathletes and 347 kJ/kg/day (83 kcal/kg/day) in Tour de France cyclists. In general, sports that emphasized aesthetics had the lowest intake, team sports were intermediate, and endurance sport the highest. It is important to note, however, that these were reported intakes and were not confirmed by objective assessment of energy expenditure. From these data, it is apparent that energy intake for aesthetic-type athletes is far below the 9.6–13.0 MJ/day (2300–3100 kcal/d) recommended for a healthy adult. Conversely, a single day in the Tour de France bike race can have an energy expenditure of close to 37.5 MJ (9,000 kcal),[29] or three to four times average energy intake.

Since doubly-labeled water is becoming more readily available, a more complete record of the energy expenditure involved in a variety of activities is developing. Recent publications have demonstrated energy expenditures of 14.7 MJ/day (3500 kcal/day) in soccer players,[47] 14.7 MJ/day (3500 kcal/day) in elite Kenyan runners,[48] 16.5 MJ/day (3950 kcal/day) female lightweight rowers,[49] 19.2 MJ/day (4600 kcal/day), 20.5 MJ/day (4900 kcal/day) for wildfire suppression,[50] and 23.5 MJ/day (5600 kcal/day) in elite female swimmers.[51] It is interesting that when self-reported energy intakes are compared with energy outputs calculated from doubly labeled water, it appears that many of these athletes should be in energy deficit. Although it may be true that some athletes maintain a chronic energy deficit, it is also likely that some athletes are underreporting actual dietary intake. A recent report on elite Kenyan runners indicates that in the period leading up to competition, these athletes may indeed be in a negative energy balance.[48] Support for the latter possibility comes from the variety of sources showing that underreporting intake is common in nutritional surveys. As doubly-labeled water measurements and carefully controlled studies of dietary intake become more feasible, we should achieve a better understanding of energy status (deficit, balance, surplus) in different physical activities.

B. CARBOHYDRATE NEEDS

Since carbohydrate depletion correlates with fatigue, maintenance of carbohydrate stores throughout and between exercise bouts is of critical importance. It is increasingly apparent that muscle (and probably liver) glycogen content has metabolic effects, for example in cell signaling[22,23] and exercise pacing,[21] which extend beyond simple energy storage. The current Institute of Medicine (IOM) recommendation for carbohydrate intake is 45–65% of daily caloric intake.[52] Recommendations based on percentages of total daily intake do not work well for athletes. Burke et al. have published evidence that energy and carbohydrate intake are only loosely correlated in men, while there is no correlation in women.[53] Therefore, basing recommendations on a percentage of caloric intake does not guarantee adequate carbohydrate intake in athletes. Current recommendations for carbohydrate intake vary based on training duration and intensity and are 5–7 g/kg/d for moderate duration/low intensity, 7–12 g/kg/day for moderate to heavy endurance training, and 10–12 g/kg/day for an extreme exercise program.[54] From an analysis of published nutritional surveys, it appears that typical male non-endurance and endurance athletes meet these recommendations, 5.5 g/kg/day and 7.5 g/kg/day, respectively, although they tend to fall on the low end of the recommendations.[53] Conversely, female non-endurance and endurance athletes report intakes of 4.7 and 5.5 g/kg/day, respectively, which indicates that the females fall below the recommendations. The values provided here have been demonstrated to achieve glycogen concentrations that approach muscle storage capacity over 24 hours of passive recovery. However, these values do not take into account the timing of post-exercise carbohydrate ingestion when in the first hour or two after exercise can result in higher rates of glycogen repletion.

C. PROTEIN NEEDS

Whether exercise increases the need for protein is a contentious topic. With endurance training, protein needs may be higher due to increased rates of amino acid oxidation during exercise. With strength/power athletes, there is speculation that protein requirements are elevated to support gains in protein mass. The current recommendation of protein intake by IOM is 0.8 g/kg/day for healthy adults. Current recommendations for endurance and strength athletes vary greatly, however recent reviews by Tarnopolsky[55] and Phillips[56] have nicely summarized much of the currently available data. For endurance athletes it was recommended that there are no additional protein requirements for low to moderate-intensity exercise. However, at the initiation of training and at top level endurance training, needs may increase to 1.6 g/kg/day.[55] For strength athletes it was recommended that 1.33 g/kg/dat represents a "safe" intake.[56] The typical protein intake in most endurance athletes exceeds the daily recommended intake and even the 1.6 g/kg/day recommendation because of the quantity of food that endurance athletes consume to maintain energy balance.[55] Retrospective analysis of the protein intake of strength athletes also demonstrates that the mean reported value of 2.05 g/kg/d greatly exceeds the extrapolated 1.33 g/kg/d "safe" recommendation.

Perhaps more than the other macronutrients, daily recommendations of protein should be treated as broad recommendations. As demonstrated in the 1980's, protein requirements are dependent on the energy status of the individual.[27] Further, it was demonstrated that exercise training may actually decrease protein requirements because of an increased efficiency of energy utilization.[57] Conversely, current protein recommendations do not account for the greatly elevated protein needs of athletes consuming restricted energy diets. But, as with carbohydrate, the timing of the protein intake relative to other stimuli (e.g., exercise) can have a large effect on the net protein balance.[58] It is even plausible to consider that the timing of protein nutrition is more important than the amount of protein consumed.

V. CONCLUSION

There are complex biologic systems that monitor energy demand and meet that demand by precisely releasing stored energy in the appropriate quantity and "quality" (blend of fuel sources). These mechanisms adhere to the basic principles of thermodynamics and function to preserve the top metabolic priorities: providing glucose for the CNS, maintaining adequate muscle glycogen stores to facilitate physical activity required to catch (or avoid becoming) dinner, and storing sufficient energy to survive periods of extended fasting. Athletes and other active individuals must conform to the same physical laws, but test the boundaries of the metabolic systems because of their high energy and carbohydrate expenditure, obligating considerably higher rates of energy and carbohydrate replacement. Although much has been elucidated about the demands that exercise puts on energy-regulating systems, and effective dietary manipulations to meet those demands, there is still much to be learned about how the systems are regulated. These key discoveries will enable sport nutritionists to craft optimal dietary strategies that maximize athletic performance.

REFERENCES

1. Krogh A and Lindhard J. The Relative Value of Fat and Carbohydrate as Sources of Muscular Energy: With Appendices on the Correlation between Standard Metabolism and the Respiratory Quotient during Rest and Work. *Biochem. J.* 14: 290–363, 1920.
2. Bergstrom J and Hultman E. Synthesis of muscle glycogen in man after glucose and fructose infusion. *Acta Med. Scand.* 182: 93–107, 1967.
3. Tipton KD, Ferrando AA, Phillips SM, Doyle D, Jr., and Wolfe RR. Postexercise net protein synthesis in human muscle from orally administered amino acids. *Am. J. Physiol* 276: E628, 1999.
4. Schulman RG. Glycogen turnover forms lactate during exercise. *Exer. Sport Sci. Rev.* 33:157–62, 2005.
5. Brooks GA. Mammalian fuel utilization during sustained exercise. *Comp. Biochem. Physiol. B: Biochem Mol. Biol.* 120: 89–107, 1998.
6. Brooks GA, Dubouchaud H, Brown M, Sicurello JP, and Butz CE. Role of mitochondrial lactate dehydrogenase and lactate oxidation in the intracellular lactate shuttle. *Proc. Natl. Acad. Sci. USA* 96: 1129, 1999.
7. Braun B and Horton T. Endocrine regulation of exercise substrate utilization in women compared to men. *Exerc. Sport Sci. Rev.* 29: 149, 2001.
8. Hashimoto T, Hussien R, and Brooks GA. Colocalization of MCT1, CD147, and LDH in mitochondrial inner membrane of L6 muscle cells: evidence of a mitochondrial lactate oxidation complex. *Am. J. Physiol. Endocrinol. Metab.* 290 E1237–1244, 2006.
9. Gladden LB. Lactate metabolism: a new paradigm for the third millennium. *J. Physiol. (London)* 558: 5–30, 2004.
10. Sahlin K, Fernstrom M, Svensson M, and Tonkonogi M. No evidence of an intracellular lactate shuttle in rat skeletal muscle. *J. Physiol.* 541: 569–574, 2002.
11. Jeukendrup A and Gleeson M. *Sport Nutrition: An introduction to energy production and performance.* Champaign, IL: Human Kinetics, 2004.
12. Bergstrom J, Hermansen L, Hultman E, and Saltin B. Diet, muscle glycogen and physical performance. *Acta Physiol. Scand.* 71: 140–150, 1967.
13. Jeukendrup AE, Saris WH, and Wagenmakers AJ. Fat metabolism during exercise: a review. Part I: fatty acid mobilization. *Int. J. Sports Med.*19: 231–244, 1998.
14. Achten J, Gleeson M, and Jeukendrup AE. Determination of the exercise intensity that elicits maximal fat oxidation. *Med. Sci. Sports Exerc.* 34: 92–97, 2002.
15. Bergman BC, Butterfield GE, Wolfel EE, Casazza GA, Lopaschuk GD, and Brooks GA. Evaluation of exercise and training on muscle lipid metabolism. *Am. J. Physiol.* 276: E106, 1999.

16. Kuo CC, Fattor JA, Henderson GC, and Brooks GA. Lipid oxidation in fit young adults during postexercise recovery. *J. Appl. Physiol.* 99: 349–356, 2005.

17. Watt MJ, Heigenhauser GJ, and Spriet LL. Intramuscular triacylglycerol utilization in human skeletal muscle during exercise: is there a controversy? *J. Appl. Physiol* 93: 1185, 2002.

18. Knapik J, Meredith C, Jones B, Fielding R, Young V, and Evans W. Leucine metabolism during fasting and exercise. *J. Appl. Physiol.* 70: 43–47, 1991.

19. Greenhaff PL, Casey A, Short AH, Harris R, Soderlund K, and Hultman E. Influence of oral creatine supplementation of muscle torque during repeated bouts of maximal voluntary exercise in man. *Clin. Sci. (London)* 84: 565–571, 1993.

20. Harris RC, Soderlund K, and Hultman E. Elevation of creatine in resting and exercised muscle of normal subjects by creatine supplementation. *Clin. Sci. (London)* 83: 367–374, 1992.

21. Rauch HG, St Clair Gibson A, Lambert EV, and Noakes TD. A signalling role for muscle glycogen in the regulation of pace during prolonged exercise. *Br. J. Sports Med.* 39: 34–38, 2005.

22. Wojtaszewski JF, MacDonald C, Nielsen JN, Hellsten Y, Hardie DG, Kemp BE, Kiens B, and Richter EA. Regulation of 5'AMP-activated protein kinase activity and substrate utilization in exercising human skeletal muscle. *Am. J. Physiol. Endocrinol. Metab.* 284: E813–822, 2003.

23. Hansen AK, Fischer CP, Plomgaard P, Andersen JL, Saltin B, and Pedersen BK. Skeletal muscle adaptation: training twice every second day vs. training once daily. *J. Appl. Physiol.* 98: 93–99, 2005.

24. Burke LM and Kiens B. "Fat adaptation" for athletic performance: the nail in the coffin? *J. Appl. Physiol.* 100:7–8, 2006.

25. Loucks AB. Energy availability, not body fatness, regulates reproductive function in women. *Exerc. Sport Sci. Rev.* 31: 144–148, 2003.

26. Loucks AB, Verdun M, and Heath EM. Low energy availability, not stress of exercise, alters LH pulsatility in exercising women. *J. Appl. Physiol.* 84: 37–46, 1998.

27. Todd KS, Butterfield GE, and Calloway DH. Nitrogen balance in men with adequate and deficient energy intake at three levels of work. *J. f Nutr.* 114: 2107–2118, 1984.

28. Jebb SA, Prentice AM, Goldberg GR, Murgatroyd PR, Black AE, and Coward WA. Changes in macronutrient balance during over- and underfeeding assessed by 12-d continuous whole-body calorimetry. *Am. J. Clin. Nutr.* 64: 259–266, 1996.

29. Saris WH, van Erp-Baart MA, Brouns F, Westerterp KR, and ten Hoor F. Study on food intake and energy expenditure during extreme sustained exercise: the Tour de France. *Int. J. Sports Med.* 10 Suppl 1: S26–31, 1989.

30. Westerterp KR. Diet induced thermogenesis. *Nutr. Metab. (London)* 1: 5, 2004.

31. Kirkwood JK. A limit to metabolisable energy intake in mammals and birds. *Comp. Biochem Physiol A: Physiol.* 75: 1, 1983.

32. Lucia A, Hoyos J, Santalla A, Earnest C, and Chicharro JL. Tour de France versus Vuelta a Espana: which is harder? *Med. Sci. Sports Exerc.* 35: 872–878, 2003.

33. Brooks GA and Mercier J. Balance of carbohydrate and lipid utilization during exercise: the "crossover" concept. *J. Appl. Physiol.* 76: 2253, 1994.

34. Horton T. and B. Braun. Sex-based differences in substrate metabolism; in: *Advances in Molecular and Cell Biology, 34: Principles of Sex-Based Differences in Physiology.* VM Miller and M Hay, eds., Elsevier Publishing Co., Amsterdam, The Netherlands, pp. 209–228, 2004.

35. Braun B and Horton T. Endocrine regulation of exercise substrate utilization in women compared to men. *Exerc. Sport Sci. Rev.* 29: 149, 2001.
36. Staron RS, Hagerman FC, Hikida RS, Murray TF, Hostler DP, Crill MT, Ragg KE, and Toma K. Fiber type composition of the vastus lateralis muscle of young men and women. *J. Histochem. Cytochem.* 48: 623, 2000.
37. Braun B, Gerson L, Hagobian T, Grow D, and Chipkin SR. No effect of short-term testosterone manipulation on exercise substrate metabolism in men. *J. Appl. Physiol.* 99: 1930–1937, 2005.
38. Febbraio MA. Alterations in energy metabolism during exercise and heat stress. *Sports Med.* 31: 47–59, 2001.
39. Brooks GA, Butterfield GE, Wolfe RR, Groves BM, Mazzeo RS, Sutton JR, Wolfel EE, and Reeves JT. Increased dependence on blood glucose after acclimatization to 4,300 m. *J. Appl. Physiol* 70: 919, 1991.
40. Hunt DG, Ding Z, and Ivy JL. Clenbuterol prevents epinephrine from antagonizing insulin-stimulated muscle glucose uptake. *J. Appl. Physiol.* 92: 1285–1292, 2002.
41. Schoeller DA and Buchholz AC. Energetics of obesity and weight control: does diet composition matter? *J. Am. Diet. Assoc.* 105: S24–28, 2005.
42. Buchholz AC and Schoeller DA. Is a calorie a calorie? *Am. J. Clin. Nutr.* 79: 899S–906S, 2004.
43. Flatt JP. Use and storage of carbohydrate and fat. *Am. J. Clin. Nutr.* 61: 952S–959S, 1995.
44. Hellerstein MK. No common energy currency: de novo lipogenesis as the road less traveled. *Am. J. Clin. Nutr.* 74: 707–708, 2001.
45. Jeukendrup AE. Carbohydrate intake during exercise and performance. *Nutrition* 20: 669–677, 2004.
46. van Erp-Baart AM, Saris WH, Binkhorst RA, Vos JA, and Elvers JW. Nationwide survey on nutritional habits in elite athletes. Part I. Energy, carbohydrate, protein, and fat intake. *Int. J. Sports Med.* 10 Suppl 1: S3–10, 1989.58. Westerterp KR, Saris WH, van Es M, and ten Hoor F. Use of the doubly labeled water technique in humans during heavy sustained exercise. *J. Appl. Physiol.* 61: 2162–2167, 1986.
47. Ebine N, Feng JY, Homma M, Saitoh S, and Jones PJ. Total energy expenditure of elite synchronized swimmers measured by the doubly labeled water method. *Eur. J. Appl. Physiol.* 83: 1–6, 2000.
48. Fudge BW, Westerterp KR, Kiplamai FK, Onywera VO, Boit MK, Kayser B, and Pitsiladis YP. Evidence of negative energy balance using doubly labelled water in elite Kenyan endurance runners prior to competition. *Br. J. Nutr.* 95: 59–66, 2006.
49. Hill RJ and Davies PS. Energy intake and energy expenditure in elite lightweight female rowers. *Med. Sci. Sports Exerc.* 34: 1823–1829, 2002.
50. Ruby BC, Shriver TC, Zderic TW, Sharkey BJ, Burks C, and Tysk S. Total energy expenditure during arduous wildfire suppression. *Med. Sci. Sports Exerc.* 34: 1048–1054, 2002.
51. Trappe TA, Gastaldelli A, Jozsi AC, Troup JP, and Wolfe RR. Energy expenditure of swimmers during high volume training. *Med. Sci. Sports Exerc.* 29: 950–954, 1997.
52. Dietary Guidelines for Americans 2005: U.S. Department of Health and Human Services and U.S. Department of Agriculture, 2005, p. 1–73.
53. Burke LM, Cox GR, Culmmings NK, and Desbrow B. Guidelines for daily carbo-hydrate intake: do athletes achieve them? *Sports Med.* 31: 267–299, 2001.
54. Burke LM, Kiens B, and Ivy JL. Carbohydrates and fat for training and recovery. *J. Sports Sci.* 22: 15–30, 2004.

55. Tarnopolsky M. Protein requirements for endurance athletes. *Nutrition* 20: 662–668, 2004.
56. Phillips SM. Protein requirements and supplementation in strength sports. *Nutrition* 20: 689–695, 2004.
57. Butterfield GE and Calloway DH. Physical activity improves protein utilization in young men. *Br. J. Nutr.* 51: 171–184, 1984.
58. Tipton KD, Borsheim E, Wolf SE, Sanford AP, and Wolfe RR. Acute response of net muscle protein balance reflects 24-h balance after exercise and amino acid ingestion. *Am. J. Physiol. Endocrinol. Metab.* 284: E76, 2003.

Section 1

Energy-Yielding Nutrients

2 Utilization of Carbohydrates in Energy Production

J. Andrew Doyle, Charilaos Papadopoulos, and Michael S. Green

CONTENTS

I. INTRODUCTION

Carbohydrates and fats are the main sources of energy during endurance exercise. Fat is the predominant fuel source at rest and during low intensity activity and exercise. The energy requirements of competitive endurance training and competition generally exceed the rate at which fat can be oxidized however, so carbohydrates are the predominant fuel source for these athletic activities. Carbohydrate is also the major source of energy for repetitive, high-intensity activities that utilize the anaerobic glycolytic energy system. It has been well established that severely reduced carbohydrate stores, i.e., muscle glycogen, liver glycogen, and blood glucose, are closely associated with fatigue and impaired performance in prolonged endurance tasks.[1] Therefore, a considerable amount of research has focused on methods of

25

manipulating endogenous carbohydrate stores and facilitating carbohydrate intake in an attempt to enhance carbohydrate oxidation and improve athletic performance in training and competition.

Research on carbohydrate manipulation has generally focused on one or more of the time periods during which its alteration may have a significant impact on endurance exercise performance, including:

1. Daily training
2. The week before a prolonged event
3. The hours (meal) before exercise
4. During the exercise task
5. The post-exercise period (4–48 hours)

The majority of this research has attempted to determine the optimal amount of carbohydrate to consume, the appropriate timing of the consumption, and within a fairly narrow focus, the appropriate type of carbohydrate. Studies of carbohydrate type have largely focused on the efficacy of different simple sugars (e.g., glucose and fructose) or polymers of glucose, and the optimal concentration of those carbohydrates in a beverage or sports drink. Comparably less attention has been given to carbohydrates in other forms, such as solid or semi-solid, or by their characterization as complex carbohydrates, and how their consumption may affect endurance exercise performance.

A relatively recent approach in sports nutrition research has been to study carbohydrates by the physiological response they provoke, particularly the blood glucose and insulin responses that result from their consumption. This categorization by glycemic response, known as the glycemic index (GI), may be a more appropriate way to examine the effectiveness of carbohydrate consumption on exercise and sports performance than a more general structural classification as simple or complex carbohydrates, because there is a wide range of glycemic responses within each general category.[2] Another recent focus in research of carbohydrates and exercise performance has been the inclusion of other nutrients such as specific amino acids along with the carbohydrate and the combination of different types of carbohydrates together to optimize the physiological response to the diet manipulation.

Athletes who are training and competing must make appropriate dietary decisions concerning carbohydrate intake: optimal amounts, timing, and types. They must consider the effect of carbohydrate intake on short-term training and competitive performance, but they must also keep in mind the potential effect of their dietary choices on long-term health and fitness. The purpose of this chapter is to examine the role of carbohydrates in exercise and sport, and to make practical recommendations by which the athlete can choose a healthy fundamental diet and can further optimize carbohydrate intake to potentially enhance exercise performance.

II. CARBOHYDRATE METABOLISM

Before exploring the manipulation of carbohydrate in the diet to improve exercise and sport performance, it is important to understand some of the fundamental concepts of carbohydrate digestion, absorption, and metabolism.

TABLE 2.1
Simple Carbohydrates

Carbohydrate	Comments
Monosaccharides:	
Glucose	Also known as dextrose; found in plant foods, fruits, honey
Fructose	Also known as fruit sugar; found in plant foods, fruits, honey
Galactose	Product of lactose digestion
Disaccharides:	
Sucrose	Also known as white or table sugar; composed of glucose and fructose; used as a sweetener
Lactose	Composed of galactose and glucose; found in milk and dairy products
Maltose	Composed of two glucose molecules; a product of starch digestion

Carbohydrates can be characterized by their structure and by the number of sugar molecules as either monosaccharides, disaccharides, or polysaccharides. Monosaccharides, such as glucose and fructose, containing one sugar molecule, are simple sugars. Disaccharides, such as sucrose, contain two sugar molecules, and are also characterized as simple carbohydrates. Simple carbohydrates and typical sources in the diet are listed in Table 2.1.

Polysaccharides, with many glucose units chained together, are considered complex carbohydrates. Starches, dextrins, fiber, and processed concentrated sugars compose complex carbohydrates. Maltodextrins are polysaccharides — glucose polymers — but contain no starch or fiber and are metabolized like simple sugars. Complex carbohydrates and typical dietary sources are listed in Table 2.2.

TABLE 2.2
Complex Carbohydrates

Carbohydrate	Comments
Polysaccharides:	
Amylopectin	Starch; found in plant foods and grains
Amylose	Starch; found in plant foods and grains
Carageenan	Soluble fiber; found in the extract of seaweed and used as food thickener and stabilizer
Cellulose	Insoluble fiber; found in the bran layers of grains, seeds, edible skins and peels
Corn Syrup	Hydrolyzed starch; found in processed foods
Dextrins	Starch; found in processed foods
Glycogen	Animal starch; found in meat, liver
Hemicellulose	Insoluble fiber; found in the bran layers of grains, seeds, edible skins and peels
Inulin	Soluble fiber; found in Jerusalem artichokes
Invert Sugar	Hydrolyzed sucrose; found in processed foods
Lignin	Insoluble fiber; found in plant cell walls
Pectins	Soluble fiber; found in apples

A. DIGESTION AND ABSORPTION

A wide variety of factors, alone and in combination, can affect the digestion and absorption of carbohydrates, including the form or structure of the carbohydrate, the type and content of fiber, the type of starch, the presence of other nutrients, the size of the food particles, and the methods of cooking and processing.[3] A brief overview is presented here.

Digestion and absorption of carbohydrates begins to a small degree in the mouth. Salivary amylases begin the process of digestion for complex carbohydrates by initiating the breakdown of starches and dextrins. Mastication, or chewing, is also an important part of the digestive process to reduce foods to smaller-sized particles. Mechanical action of the stomach continues this process of size reduction, which influences both rate of gastric emptying of food from the stomach into the small intestine and the surface area of the food particles made accessible to intestinal enzymes.

The majority of carbohydrate digestion and absorption occurs in the small intestine. After moving into the small intestine, the monosaccharides (glucose, fructose, and galactose) are absorbed directly into the blood via the capillaries within the intestinal villi. The disaccharides (sucrose, lactose, and maltose) are split into their constituent monosaccharides by disaccharidases, which are then absorbed directly into the blood. The complex carbohydrates are acted upon by pancreatic amylase and brush border enzymes that reduce polysaccharides to monosaccharides, which are then absorbed as described above. The monosaccharides that are absorbed into the intestinal circulation are transported to the liver via the hepatic portal vein. From this point forward, carbohydrate is mostly utilized by the body either as glucose, or in its storage form as glycogen.

Not all of the carbohydrate content of foods that are consumed is digested and absorbed. The carbohydrate that is not absorbed may be related to the form of the food, the type of starch, or the amount of fiber present in the food. Undigested and unabsorbed carbohydrates go to the large intestine, where they may be digested by colonic bacteria or excreted in the feces. Large amounts of indigestible carbohydrates or excessive amounts of simple sugars consumed rapidly may result in excessive gas production or gastrointestinal disturbances such as cramping and diarrhea. The fiber content of carbohydrate foods, which is largely indigestible by humans, plays an important role in maintaining appropriate gastric transit, may influence the eventual glycemic response to the foods consumed, and has important long-term health implications.

B. METABOLISM OF GLUCOSE AND GLYCOGEN

The major function of carbohydrates in human metabolism is to supply energy. Brain, retina, and red blood cells are totally dependent on glucose for energy.[4] Carbohydrates are also the most important energy source during exercise. During high-intensity exercise, carbohydrates are the preferred fuel and are almost exclusively utilized during maximal- or supramaximal-intensity exercise. Carbohydrate supplementation has been shown in a number of studies to improve endurance performance[5–12] The physiological source of carbohydrate used during endurance performance can be partitioned between endogenous and exogenous sources. Endogenous carbohydrate can be thought of as that present in the body prior to any form of supplementation (e.g., liver and muscle glycogen, circulating blood glucose, and glucose derived via gluconeogenesis). Our bodies, however, have a limited ability to store carbohydrates. The greatest amount of carbohydrate is stored in the form of muscle glycogen, between 300–400 grams, or 1,200–1,600 kilocalories. Glucose found in the blood totals approximately 5 grams, which is the equivalent of 20 kcals, while the liver contains about 75–100 grams of glycogen, or about 300–400 kcals.[4] Therefore, the total body storage of carbohydrate is approximately 1,600–2,000 kcals. Exogenous carbohydrate refers to that provided via ingested carbohydrate during or just prior to exercise.

The primary carbohydrate source of energy for physical exertion is muscle glycogen. As muscle glycogen is being used, blood glucose enters the muscle to maintain the energy requirements of the active tissue. Consequently, the liver will release some of its glucose to maintain blood glucose and prevent hypoglycemia (low blood glucose levels). Blood glucose is in short supply, so as it is being used during exercise it has to be replenished by liver glycogen stores. A depletion of glycogen stores may lead to hypoglycemia. Liver glycogen content can be decreased by starvation or exercise, or increased by a carbohydrate-rich diet. One hour of moderate-intensity exercise can reduce about half of the liver glycogen supply, whereas fifteen or more hours of starvation (such as an overnight fast) can virtually deplete liver glycogen. Hypoglycemia has been shown to impair the functioning of the central nervous system and is accompanied by feelings of dizziness, muscular weakness, and fatigue.

Normal concentration of blood glucose ranges between 4.0–5.5 mmol/L (80–100 mg/100 mL). Blood glucose concentration can increase after a carbohydrate meal or decrease after fasting. Maintenance of normal blood glucose is vital to human metabolism, thus blood glucose concentration is closely regulated. An increase in blood glucose stimulates the beta cells of the pancreas to secrete insulin into the blood. Insulin acts to lower blood glucose by facilitating its entrance into insulin-sensitive tissues, most notably muscle and adipose tissue, and the liver. On the other hand, low blood glucose levels cause other regulatory hormones to be secreted. Glucagon, secreted by the alpha cells in the pancreas, acts on the hepatic cells of the liver to cause the breakdown of glycogen. Epinephrine, the "fight or flight" hormone, acts on liver and muscle, causing glycogenolysis by stimulating glycogen phosphorylase, thus releasing glucose for muscle metabolism. Glucose can also be formed in the liver via a process called gluconeogenesis. During starvation, some amino acids like alanine can be converted to glucose. Muscle and red blood cells oxidize glucose to form lactate. Lactate can then enter the liver and be converted to glucose. This cyclic conversion, known as the Cori Cycle, allows this "new" glucose to circulate back to the tissue, and may account for approximately 40% of the normal glucose turnover.

Glucose enters the cells by facilitative glucose transporters (GLUT). These are integral membrane proteins that transport glucose down its concentration gradient via a process known as facilitated diffusion. Five hexose transporters have been identified and cloned. GLUT 1 (erythroid-brain barrier) is the glucose transporter in the human red cell. It is found in many tissues including heart, kidney, adipose cells, retina, and brain, but not in muscle or liver. Since it has a high expression in the brain, it forms part of the blood-brain barrier. GLUT 2 (liver glucose transporter) is expressed in liver, kidney, small intestine, and pancreas. GLUT 3 (brain glucose transporter) is 64% identical to GLUT 1 and appears to be present in all tissues, but its highest expression is in adult brain, kidney, and placenta. GLUT 4 (insulin-responsive glucose transporter) is a protein transporter that is 50%–65% identical to the other three glucose transporters. It is the major glucose transporter of insulin-sensitive tissue such as brown and white fat, skeletal, and cardiac muscle. Finally, GLUT 5 (the fructose transporter) has only 40% identity with the other glucose transporters and appears to transport glucose poorly. It is believed to transport fructose because it is found in high concentrations in human spermatozoa, which use fructose as an energy source.

One of the main sources of energy for competitive endurance activities is acquired via the oxidation of carbohydrate. Carbohydrate supplementation has been shown in a number of studies to improve endurance performance,[5-12] and numerous available reviews reiterate this information.[7,13] During endurance exercise at approximately 70% of $\dot{V}O_{2max}$, research suggests that muscle glycogen is primarily utilized for muscle ATP synthesis.[7,14]

C. Glycemic Index

Under normal circumstances, the physiological result of carbohydrate consumption, digestion, and absorption is a postprandial increase in blood glucose, followed by an increase in glucose uptake by tissues in the body that is facilitated by insulin secretion by the pancreas. The time course and magnitude of this glycemic response are highly variable with different foods and do not follow the basic structural characterization of carbohydrates as simple or complex. For example, the consumption of identical amounts of two simple sugars, glucose and fructose, result in very different blood glucose responses. Glucose ingestion provokes a rapid and large increase in blood glucose, which in turn rapidly returns to baseline levels. Fructose consumption, on the other hand, results in a much slower and lower glycemic response. This variability in postprandial glycemic response with different foods has important implications, particularly for those people who must carefully control their blood glucose level, such as people with diabetes. Because the glycemic response to carbohydrate consumption is not easily predictable by their characterization as simple or complex, the concept of the GI was created, tested on a variety of foods, and initially published by Jenkins, et al. in 1981.[2]

The GI is a ranking based upon the postprandial blood glucose response of a particular food compared with a reference food. Specifically, the GI is a percentage of the area under the glucose response curve for a specific food compared with the area under the glucose response curve for the reference food:[15]

$$GI = \left(\frac{\text{Blood glucose area of test food}}{\text{Blood glucose area of reference food}} \right) \times 100$$

Glucose or white bread containing 50 g of carbohydrate is typically used as the reference food. Test foods contain an identical amount of carbohydrate, and the blood glucose response is determined for either two or three hours after consumption of the meal.[16] Extensive testing of foods has resulted in the publication of tables of glycemic indices for a wide variety of foods.[17] Use of the GI has become an important reference tool for prescribing appropriate diets for clinical populations that have a need for close regulation of blood glucose, such as people with diabetes. Based as it is on physiological measurement, a high degree of precision cannot be expected from the GI. However, reviews of numerous GI studies indicate a high degree of consistency of response with the same foods, within approximately 10–15 units of measurement for most foods.[16] The GI of glucose (GI = 100) and fructose (GI = 23) clearly demonstrates the vast difference in glycemic response that can occur with the consumption of these two structurally similar monosaccharides.

Athletes may also benefit from considering the GI of the carbohydrates they consume as well as whether they are categorized as simple or complex carbohydrates. There may be specific situations where an athlete would want to consume high glycemic index foods and provoke a large blood glucose and insulin response, e.g., when attempting to synthesize muscle glycogen quickly.[18] Conversely, there may be occasions when the athlete may want to consume lower GI foods and avoid large increases in glucose and insulin. There is controversial evidence that the hyperglycemia and hyperinsulinemia associated with high GI foods consumed shortly before the onset of endurance exercise suppresses fat oxidation and may have a negative impact upon subsequent performance.[19] Therefore, the concept of the GI will be revisited in the sections on carbohydrate manipulation that follow.

III. CRITICAL PERIODS FOR CARBOHYDRATE MANIPULATION

Substantial research on the effect of carbohydrate intake on exercise performance has been published. In general, carbohydrate manipulation has been shown to be most effective for prolonged endurance activities (>2 hours) where carbohydrate stores and oxidation may limit performance, or is related to fatigue. A few studies have indicated a potential ergogenic effect of carbohydrate loading, pre-exercise meals, or intake during exercise on shorter-duration high-intensity activity, but the evidence is not sufficiently strong to definitively recommend carbohydrate use for improving performance in these types of activities.[20]

There are two major considerations athletes must contemplate when making dietary plans concerning carbohydrate intake. First, for maintenance of long-term health, most major health organizations recommend that carbohydrate make up the majority of energy intake.[21–23] Second, athletes must consider the demands of their sport or activity, and determine if it is appropriate to further manipulate carbohydrate intake in order to positively influence physical performance in training or competition.

Research of carbohydrate manipulation has typically used simple carbohydrates in beverages, when consumption of other forms of carbohydrate (e.g., solid food) may be difficult or poorly tolerated. Use of complex/solid carbohydrate during exercise may not be necessary, unless the exercise task is very prolonged, to the point that satiety and satisfaction are improved with solid food intake (e.g., ultra-marathons). An examination of the critical dietary periods for carbohydrate intake follows, with reference where applicable, to recommendations about complex versus simple carbohydrate intake.

A. THE DAILY TRAINING DIET

The first consideration for an athlete's daily training diet is to conform to recommendations for a long-term healthy dietary intake. Carbohydrates should make up the bulk of total energy intake, primarily in the form of grain products, vegetables, and fruits. Individuals should further seek to limit total fat, saturated fat, and cholesterol in their diets. The Dietary Guidelines for Americans further recommends that people choose a diet that is moderate in sugars.[21] The implication of this recommendation is an emphasis on complex carbohydrates and some simple sugars as consumed in grains, vegetables, and fruits, and a reduction in the intake of simple sugars that are typically consumed in soft drinks and snack foods. There is an emphasis on complex carbohydrates because a number of studies have shown an increased risk of chronic disease, particularly non-insulin-dependent diabetes mellitus (NIDDM), with a long-term dietary intake of foods with a high glycemic load, especially in conjunction with low fiber consumption.[24,25] By emphasizing a broad variety of food choices, athletes can easily consume a diet that is adequate in carbohydrate and also contains sufficient vitamins, minerals, and fiber.

To reduce the risk of chronic disease and to promote long-term health, a number of health organizations make basic dietary recommendations that are applicable to athletes. For reduced risk of heart disease, the American Heart Association recommends that the diet consist of 55–60% or more of energy intake from carbohydrates, with an emphasis on complex carbohydrates. They further recommend that fat compose 30% or less of the diet, with 8–10% from saturated fats.[23] To reduce one's risk of various common forms of cancer, the American Cancer Society recommends that the diet be mainly composed of foods from plant sources, with a minimum of five servings of fruits or vegetables each day, coupled with a limited intake of high-fat foods.[22] These dietary guidelines are well suited for active and athletic populations, giving a dietary foundation for long-term health, as well as providing a varied diet that is predominately composed of carbohydrates for fueling exercise.

Athletes must further consider whether the carbohydrate content of their diets is sufficient to support optimal performance in training and competition. The recommendation of The American Dietetic Association and The Canadian Dietetic Association is that, in general, the diet should be 60–65% carbohydrate, and elevated to 65–70% if the individual is currently engaged in exhaustive training.[26] It is important to note that total energy intake must be sufficient in order to obtain the necessary amount of carbohydrate. If total caloric intake is too low, even a diet that is >70% carbohydrate may yield an inadequate number of grams of carbohydrate. Therefore, carbohydrate consumption should be considered on an absolute basis (number of grams for each kilogram of body weight) to ensure adequate intake.

Carbohydrate content of the diet should be sufficient to maintain muscle glycogen stores during periods of intense training, or muscle glycogen concentrations will progressively decline.[27] Inadequate muscle glycogen levels may be associated with diminished training and competitive performance.[28] For those athletes engaged in exhaustive training, it is apparent that the diet may need to contain up to 10 grams of carbohydrate per kilogram of body weight each day to adequately replace the muscle glycogen they utilize during their daily training.[29] People involved in activities or training of lesser intensity and duration do not need to consume this much carbohydrate, but should maintain their carbohydrate intake at 7 grams per kilogram of body weight or more, depending on their level (intensity and duration) of activity. It may be difficult to consume this large amount of carbohydrate as food, and athletes may want to consider using carbohydrate supplements, particularly in liquid form, to increase their intake. Liquid carbohydrate supplements have the added advantage of increasing fluid intake, thus helping the athlete maintain adequate hydration levels.

B. THE WEEK BEFORE A PROLONGED ENDURANCE EVENT

Manipulation of exercise and carbohydrate content of the diet over a week's time has been shown to result in supranormal levels of muscle glycogen, which in turn enhances carbohydrate oxidation and improves endurance capacity in prolonged endurance activities such as cycling and running.[28,30] This strategy is known as "carbohydrate loading," or "muscle glycogen supercompensation." Most studies of muscle glycogen supercompensation have shown an increase in "time to exhaustion" during exercise at a moderate to high intensity, but few have assessed the effect on more valid and reliable measures of endurance performance such as actual competitive performance, time trials, time to perform a set amount of work, or use of protocols that more accurately mimic competitive events. Additionally, some studies lack placebo controls and utilize procedures such as overnight fasting, consumption of non-carbohydrate beverages during the exercise test, and other practices not typical of real-world conditions. A recent study, controlling for many of these variables (placebo-controlled and reliable laboratory cycle protocol), found no discernible effect of supercompensation on cycling performance.[31] Further research is needed to determine the potential beneficial effect of muscle glycogen supercompensation on performance.

Early studies showed a near doubling of muscle glycogen following the strategy referred to as the "classical" carbohydrate loading method.[28] However, this method has some onerous exercise and dietary demands that may be unacceptable to the athlete preparing for an important competition. Muscle glycogen is depleted with prolonged, exhaustive exercise and is maintained in a suppressed state for the next three days with a virtually carbohydrate-free diet. Depleting exercise is performed again to further reduce glycogen stores, after which the athlete rests and consumes a carbohydrate-rich diet for the three days before the event. While resulting in the highest muscle glycogen stores, this method of carbohydrate loading may have other adverse physical and psychological effects that may not be advantageous for subsequent performance.

Because of the extreme exercise and dietary manipulations of the classical carbohydrate loading method, many athletes may choose a more palatable method

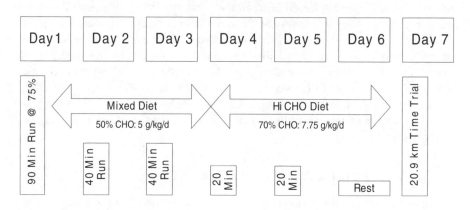

FIGURE 2.1 The modified carbohydrate loading strategy. (Adapted from Sherman, W.M. et al. Effect of exercise–diet manipulation on muscle glycogen and its subsequent utilization during performance. *Int. J. Sports Med.*, 2, 1981.With permission.)

referred to as "modified" carbohydrate loading (Figure 2.1).[30] In this method, athletes taper their training, following a more realistic exercise preparation during the week before an important event. Early in the week when the athlete is exercising for longer duration, the diet is manipulated to include a higher percentage of fat and protein, and less carbohydrate (approximately 50% of total calories). The final three days before the event, when the athlete is exercising the least, the amount of carbohydrate in the diet is increased to 70% or more, stimulating muscle glycogen storage. The amount of muscle glycogen synthesis following this modification is nearly as great as with the classical method, but the difficulties associated with exhaustive exercise and a period of very low carbohydrate diet are avoided.

The earliest studies did not have a detailed description of the composition of the diet used, but the carbohydrate content apparently consisted of a combination of complex and simple carbohydrates.[28,30] Two more-recent studies have investigated the efficacy of one type of carbohydrate over the other, and both concluded there was no advantage of either a predominately simple or a predominately complex carbohydrate diet in the three-day high carbohydrate period of the loading phase.[24,32] Both types of carbohydrate in the diet increased muscle glycogen similarly, and had a similarly positive impact on subsequent endurance exercise. Carbohydrate loading is a short-term, relatively infrequent manipulation of diet and exercise, and the incorporation of simple sugars during this period should not pose any significant dietary health risk for the athlete. It is recommended, however, that long-term dietary composition be composed mostly of complex carbohydrates with a lower glycemic load because of the relationship of chronic low-fiber, high-glycemic diets to increased risk of NIDDM.[25–33]

C. THE MEAL BEFORE EXERCISE

The meal consumed just prior to a training bout or competitive event may also be used to maximize carbohydrate stores in an attempt to improve performance. If these meals consist primarily of carbohydrate, they act to maximize muscle and liver glycogen stores before the onset of exercise. It has been conclusively demonstrated that fasting before prolonged endurance events results in diminished performance, so it is important for the athlete to consume a meal in the hours before long-duration training sessions or competitive efforts.[34] The meal should provide adequate energy and carbohydrate to support the metabolic demands of the exercise, be consumed in adequate time before the onset of exercise to allow for gastric emptying, digestion, and absorption, and also be palatable and acceptable to the athlete.

Carbohydrate meals of 1–2 grams per kilogram body weight eaten 1 hour before exercise, and meals containing up to 4.5 grams of carbohydrate per kilogram body weight consumed 3–4 hours before exercise have been shown to improve endurance performance.[12,35,36] There appears to be a positive additive effect when pre-exercise meals are consumed in conjunction with carbohydrate intake during exercise, leading to substantially better performance than when no carbohydrate is consumed, or when carbohydrate is consumed only before, or only during exercise.[12]

A current area of investigation is the possible effect that foods of differing glycemic indices may have on subsequent performance because of the potential for hyperglycemia and hyperinsulinemia at the onset of exercise.[19] Meals high in carbohydrate, particularly high glycemic foods, consumed in the hour or so before exercise, result in high insulin and decreasing blood glucose at the time that exercise begins. It has been hypothesized that this glycemic response, coupled with the enhanced glucose uptake by exercising muscle, may result in a "rebound" hypoglycemia, inhibition of FFA oxidation, and may impair endurance exercise performance. This concern has stimulated a considerable amount of recent research, and has led to recommendations to consume only low glycemic index foods prior to exercise.[19,37]

Studies generally show that consuming high GI foods within an hour of the onset of exercise results in hyperglycemia and hyperinsulinemia before exercise compared to low GI foods. At the onset of exercise, this results in a lowering of blood glucose, a decrease in free fatty acid (FFA) release and oxidation, and a greater reliance on carbohydrate oxidation during the exercise. However, there are two major reasons that this should not be of concern to the athlete. First, most studies show a decrease in blood glucose in the first 30–60 minutes of exercise, but blood glucose does not decrease to the low levels at which symptoms of hypoglycemia are experienced (neuroglucopenia), and very few studies have shown an impairment in subsequent performance.[38] If the exercise is continued for sufficient duration, blood glucose and insulin generally return to normally expected levels, and most studies show that carbohydrate consumption 1 hour before exercise improves performance regardless of the glycemic index.[20,38–45]

Second, from a practical perspective, most athletes would not choose to eat within an hour of beginning a long exercise bout. To allow time for adequate gastric emptying and to avoid gastrointestinal discomfort, most people would tend to eat 3–4 hours before exercise. This additional time allows for the return of glucose and insulin toward baseline levels and diminishes any lingering effects of the GI of the meal consumed.[46] Athletes should pay careful attention to their pre-training and competition diet to ensure they understand their body's response to the composition, amount, and timing of their pre-event meal.

In summary, it is important for an athlete to consume a meal before prolonged exercise in order to maximize endogenous carbohydrate stores. The meal should be timed so that it is largely cleared from the gastrointestinal tract before the onset of exercise, usually 3–4 hours, to minimize the possibility of gastric upset. The meal should be largely composed of carbohydrate, and should consist of food(s) the athlete is used to eating. This strategy should be employed consistently in training; new foods or meal patterns should not be instituted before important competitive events. The glycemic index of the foods consumed is not as important as the familiarity with, tolerance of, and timing of the meal. For example, in the early morning hours before a marathon, it would be more practical for a runner to consume a familiar high carbohydrate breakfast food such as oatmeal (GI = 61), rather than attempting to meet an unwarranted recommendation to consume a low glycemic index meal by consuming a bowl full of lentils (GI = 30).

D. DURING PROLONGED ENDURANCE EXERCISE

Endogenous stores of carbohydrate will eventually become depleted during prolonged moderate- to high-intensity exercise. Therefore, carbohydrate must be consumed in order to maintain a high rate of carbohydrate oxidation. A large body of research provides evidence that consumption of carbohydrate during exercise maintains blood glucose levels and carbohydrate oxidation and significantly improves both endurance capacity and performance.[7] Carbohydrate consumption during cycling exercise apparently does not reduce reliance on muscle glycogen, but maintains blood glucose as a fuel source for oxidation late in exercise, and clearly results in enhanced endurance capacity.[9] A study of runners utilizing an endurance performance protocol with published reliability showed a significant improvement in time trial performance when a carbohydrate beverage was consumed.[47]

Improvements in endurance capacity or performance have been seen when 0.5 to 1.0 grams of carbohydrate are consumed per kilogram of body weight every hour during exercise. Most studies have focused on carbohydrate intake as simple sugars or maltodextrins in beverages, while few studies have investigated complex carbohydrate or solid food consumption during exercise. Glucose and glucose polymers (maltodextrins) have been shown to be effective, particularly compared with low-GI carbohydrates such as fructose.[48]

Consuming carbohydrate in the form of a liquid beverage, or sports drink, is common during exercise. The consumption of other forms of carbohydrate, e.g., solid food, may be difficult or poorly tolerated during activities such as running. Other activities, such as cycling, may provide the opportunity for consumption of solid food with less discomfort. The few studies of solid food consumption during endurance exercise show improvements in performance compared with a placebo, but there is no evidence that solid or semi-solid carbohydrate consumption has any physiological or performance advantage over carbohydrate intake in liquid form.[49–52]

There may be circumstances, such as during ultra endurance events, when the consumption of solid food may enhance the feelings of satiety.

Drinking carbohydrate beverages conveys an additional benefit of aiding fluid replacement and thermoregulation if exercise is performed in a thermally challenging environment. The beverage must be formulated to reach a balance between carbohydrate energy delivery and gastric emptying and absorption. Beverages of higher concentration deliver more energy, but empty from the stomach more slowly.[53] It is apparent, however, that athletes may consume carbohydrate beverages in concentrations up to 10% without impairing thermoregulation.[54] Popular commercially available sports drinks typically contain between 6% and 8% carbohydrate, and can therefore be used effectively during endurance exercise. As with pre-exercise meals, athletes should incorporate this feeding strategy during their regular training, particularly during training sessions of long duration, to become accustomed to carbohydrate intake during exercise, and to determine their individually appropriate volume of consumption. Sudden introduction of unfamiliar carbohydrate feeding during exercise may result in gastrointestinal distress, cramping, diarrhea, or vomiting, which would likely result in poorer, rather than improved performance.

To date, most endurance performance studies have used glucose or glucose polymers to assess the benefits of performance during endurance exercise.[9,10,14] Additionally, different types of carbohydrates (such as fructose and the disaccharide sucrose) have been compared with each other.[48,55] Although many of these studies have demonstrated a beneficial effect of carbohydrate supplementation, many have also found there is an upper limit to the amount of carbohydrate that can actually be absorbed and utilized (i.e., oxidized) by the body during exercise. Due to factors related to the saturation of intestinal sodium-dependent glucose transporters (SGLT-1), as well as possible limitations exerted by the liver, it appears that exogenous glucose oxidation peaks at 1.0–1.1 g/min.[11,56] Similar investigations utilizing fructose have demonstrated oxidation rates 20–25% lower (peaking at ~0.7 g/min) when compared with glucose, thus suggesting the fructose intestinal transporter (GLUT-5) may act as a limiting factor, with the added possibility that conversion of fructose to glucose in the liver may also limit its oxidation.[55–57] The disaccharide sucrose (composed of equal amounts of glucose and fructose) also exhibits oxidation rates (~1.0 g/min) similar to glucose when provided in equal amounts.[58] An intriguing step is to thus combine mono- and disaccharides of various types in an attempt to overcome the saturation limitation of their individual intestinal transport mechanisms, with a resultant increase in oxidation rates (and presumably endurance performance).

A progressive series of studies have recently investigated the oxidation rates of various combinations of mono- and disaccharides in well-trained cyclists exercising for 120–150 min at 50% of maximum power (60–63% of $\dot{V}O_{2max}$).[59–62] A mixture of glucose and fructose (1.2 g/min glucose and 0.6 g/min fructose) was shown to have a peak exogenous oxidation rate of 1.26 g/min, a value 55% higher than that found with a solution of glucose alone.[60] Possibly substantiating the concept of intestinal saturation, this study also showed that there were no increases in oxidation rates when glucose-only solutions providing 1.2 or 1.8 g/min were used.[60] Likewise, no increases in exogenous carbohydrate oxidation significantly above 1.0 g/min have been achieved by supplementing either 2.4 g/min of glucose or 1.2 g/min of glucose combined with 0.6 g/min of the disaccharide maltose.[59,61] These findings suggest that additional amounts of carbohydrate in the form of glucose ingested above a rate of 1.2 g/min will not further increase oxidation rates.

Building on the findings of the above studies, and the apparent ceiling of exogenous carbohydrate oxidation that is reached at a glucose intake of 1.2 g/min, the effects of various glucose, sucrose, and fructose combinations and amounts has continued to provide interesting findings. High peak oxidation rates of 1.70 g/min have been found as a result of ingestion of a mixture providing 1.2 g/min glucose, 0.6 g/min sucrose, and 0.6 g/min fructose (for a total of 2.4 g/min of carbohydrate).[61] Of particular note, ingesting a total of 2.4 g/min of carbohydrate in the form of 1.2 g/min glucose and 1.2 g/min fructose has resulted in some of the highest oxidation measurements to date, resulting in peak oxidation rates of 1.75 g/min.[62]

Oxidation rates for exogenous carbohydrate have thus been shown to be highest when a prudent mixture of glucose and fructose (1.2 g/min of each) are combined together in a beverage consumed during prolonged exercise. It also appears that a mixture of glucose (1.2 g/min), sucrose (0.6 g/min), and fructose (0.6 g/min) can provide similar oxidation maximums. It seems that glucose consumed in isolation cannot sustain oxidation rates above 1.0 g/min, and if used in isolation does not need to be consumed in amounts higher than 1.2 g/min, which comes conveniently close to the recommended amount of 60–70 g of carbohydrate per hour typically recommended during prolonged endurance performance. The studies discussed above provide a strong theoretical basis for enhancing endurance performance via supplementation with a mixture of specific mono- or disaccharides. The ability to utilize greater levels of exogenous carbohydrate, especially in the latter stages of an endurance event, while possibly minimizing the use of endogenous carbohydrate sources, would seem to hold great potential for maintaining high levels of endurance performance. Further research is warranted to determine whether higher carbohydrate oxidation rates indeed translate into improved endurance performance.

E. IMMEDIATELY AFTER EXERCISE

Rapid replacement of carbohydrate stores, especially muscle and liver glycogen, may be important for many athletes. The athlete that competes in the occasional prolonged endurance event such as the marathon may not have the need for resynthesizing muscle glycogen rapidly, but one who participates in multiple, frequent activities that tax carbohydrates stores, such as weekend soccer tournaments, may require fast recovery. Rapid replacement of the body's carbohydrate stores can be achieved if carbohydrate is consumed quickly after depleting exercise. Delay for as little as 2 hours may result in significantly less muscle glycogen synthesis.[63] Therefore, the athlete seeking fast recovery should consume carbohydrates as soon as feasible after the depleting exercise.

Studies of muscle glycogen synthesis rates in the hours after exhaustive exercise have shown very rapid resynthesis when carbohydrates in amounts from 0.75 to 1.6 grams per kilogram body weight are consumed every hour for 4 hours.[64,65] When carbohydrate is consumed in a large meal every 2 hours, several studies indicate the larger amount of carbohydrate intake does not increase the glycogen synthesis rate any further.[65,66] However, at least one study has shown higher rates of synthesis when smaller carbohydrate meals were consumed more frequently (every 15 minutes).[64]

Although rapid muscle glycogen synthesis was seen with this feeding amount and strategy, athletes should be aware that the rapid consumption of large amounts of carbohydrates after exercise may cause gastrointestinal upset.

The form in which the carbohydrate is consumed after exercise may have some effect on the muscle glycogen replenishment rate. Although classified as a simple sugar, fructose has a low glycemic response, and its consumption has been shown to result in a slower rate of muscle glycogen synthesis than glucose.[66] Carbohydrate consumed in equivalent amounts in liquid and solid form appears to result in similar replacement rates for muscle glycogen.[67,68] Studies of simple versus complex carbohydrates have shown there to be no difference in the amount of muscle glycogen resynthesized in the first 24 hours after exhaustive exercise, but a diet in which the carbohydrate content was 70% complex carbohydrates resulted in greater muscle glycogen content 48 hours after exhaustive running.[69] In a study emphasizing the glycemic index of foods, Burke et al. demonstrated that high GI foods resulted in significantly greater muscle glycogen synthesis in the 24 hours after exhaustive cycling than low GI foods. The increased insulin and blood glucose response seen after consumption of high GI foods may stimulate a greater short-term synthesis of muscle glycogen, but there doesn't appear to be any advantage to their consumption after the first 24 hours.[18]

Another consideration is the inclusion of nutrients other than carbohydrate in the post-exercise meal. The inclusion of large amounts of fat in the meal is not advisable, as gastric emptying may be slowed and fat consumption provides neither the substrate nor the hormonal environment for optimal glycogen synthesis. A number of studies have examined the efficacy of including protein or specific amino acids in the post-exercise meal because of the effect they may have on increasing insulin secretion. When a mixture of wheat protein hydrolysate and the free amino acids leucine and phenylalanine was added to a post-exercise carbohydrate beverage, higher blood insulin levels and higher muscle glycogen synthesis were found compared with a carbohydrate-only beverage.[70,71] The inclusion of protein and amino acids apparently aids muscle glycogen synthesis when the amount of carbohydrate consumed is limited, but not when large amounts of carbohydrate are ingested. The consumption of 1.2 g/kg/h of carbohydrate stimulates a rate of muscle glycogen synthesis that is not exceeded when protein and amino acids are added.[71,72] The addition of protein and amino acids may have an additional benefit after exercise by stimulating protein synthesis and improving net protein balance.[73,74]

Athletes requiring rapid replacement of carbohydrate stores should eat or drink as soon as possible after depleting exercise. They should choose carbohydrates with a high glycemic index, and preferably consume them in small, more frequent meals rather in large amounts at one time. After this initial replacement period, the normal predominately complex carbohydrate diet can be resumed.

IV. PRACTICAL RECOMMENDATIONS

1. The basic diet should be consistent with the recommendations for chronic disease prevention and long-term health promotion. This diet is high in carbohydrate (>55% of total calories), low in fat (≤30% of total calories), and emphasizes a wide variety of foods.

TABLE 2.3
Practical Recommendations for Manipulation of Carbohydrate Intake

Time Period	Carbohydrate	Comments
Daily Training	7–10 g·kg⁻¹·day⁻¹ (3.2–4.5 grams per pound)	Amount depends upon duration and intensity of daily training; may need to supplement
Carbohydrate Loading	5 g·kg⁻¹·day⁻¹ for 3 days, then 8 + g·kg⁻¹·day⁻¹ for 3 days (2.3 then 3.6+ grams per pound)	For prolonged events (>2 hours); depleting exercise bout followed by tapered training for 6 days
Pre-exercise Meal	1–2 g·kg⁻¹ 1 to 2 hours before, or up to 4–5 g·kg⁻¹ 3 to 4 hours before (0.45–0.90 or 1.8–2.3 grams per pound)	Consume familiar foods; time meal before exercise to insure complete digestion
During Exercise	0.5–1.0 g·kg⁻¹·hour⁻¹ (0.23–0.45 grams per pound)	For prolonged events (>2 hours); sports drinks up to 10% concentration; may consider mixed carbohydrate types (glucose and fructose)
After Exercise	0.75–1.5 g·kg⁻¹·hour⁻¹ (0.34–0.68 grams per pound)	Evaluate need for rapid replacement of muscle glycogen; small, frequent feedings beginning as soon as possible for 2 to 4 hours; may consider addition of amino acids or protein

2. Evaluate the demands of the sporting or athletic activity, both for training and for competition. If the activity is of high intensity and is repeated frequently, or it is of prolonged duration, additional manipulation of carbohydrate in the diet may be called for during appropriate time periods.

3. Carbohydrate intake should be determined as an absolute amount based on the athlete's body weight, i.e., grams of carbohydrate per kilogram or pound of body weight (see recommended amounts in Table 2.3). A diet containing a high percentage of carbohydrate may be too low in actual grams of carbohydrate if the total energy intake is insufficient.

4. The majority of carbohydrate intake should be from a variety of foods, particularly fruits, vegetables, and whole grains. However, if carbohydrate intake needs are extreme, as with intense, prolonged training, consider the use of carbohydrate supplements.

5. Consider manipulation of carbohydrates during each of the critical time periods for training and competition. Practice these strategies during training; don't introduce any new foods or dietary practices before important competitive events.

V. FUTURE DIRECTIONS FOR RESEARCH

1. Studies of carbohydrate manipulation have predominately used exercise protocols that measure time to exhaustion at a fixed exercise intensity as a measure of endurance capacity. Few studies have determined the effects of carbohydrate consumption on valid and reliable measures of endurance performance.[47] Additional research is needed to confirm the ergogenic advantage of carbohydrate consumption using exercise protocols that more closely mimic the demands of competitive athletic performance.
2. Further research is needed to clarify whether the glycemic index of pre-exercise meals is an important determinant of subsequent performance. Recommendations to avoid high GI foods before exercise are based on what are perceived to be the adverse metabolic responses to these meals, while few studies have assessed their impact on endurance performance using valid and reliable protocols.
3. Mixing carbohydrate types in a beverage has the potential to increase carbohydrate uptake and oxidation during exercise. Additional research is required to determine if this enhanced carbohydrate availability can lead to improved endurance performance.

REFERENCES

1. Bergstrom, J. and Hultman, E. A study of the glycogen metabolism during exercise in man. *Scand. J. Clin. Lab. Invest.*, 19, 218–228, 1967.
2. Jenkins, D.J., Wolever, T.M., Taylor, R.H., Barker, H., Fielden, H., Baldwin, J.M., Bowling, A.C., Newman, H.C., Jenkins, A.L., and Goff, D.V. Glycemic index of foods: a physiological basis for carbohydrate exchange. *Am. J. Clin. Nutr.*, 34, 362–366, 1981.
3. Christian, J.L. and Greger, J.L. *Nutrition for Living;* The Benjamin/Cummings Publishing Company, Inc.: Redwood City, CA, 1991.
4. Shils, M.E., Olson, J.A., Shike, M., and Ross, A.C. *Modern Nutrition in Health and Disease;* 9th ed.; Williams and Wilkins: Baltimore, MD, 1999.
5. Below, P.R., Mora-Rodriguez, R., Gonzalez-Alonso, J., and Coyle, E.F. Fluid and carbohydrate ingestion independently improve performance during 1 h of intense exercise. *Med. Sci. Sports. Exerc.*, 27, 200–210, 1995.
6. Coggan, A.R. and Coyle, E.F. Reversal of fatigue during prolonged exercise by carbohydrate infusion or ingestion. *J. Appl. Physiol.*, 63, 2388–2395, 1987.
7. Coggan, A.R. and Coyle, E.F. Carbohydrate ingestion during prolonged exercise: Effects on metabolism and performance. In *Exercise and Sport Science Reviews*, John O.Holloszy, Ed.; Williams & Wilkins: Baltimore, 1991; p. 1.
8. Coyle, E.F., Hagberg, J.M., Hurley, B.F., Martin, W.H., Ehsani, A.A., and Holloszy, J.O. Carbohydrate feeding during prolonged strenuous exercise can delay fatigue. *J. Appl. Physiol.*, 55, 230–235, 1983.
9. Coyle, E.F., Coggan, A.R., Hemmert, M.K., and Ivy, J.L. Muscle glycogen utilization during prolonged strenuous exercise when fed carbohydrate. *J. Appl. Physiol.*, 61, 165–172, 1986.

10. Jeukendrup, A., Brouns, F., Wagenmakers, A.J., and Saris, W.H. Carbohydrate-electrolyte feedings improve 1 h time trial cycling performance. *Int. J. Sports Med.*, 18, 125–129, 1997.

11. Jeukendrup, A.E., Mensink, M., Saris, W.H., and Wagenmakers, A.J. Exogenous glucose oxidation during exercise in endurance-trained and untrained subjects. *J. Appl. Physiol.*, 82, 835–840, 1997.

12. Wright, D.A., Sherman, W.M., and Dernbach, A.R. Carbohydrate feedings before, during, or in combination improve cycling endurance performance. *J. Appl. Physiol.*, 71, 1082–1088, 1991.

13. Jeukendrup, A.E. Carbohydrate intake during exercise and performance. *Nutrition*, 20, 669–677, 2004.

14. Angus, D.J., Febbraio, M.A., and Hargreaves, M. Plasma glucose kinetics during prolonged exercise in trained humans when fed carbohydrate. *Am. J. Physiol. Endocrinol. Metab.*, 283, E573–E577, 2002.

15. Jenkins, D.J., Wolever, T.M., Jenkins, A.L., Josse, R.G., and Wong, G.S. The glycaemic response to carbohydrate foods. *Lancet*, 2, 388–391, 1984.

16. Wolever, T.M., Jenkins, D.J., Jenkins, A.L., and Josse, R.G. The glycemic index: methodology and clinical implications. *Am. J. Clin. Nutr.*, 54, 846–854, 1991.

17. Foster-Powell, K. and Miller, J.B. International tables of glycemic index. *Am. J. Clin. Nutr.*, 62, 871S–890S, 1995.

18. Burke, L.M., Collier, G.R., and Hargreaves, M. Muscle glycogen storage after prolonged exercise: effect of the glycemic index of carbohydrate feedings. *J. Appl. Physiol.*, 75, 1019–1023, 1993.

19. Walton, P. and Rhodes, E.C. Glycaemic index and optimal performance. *Sports Med.*, 23, 164–172, 1997.

20. Neufer, P.D., Costill, D.L., Flynn, M.G., Kirwan, J.P., Mitchell, J.B., and Houmard, J. Improvements in exercise performance: effects of carbohydrate feedings and diet. *J. Appl. Physiol.*, 62, 983–988, 1987.

21. *Dietary Guidelines for Americans, 2005*;001-000-04719-1; US Government Printing Office: Washington, DC, 05.

22. Kushi, L.H., Byers, T., Doyle, C., Bandera, E.V., McCullough, M., Gansler, T., Andrews, K.S., and Thun, M.J. The American Cancer Society Guidelines on Nutrition and Physical Activity for Cancer Prevention: Reducing the Risk of Cancer With Healthy Food Choices and Physical Activity. *CA Cancer J. Clin.*, 56, 254–281, 2006.

23. Lichtenstein, A.H., Appel, L.J., Brands, M., Carnethon, M., Daniels, S., Franch, H.A. Franklin, B., Kris-Etherton, P., Harris, W. S., Howard, B., Karanja, N., Lefevre, M., Rudel, L., Sacks, F., Van Horn, L., Winston, M., and Wylie-Rosett, J. Diet and Lifestyle Recommendations Revision 2006: A Scientific Statement From the American Heart Association Nutrition Committee. *Circulation*, 114, 82–96, 2006.

24. Roberts, K.M., Noble, E.G., Hayden, D.B., and Taylor, A.W. Simple and complex carbohydrate-rich diets and muscle glycogen content of marathon runners. *Eur. J. Appl. Physiol. Occup. Physiol.*, 57, 70–74, 1988.

25. Salmeron, J., Manson, J.E., Stampfer, M.J., Colditz, G.A., Wing, A.L., and Willett, W.C. Dietary fiber, glycemic load, and risk of non-insulin-dependent diabetes mellitus in women. *JAMA*, 277, 472-477, 1997.

26. Position of the American Dietetic Association and the Canadian Dietetic Association: nutrition for physical fitness and athletic performance for adults. *J. Am. Diet. Assoc.*, 93, 691–696, 1993.

27. Costill, D.L., Bowers, R., Branam, G., and Sparks, K. Muscle glycogen utilization during prolonged exercise on successive days. *J. Appl. Physiol.*, 31, 834–838, 1971.

28. Bergstrom, J., Hermansen, L., Hultman, E., and Saltin, B. Diet, muscle glycogen and physical performance. *Acta. Physiol. Scand.*, 71, 140–150, 1967.

29. Sherman, W.M., Doyle, J.A., Lamb, D.R., and Strauss, R.H. Dietary carbohydrate, muscle glycogen, and exercise performance during 7 d of training. *Am. J. Clin. Nutr.*, 57, 27–31, 1993.

30. Sherman, W.M., Costill, D.L., Fink, W.J., and Miller, J.M. Effect of exercise–diet manipulation on muscle glycogen and its subsequent utilization during performance. *Int. J. Sports Med.*, 2, 114–118, 1981.

31. Burke, L.M., Hawley, J.A., Schabort, E.J., St. Clair, G.A., Mujika, I., and Noakes, T.D. Carbohydrate loading failed to improve 100-km cycling performance in a placebo-controlled trial. *J. Appl. Physiol.*, 88 (4), 1284–1290, 2000.

32. Brewer, J., Williams, C., and Patton, A. The influence of high carbohydrate diets on endurance running performance. *Eur. J. Appl. Physiol. Occup. Physiol.*, 57, 698–706, 1988.

33. Salmeron, J., Ascherio, A., Rimm, E.B., Colditz, G.A., Spiegelman, D., Jenkins, D.J., Stampfer, M.J., Wing, A.L., and Willett, W.C. Dietary fiber, glycemic load, and risk of NIDDM in men. *Diabetes Care*, 20, 545–550, 1997.

34. Dohm, G.L., Beeker, R.T., Israel, R.G., and Tapscott, E.B. Metabolic responses to exercise after fasting. *J. Appl. Physiol.*, 61, 1363–1368, 1986.

35. Sherman, W.M., Brodowicz, G., Wright, D.A., Allen, W.K., Simonsen, J., and Dernbach, A. Effects of 4 h preexercise carbohydrate feedings on cycling performance. *Med. Sci. Sports Exerc.*, 21, 598–604, 1989.

36. Sherman, W.M., Peden, M.C., and Wright, D.A. Carbohydrate feedings 1 h before exercise improves cycling performance. *Am. J. Clin Nutr.*, 54, 866–870, 1991.

37. Guezennec, C.Y. Oxidation rates, complex carbohydrates and exercise. Practical recommendations. *Sports Med.*, 19, 365–372, 1995.

38. Thomas, D.E., Brotherhood, J.R., and Brand, J.C. Carbohydrate feeding before exercise: effect of glycemic index. *Int. J. Sports Med.*, 12, 180–186, 1991.

39. Febbraio, M.A. and Stewart, K.L. CHO feeding before prolonged exercise: effect of glycemic index on muscle glycogenolysis and exercise performance. *J. Appl. Physiol.*, 81, 1115–1120, 1996.

40. Goodpaster, B.H., Costill, D.L., Fink, W.J., Trappe, T.A., Jozsi, A.C., Starling, R.D., and Trappe, S.W. The effects of pre-exercise starch ingestion on endurance performance. *Int. J. Sports Med.*, 17, 366–372, 1996.

41. Guezennec, C.Y., Satabin, P., Duforez, F., Koziet, J., and Antoine, J.M. The role of type and structure of complex carbohydrates response to physical exercise. *Int. J. Sports Med.*, 14, 224–231, 1993.

42. Horowitz, J.F. and Coyle, E.F. Metabolic responses to preexercise meals containing various carbohydrates and fat. *Am. J. Clin. Nutr.*, 58, 235–241, 1993.

43. Jarvis, J.K., Pearsall, D., Oliner, C.M., and Schoeller, D.A. The effect of food matrix on carbohydrate utilization during moderate exercise. *Med. Sci. Sports Exerc.*, 24, 320–326, 1992.

44. Sparks, M.J., Selig, S.S., and Febbraio, M.A. Pre-exercise carbohydrate ingestion: effect of the glycemic index on endurance exercise performance. *Med. Sci. Sports Exerc.*, 30, 844–849, 1998.

45. Thomas, D.E., Brotherhood, J.R., and Miller, J.B. Plasma glucose levels after prolonged strenuous exercise correlate inversely with glycemic response to food consumed before exercise. *Int. J. Sport Nutr.*, 4, 361–373, 1994.

46. Coyle, E.F. Substrate utilization during exercise in active people. *Am. J. Clin. Nutr.*, 61, 968S–979S, 1995.

47. Doyle, J.A. and Martinez, A. L. Reliability of a protocol for testing endurance performance in runners and cyclists. *Res. Q. Exerc. Sport*, 69, 304–307, 1998.
48. Murray, R., Paul, G.L., Seifert, J.G., Eddy, D.E., and Halaby, G.A. The effects of glucose, fructose, and sucrose ingestion during exercise. *Med. Sci. Sports Exerc.*, 21, 275–282, 1989.
49. Fielding, R.A., Costill, D.L., Fink, W.J., King, D.S., Hargreaves, M., and Kovaleski, J.E. Effect of carbohydrate feeding frequencies and dosage on muscle glycogen use during exercise. *Med. Sci. Sports Exerc.*, 17, 472–476, 1985.
50. Hargreaves, M., Costill, D.L., Coggan, A., Fink, W.J., and Nishibata, I. Effect of carbohydrate feedings on muscle glycogen utilization and *exercise* performance. *Med. Sci. Sports Exerc.*, 16, 219–222, 1984.
51. Mason, W.L., McConell, G., and Hargreaves, M. Carbohydrate ingestion during exercise: liquid vs solid feedings. *Med. Sci. Sports Exerc.*, 25, 966–969, 1993.
52. Peters, H.P., van Schelven, W.F., Verstappen, P.A., de Boer, R.W., Bol, E., Erich, W.B., van der Togt, C.R., and de Vries, W.R. Exercise performance as a function of semi-solid and liquid carbohydrate feedings during prolonged exercise. *Int. J. Sports Med.*, 16, 105–113, 1995.
53. Murray, R. The effects of consuming carbohydrate-electrolyte beverages on gastric emptying and fluid absorption during and following exercise. *Sports Med.*, 4, 322–351, 1987.
54. Owen, M.D., Kregel, K.C., Wall, P.T., and Gisolfi, C.V. Effects of ingesting carbohydrate beverages during exercise in the heat. *Med. Sci. Sports Exerc.*, 18, 568–575, 1986.
55. Massicotte, D., Peronnet, F., Allah, C., Hillaire-Marcel, C., Ledoux, M., and Brisson, G. Metabolic response to [^{13}C]glucose and [^{13}C]fructose ingestion during exercise. *J. Appl. Physiol.*, 61, 1180–1184, 1986.
56. Jeukendrup, A.E. and Jentjens, R. Oxidation of carbohydrate feedings during prolonged exercise: current thoughts, guidelines and directions for future research. *Sports Med.*, 29, 407–424, 2000.
57. Massicotte, D., Peronnet, F., Brisson, G., Bakkouch, K., and Hillaire-Marcel, C. Oxidation of a glucose polymer during exercise: comparison with glucose and fructose. *J. Appl. Physiol.*, 66, 179–183, 1989.
58. Wagenmakers, A.J., Brouns, F., Saris, W.H., and Halliday, D. Oxidation rates of orally ingested carbohydrates during prolonged exercise in men. *J. Appl. Physiol.*, 75, 2774–2780, 1993.
59. Jentjens, R.L., Venables, M.C., and Jeukendrup, A.E. Oxidation of exogenous glucose, sucrose, and maltose during prolonged cycling exercise. *J. Appl. Physiol.*, 96, 1285–1291, 2004.
60. Jentjens, R. L., Moseley, L., Waring, R. H., Harding, L. K., and Jeukendrup, A.E. Oxidation of combined ingestion of glucose and fructose during exercise. *J. Appl. Physiol.*, 96, 1277–1284, 2004.
61. Jentjens, R.L., Achten, J., and Jeukendrup, A.E. High oxidation rates from combined carbohydrates ingested during exercise. *Med. Sci. Sports Exerc.*, 36, 1551–1558, 2004.
62. Jentjens, R.L. and Jeukendrup, A.E. High rates of exogenous carbohydrate oxidation from a mixture of glucose and fructose ingested during prolonged cycling exercise. *Br. J. Nutr.*, 93, 485–492, 2005.
63. Ivy, J.L., Katz, A.L., Cutler, C.L., Sherman, W.M., and Coyle, E.F. Muscle glycogen synthesis after exercise: effect of time of carbohydrate ingestion. *J. Appl. Physiol.*, 64, 1480–1485, 1988.

64. Doyle, J.A., Sherman, W.M., and Strauss, R.L. Effects of eccentric and concentric exercise on muscle glycogen replenishment. *J. Appl. Physiol.*, 74, 1848–1855, 1993.
65. Ivy, J.L., Lee, M.C., Brozinick, J.T., Jr., and Reed, M.J. Muscle glycogen storage after different amounts of carbohydrate ingestion. *J. Appl. Physiol.*, 65, 2018–2023, 1988.
66. Blom, P.C., Costill, D.L., and Vollestad, N.K. Exhaustive running: inappropriate as a stimulus of muscle glycogen super-compensation. *Med. Sci. Sports Exerc.*, 19, 398–403, 1987.
67. Keizer, H.A., Kuipers, H., van Kranenburg, G., and Geurten, P. Influence of liquid and solid meals on muscle glycogen resynthesis, plasma fuel hormone response, and maximal physical working capacity. *Int. J. Sports Med.*, 8, 99–104, 1987.
68. Reed, M.J., Brozinick, J.T., Jr., Lee, M.C., and Ivy, J.L. Muscle glycogen storage postexercise: effect of mode of carbohydrate administration. *J. Appl. Physiol.*, 66, 720–726, 1989.
69. Costill, D.L., Sherman, W.M., Fink, W.J., Maresh, C., Witten, M., and Miller, J.M. The role of dietary carbohydrates in muscle glycogen resynthesis after strenuous running. *Am. J. Clin. Nutr.*, 34, 1831–1836, 1981.
70. van Loon, L.J., Kruijshoop, M., Verhagen, H., Saris, W.H., and Wagenmakers, A.J. Ingestion of protein hydrolysate and amino acid-carbohydrate mixtures increases postexercise plasma insulin responses in men. *J. Nutr.*, 130, 2508–2513, 2000.
71. van Loon, L.J., Saris, W.H., Kruijshoop, M., and Wagenmakers, A.J. Maximizing postexercise muscle glycogen synthesis: carbohydrate supplementation and the application of amino acid or protein hydrolysate mixtures. *Am. J. Clin. Nutr.*, 72, 106–111, 2000.
72. Jentjens, R.L., van Loon, L.J., Mann, C.H., Wagenmakers, A.J., and Jeukendrup, A.E. Addition of protein and amino acids to carbohydrates does not enhance postexercise muscle glycogen synthesis. *J. Appl. Physiol.*, 91, 839–846, 2001.
73. Tipton, K. D., Ferrando, A.A., Phillips, S.M., Doyle, D., Jr., and Wolfe, R.R. Postexercise net protein synthesis in human muscle from orally administered amino acids. *Am. J. Physiol.*, 276, E628–E634, 1999.
74. Rasmussen, B. B., Tipton, K.D., Miller, S.L., Wolf, S.E., and Wolfe, R.R. An oral essential amino acid-carbohydrate supplement enhances muscle protein anabolism after resistance exercise. *J. Appl. Physiol.*, 88, 386–392, 2000.

3 Utilization of Fats in Energy Production

Serge P. von Duvillard, Jena Hamra, G. William Lyerly, Jonathan A. Moore, and J. Larry Durstine

CONTENTS

I. INTRODUCTION

Energy sources for skeletal muscle metabolism are fats and carbohydrates; however, energy fuel mobilization and utilization are largely determined by the duration and intensity of the activity. During prolonged lower-intensity exercise performance, lipid oxidation becomes predominant, while high-intensity exercise utilizes carbohydrate metabolism. Triacylglycerols represent the largest fuel reserve in the body, with most stored in adipose tissue (~17,500 mM) and to a lesser extent, skeletal muscle (~300 mM) and plasma (~0.5 mM).[1] Furthermore, the amount of lipid stored in the body exceeds glycogen stores by approximately 50 times.[1]

Fatty acid oxidation during sustained prolonged physical activity delays glycogen depletion and hypoglycemia. Utilization of fatty acids requires the hydrolysis
of triacylglycerols from adipose tissue, muscle, and plasma. The increased hydrolysis
from adipose tissue requires the delivery of fatty acids to skeletal muscle mitochondria for oxidation.[1] However, the release of free fatty acids (FFAs) into blood and
the concentration of plasma FFAs are not closely matched to energy need.[2] While
vigorous exercise results in an initial fall of plasma FFA usage, a progressive increase
in the release of FFAs is seen following prolonged exercise as a result of increased
rates of lipolysis.[2] Exercise-induced increases in catecholamine levels and concurrent
decreases in plasma insulin concentrations mediate the increased lipolysis rates and
therefore FFA release. Therefore, working muscles progressively increase the uptake
and oxidation of FFAs due to increasing plasma concentrations. Surprisingly, intramuscular triacylglycerol stores still provide more than half of the oxidized fat,
although the contributions of fats from muscle decrease as they are depleted.[2]

The use of triacylglycerols as an energy source requires the coordination and
regulation of lipolysis in adipocytes, adipose tissue blood flow, and skeletal muscle
blood flow. However, triacylglycerol's role as an energy substrate is dependent not
only on exercise intensity and duration but is also modulated by other factors, such
as endurance training, diet, age, and gender. As carbohydrate storage is limited and
fat yields more than twice the energy of carbohydrates, bodily actions that increase
fat utilization will ultimately improve exercise endurance. Therefore, this chapter
examines some of the recent advances and current evidence that address the issues
of fat metabolism associated with exercise and human performance.

II. OVERVIEW OF FAT METABOLISM

A. SYNTHESIS OF TRIACYLGLYCEROLS (TGS)

Lipid storage sites are found in all tissue including muscle but are most apparent in fat
cells or adipocytes. Lipid fuel sources during exercise include circulating plasma triacylglycerol and free fatty acids, as well as muscle triacylglycerol. TGs, nonpolar, non-
water-soluble molecules composed of three fatty acid chains esterified to a glycerol
molecule, represent a non-ionic storage form of FFAs. Exogenous TGs are broken down
into two FFAs and one 2-monoacylglycerol molecule. Short-chain FFAs are water
soluble and can be freely absorbed and transported to the liver. However, long-chain
FFAs are not water soluble and must be resynthesized to TGs in the mucosal cells of
the intestinal tract. From there, TGs are incorporated into chylomicrons that absorb TGs
into the general circulation via intestinal lymph, thus bypassing the liver. Endogenous
TGs are synthesized in the liver from plasma FFAs or glucose and are then transported
in the plasma by VLDL (very low density lipoproteins).[3] Due to their nonpolar nature,
TGs can be stored compactly as fat droplets in adipocytes and muscle cells.[4]

B. ADIPOSE LIPOLYSIS

Hydrolysis of TGs in adipocytes results in three molecules of non-esterified FFAs
(NEFA) and one molecule of glycerol. Re-esterification of NEFA does not occur in
adipocytes as they lack the enzyme glycerol kinase, which controls the esterification of

NEFA and glycerol into TGs.[8] Hydrolysis of TGs is controlled by the rate-limiting enzyme, hormone-sensitive lipase (HSL). HSL, acting on TGs in adipose tissue, results in the formation of 2 FFAs and one monoacylglycerol molecule. Monoacylglycerol lipase then metabolizes the monoacylglycerol molecule to one FFA and one glycerol molecule.[4]

Phosphorylation activates HSL, which then shifts from the cytosol to the surface of the lipid storage droplet. HSL works at the cytosol–lipid droplet interface. The substrate concentration at the interface not only influences the rate of lipolysis, but also the specific fatty acids generated (Figure 3.1). Specifically, fatty acids mobilized from lipid droplets contain a higher concentration of highly unsaturated fatty acids in relation to long-chain saturated and monounsaturated fatty acids and this ratio may be determined by the overall shape of the binding pocket in HSL.[5,6]

HSL is regulated by several hormones, primarily the two catecholamines norepinephrine and epinephrine, and also by insulin. Catecholamines regulate the activity of HSL through activation of adrenergic receptors on adipocyte membranes. Activation of β_1 and β_2 adrenoreceptors activates HSL, thereby stimulating lipolysis, while activation of α_2 adrenoreceptors is inhibitory. Adrenergic receptors are G protein coupled receptors. β-adrenoreceptors are coupled to the G_s protein, with activation resulting in the formation of cyclic adenosine monophosphate (cAMP), while α-adrenoreceptors are coupled to the G_i protein, which inhibits the formation of cAMP.

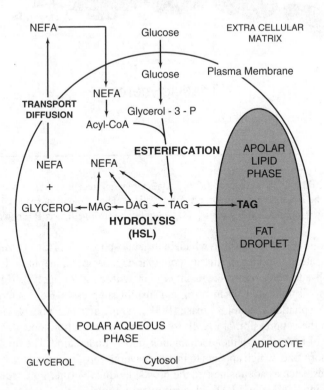

FIGURE 3.1 Simplified diagram of lipid mobilization into and from adipose tissue (DAG = diacylglycerol; HSL = hormone-sensitive lipase; MAG = monocylglycerol; NEFA = nonesterified fatty acids; TAG = tricylglycerol).

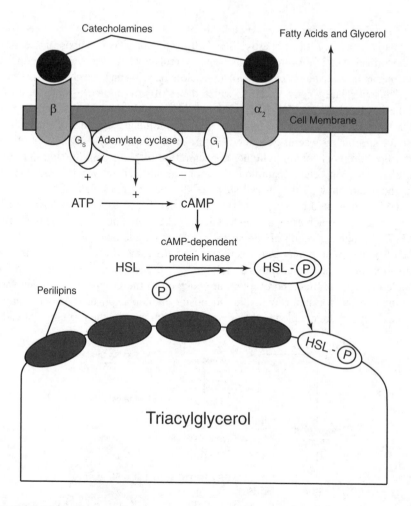

FIGURE 3.2 The lipolytic cascade (a2 = alpha2-adrenergic receptor; ATP = adenosine triphosphate; B = beta-adrenergic receptor; cAMP = cyclic adenosine monophospate; Gi = inhibitory G protein; Gs = stimulatory G protein; HSL = hormone-sensitive lipase; P = phospate group).

cAMP activates protein kinase A, which in turn phosphorylates HSL. During exercise, circulating catecholamines, primarily epinephrine, rise. As epinephrine has a higher affinity for β-adrenoreceptors, the result is an increased rate of lipolysis (Figure 3.2).[7]

Lipolysis is inhibited by insulin, and insulin suppresses HSL activity. Insulin activates phosphatidylinositol 3-kinase (PI3K), which activates phosphodiesterase-3, resulting in the suppression of cAMP formation.[7,8] Growth hormone also stimulates the activity of HSL, though the mechanism is poorly understood. The lipolytic action of growth hormone, which appears to involve several steps, is modulated by a number of paracrines, such as adenosine and the prostaglandins. Furthermore, several cytokines, including TNF-α and IL-6, also stimulate lipolysis.[8]

Under normal physiological conditions, lipolysis is controlled primarily by hormonal signaling and energy needs (see Table 3.1). The response to a given hormone

TABLE 3.1
Lipolytic Regulators and Their Proposed Mechanisms of Action

Factor	Proposed Mechanism of Action
Lipolytic Stimulators	
Catecholamines (Epinephrine and Norepinephrine)	• Stimulate β-adrenergic receptors and interact with G_s proteins on plasma membrane • Activate adenylate cyclase, initiating a cascade of signals culminating in the activation of HSL
Growth Hormone (GH)	• Increases catecholamine-stimulated lypolysis • Increases in secretion overnight, and thus may be important for regulating nocturnal lypolysis • Apparently modifies lipolytic rate over several hours and thus may have little or no acute effect on lipolysis during acute exercise
Cortisol	• Increases posttranscriptional β-adrenergic receptor expression • Increases the lipolytic response to catecholamines
Thyroid Hormones	• Upregulate adipocyte β-adrenergic receptor expression • Decrease phosphodiesterase
Cytokines	• Tumor necrosis factor α (TNFα) increases lipolysis by downregulating G_i proteins
Leptin	• Stimulates lipolysis independently of the adenylate cyclase cascade • Perhaps acts through inhibition of phosphodiesterase • May involve NO • Enhances glycerol release without a proportional increase in fatty acids
Testosterone	• Increases catecholamine-stimulated lipolysis via increased β-receptor expression and enhanced adenylate cyclase activity • May require GH for action
Lipolytic Inhibitors	
Insulin Catecholamines (Epinephrine and Norepinephrine) Insulin-like growth factor-1 (IGF-1) Adenosine Prostaglandin Neuropeptide Y (NPY)	• Increases phosphodiesterase activity, which leads to a reduction in cAMP • Stimulate $α_2$-adrenergic receptors and interact with G_i proteins on plasma membrane, which inhibits adenylate cyclase • Likely inhibits lipolysis in a manner similar to insulin (via phosphorylation of phosphodiesterase) • May interfere with lipolysis induced by growth hormone • Stimulates adenosine receptors, which inhibit adenylate cyclase by interacting with G_i proteins on the plasma membrane (similar to $α_2$-adrenergic receptors) • Prostaglandin E_1 and E_2 inhibits lipolysis via interaction with G_i proteins • Inhibits adenylate cyclase through interaction with G_i proteins

is determined not only by hormone concentration, but also by receptor densities and responsiveness, of which the location of adipose tissue plays a major role. This results in significantly different lipolytic rates, and therefore NEFA availability, depending on the location of adipose tissue.

Physiological conditions affect the energy needs and hormonal signaling that control lipolysis and NEFA release, i.e., resting post-absorptive state, resting post-prandial state, and exercise, etc. The post-absorptive phase, which is a short-term period of fasting, results in mobilization of energy stores, release of NEFA, and the increase in lipolysis in adipocytes via HSL. A reduction in plasma insulin is the primary stimulus for the increase in lipolysis.[9] In contrast, in the postprandial state there is a reduction in HSL activity and therefore lipolytic rate. Elevation of insulin levels is the primary signal mediating suppression of lipolysis after a mixed meal. Moreover, re-esterification of NEFA, resulting in the formation of TGs, is also mediated by insulin.[10] However, after a high-fat meal, most circulatory NEFA is derived from intravascular lipolysis as a result of lipoprotein lipase activity.[11]

III. NUTRITIONAL INSIGHTS

A. DIETARY SOURCES

As previously mentioned, the length of fatty acid chains influences their metabolism in the body. While all fatty acids are bonded to a single glycerol molecule, they may have one or more double bonds between carbon atoms; those fatty acids with one double bond are referred to as monounsaturated fats, and fatty acids with more than one double bond are known as polyunsaturated fats. If there are no double bonds, the fat (fatty acids) is said to be saturated. The degree of saturation in fatty acids, together with the length of the chains, determines the kind of fat. Saturated fats, which have no double bonds and tend to have longer fatty acid chains, are geometrically more linear and are usually solid at room temperature. These saturated fats are derived primarily from animal sources, in such products as meats and dairy (milk, butter). Unsaturated fats, however, are almost never solid at room temperature, due to the double bonds and shorter length of the fatty acids. The double bonds cause a slight change or twist in the molecular shape of the chain, and as a result the triglyceride molecules cannot associate as well with each other. The result is an oily, rather than solid, consistency. Unsaturated (both mono- and polyunsaturated) fats that are commonly found are almost exclusively derived from plant sources, e.g., olive oil. Research has demonstrated a strong positive association between the unsaturated fat variety and better health, especially health of the cardiovascular system.

Another type of fat is called "trans fat." Trans fats are synthetic fats produced by infusing unsaturated fats with H ions at the double bond sites, creating a newly saturated molecule. This process, however, results in a different orientation of the hydrogen atoms around the carbon atoms when compared with naturally occurring saturated fats (e.g., elaidic acid). Trans fats are hydrogenated or partially hydrogenated vegetable oils, most margarines, and shortening. They are extensively used by the fast-food industry. Several Western countries (e.g., Denmark and Canada) tightly regulate human consumption of trans fats. Several have requested better labeling and content identity of trans fats for human consumption. Trans fats have received attention as increasing the risk of cardiovascular disease even more than the natural saturated fats. In contrast, certain unsaturated fats contain omega-3 fatty acids (unsaturated fatty acids with a double bond at the omega-3 carbon), which may decrease the risk of cardiovascular disease by mitigating inflammatory processes.[58]

B. SUPPLEMENTATION

Research has addressed the question of whether there are physiologically feasible supplements that could increase lipid metabolism. One such supplement that has received attention is L-carnitine. In the body's cells, carnitine is an important protein responsible for shuttling fatty acyl-coA across the inner mitochondrial membrane into the mitochondrial matrix to undergo oxidative metabolism. The enzymes that catalyze this reaction are known collectively as carnitine acyl transferase 1, or CAT1.[12] When taken as a supplement, however, L-carnitine in the muscle has been shown to remain unchanged following supplementation,[13] and does not decrease following a single prolonged exercise session.[14] A recent study also concluded that L-carnitine taken as a supplement with exercise in untrained individuals does not have a positive effect on lipid metabolism.[15]

Diet is also a regulatory factor for fatty acid oxidation. High carbohydrate availability is associated with a decrease in lipid oxidation. Conversely, both short-term and long-term high-fat diets are associated with a decrease in carbohydrate reserves that results in increased utilization of fats as an energy source. Moreover, long-term high-fat diets may induce mitochondrial adaptations that increase fat oxidation.[16] Although primarily linked with decreased adipose lipolysis resulting from increased insulin levels, decreased fat oxidation, present knowledge suggests, results in part from decreased long-chain fatty acid entry into mitochondria.[16,17] For example, several investigations report that fat oxidation by skeletal muscle during exercise is the primary factor for increased fat oxidation following a high-fat diet.[18,19] In addition, Rowlands and Hopkins[20] found that a 2-week high-fat diet also increased fat oxidation during exercise and enhanced ultra-endurance cycling performance compared with a high carbohydrate diet. However, carbohydrate loading prior to exercise did not enhance the effects of the high-fat diet on performance.[20] Conversely, Coyle and coworkers have reported that an extremely low fat, high carbohydrate diet resulted in a reduction in fat oxidation and intramuscular triacylglycerol concentrations during exercise.[21]

Increased availability of plasma FFAs increases utilization of fat and thus spares muscle and liver glycogen. While long-chain (C_{16-22}) TGs are usually not available while one is exercising, medium-chain (C_{8-10}) TGs are quickly oxidized.[22] Lambert et al.[22] report that consumption of medium-chain TGs combined with carbohydrate spares muscle carbohydrate stores during 2 hours of submaximal cycling exercise ($<70\%$ $\dot{V}O_{2Peak}$) and improves 40 km time trial performance.[22] In addition, the same investigators examined chronic exercise training metabolic adaptations and their effects on substrate utilization and prolonged performance when athletes ingest a diet high in fat ($<70\%$ by energy). Their data showed that the body adapted to the fat diet, and after 2–4 weeks gained a nearly 2-fold increase in resistance to fatigue during prolonged, low- to moderate-intensity cycling ($<70\%$ $\dot{V}O_{2Peak}$).[22] Similarly, Helge and coworkers found that a fat-rich diet resulted in increased fat oxidation and decreased carbohydrate oxidation.[23] Lean body mass has a profound effect on fat oxidation.

Although diet has a major effect on substrate oxidation, prior athletic training does not have an effect on substrate oxidation in a controlled respiration chamber. [29]

A high-fat diet with carbohydrate restoration may affect metabolism and performance during ultra-endurance exercise.[24] Six days of exposure to a high-fat, low-carbohydrate diet followed by 1 day of carbohydrate restoration increased fat oxidation during 5 hours of submaximal cycling exercise in seven competitive athletes. The study failed to detect a significant performance benefit in a 1-hour time trial after 4 hours of continuous cycling.[24]

C. Body Reserves

Humans, like all animals, store the majority of their energy as fatty acids. These fatty acids are esterified to TG. TG, an efficient energy storage molecule, is packaged into lipid droplets similar to lipoproteins. Storing fat as TGs plays an integral part in the body's energy homeostasis. Almost every adult has TG stores that equal over 80,000 kcal of potential energy. This amount is over 40 times greater than the amount of energy that is stored in both skeletal muscle and the liver. To put this in perspective, the available energy stores of TG are enough to fuel a person to complete over 25 marathon races.[25] However, to use this energy, TGs must first be hydrolyzed. This will result in the release of fatty acids that must be delivered to the tissues where they will be oxidized. This process requires the coordinated regulation of lipolysis, blood flow and fatty acid transport in skeletal muscle to enhance the delivery of released fatty acids from adipose tissue to the mitochondria of working muscle.[25]

D. Toxicity

An excess of fatty acids, especially nonesterified fatty acids (NEFA), can accumulate in the parenchymal cells of many non-adipose tissues, including skeletal and cardiac myocytes, hepatocytes, and pancreatic -cells.[26] This excess of fatty acids is termed lipotoxicity. The accumulation of fatty acids can result in chronic cellular dysfunction and injury that has been associated with several diseases. These include insulin resistance, pancreatic -cell dysfunction, cardiomyopathy, steatohepatitis, dyslipidemia, and hypertension.[26,27] This negative effect is usually seen in the obese and not trained individuals.

Exercise seems to have positive effects on TG stores as compared with the negative effects that occur in the obese. The major difference proposed is that there is a higher skeletal muscle contractile activity in trained individuals than in the obese. This increased muscle activity results in an increased β-oxidation capacity, which results in a higher turnover rate of TGs and leads to a reduction of peroxidation.[28] In the obese, this decreased skeletal muscle activity results in a decreased β-oxidation capacity and an aggregation of TGs leading to an increase of peroxidation.[28]

IV. EFFECTS OF PHYSICAL PERFORMANCE

A. FFA Release from Adipose Tissue and Delivery to Muscle

FFA availability is a critical factor in the regulation of FFAs as an energy source. Plasma FFAs, bound to albumin, are stored as fat droplets in most tissue, but the fat must be transported to muscle cells in order for oxidation to occur. FFAs are primarily mobilized from adipose tissue; this process is dependent on the rate of lipolysis.[4] Movement of FFAs across muscle cell membranes is mediated and facilitated by the transport protein fatty acid-binding protein ($FABP_{PM}$). Once inside the cell, the cytoplasmic fatty acid binding proteins ($FABP_C$) regulate the intracellular transport of FFAs to the mitochondria. Entry into the mitochondria is another site of regulation. Long-chain fatty acids (LCFA), unlike medium-chain fatty acids (MCFA), require a transporter to enter the mitochondria, which may limit LCFA oxidation during high-intensity exercise. Finally, oxidative capacity, which is dependent primarily on β-oxidative and Krebs cycle enzymes, may also modulate FFA oxidation rates.[16] A recent study corroborated the primary importance of these myocellular mechanisms rather than the vascular delivery of plasma FFA; net leg total FFA was measured in subjects before and after different exercise intensities and durations, and FFA uptake was found to be unaffected.[30] Although exercise is an important regulator of energy balance, chronic exercise training has little effect on substrate oxidation in adipose tissue.[29]

B. LIPOLYSIS DURING EXERCISE

Many studies have addressed the effect of various exercise intensities and duration on lipolysis of adipose tissue in both men and women. Low-intensity exercise (25% $\dot{V}O_{2Max}$) increases adipose tissue TG lipolysis, resulting in increased levels of FFAs available for oxidation by exercising skeletal muscle.[31,32] Lipolysis in adipose tissue appears to be highest during low-intensity exercise (25% $\dot{V}O_{2Max}$) and does not increase over extended time periods. Although lipolysis in peripheral adipocytes does not increase with moderate exercise intensity (65% $\dot{V}O_{2Max}$), there is an increase in oxidation of plasma FFAs along with a decrease in oxidation of muscle glycogen and TGs over time. In contrast, plasma FFAs decrease as exercise intensity increases to 85% $\dot{V}O_{2Max}$, suggesting that reduced availability of plasma FFAs contributes to the decline in lipid oxidation as exercise intensity increases from 65% to 85% $\dot{V}O_{2Max}$.[33]

Endurance exercise training results in adaptations in fat and carbohydrate metabolism. When compared with untrained healthy controls, endurance-trained cyclists have an increased resting rate of TG lipolysis and an increased appearance of plasma FFAs, FFA oxidation rate, and TG-FFA cycling. Therefore, endurance exercise training results in an increased lipid kinetic profile at rest.[34] Furthermore, Phillips and coworkers demonstrated that endurance training resulted in increased fat oxidation during moderate-intensity exercise after only 5 days of training. Moreover, long-term training (31 days) resulted in greater utilization of intramuscular TGs (IMTGs) and reduced oxidation of glucose.[35] In support of these data, Schrauwen et al.[36] showed that a 3-month low-intensity endurance-training program increases resting and exercise-induced oxidation of IMTGs and plasma FFAs.[36] Moreover, these changes appear to be mediated by the up-regulation of lipoprotein lipase mRNA expression and down-regulation of acetyl-CoA carboxylase-2 mRNA expression.[36]

Fat metabolism in endurance-trained individuals is altered even as exercise intensity increases when compared with untrained individuals. Using tracer methods,

Coggan and coworkers demonstrated that endurance-trained athletes have higher levels of lipid oxidation following 30 minutes of high-intensity exercise (75–80% VO_{2max}) than untrained men.[37] Moreover, the additional FFAs utilized appear to be derived from both adipose tissue and IMTGs.[37] In contrast, a high-intensity intermittent-training program (HIIT) resulted in greater β-oxidation activity when compared with an endurance-training program. In addition, the HIIT program resulted in a greater loss of subcutaneous fat, possibly by enhancing post-exercise lipid utilization.[38]

Endurance exercise training increases adipose lipolysis regulation in part by circulating epinephrine via β-adrenoreceptors. *In vitro* studies suggest that the sensitivity of adipose tissue to epinephrine is increased in untrained individuals following exercise.[39] In endurance-trained individuals, however, a single exercise session (1 hour at 70% $\dot{V}O_{2Max}$) did not increase *in vivo* sensitivity of adipose β-adrenergic receptors to epinephrine.[40] Furthermore, endurance exercise training does not alter lipolysis or adipose tissue blood flow following an epinephrine infusion during resting conditions.[41]

While lipid metabolism has been well characterized in men, less work has been completed in women. At the same exercise intensity, women utilize a higher ratio of lipids to carbohydrates than men. Horton and coworkers[42] evaluated fuel oxidation before, during and after exercise (2 h at 40% $\dot{V}O_{2Max}$) as well as on a control day. Under resting conditions (before and after exercise, and a control day), there were no differences based on sex in substrate oxidation. During exercise, however, women utilized more fat and fewer carbohydrates as a fuel source than men.[42] Horowitz et al.[43] examined whole-body and regional lipolytic activity, and whole-body and plasma fatty acid oxidation in six women during 90 minutes of cycle exercise at 50% of pre-training $\dot{V}O_{2Peak}$.[43] These measurements were completed before and after 12 weeks of endurance training. During this experiment, skeletal muscle content for peroxisome proliferator-activated receptor-α and its target proteins, and medium-chain and very long-chain acyl-CoA dehydrogenase was measured. A 25% increase in whole body fatty acid oxidation during exercise after the 12-week exercise training period was found; exercise training, however, did not change adipose tissue lipolysis. Furthermore, exercise training doubled the levels of muscle peroxisome proliferator-activated receptor-α and its target proteins: medium-chain and very long-chain acyl-CoA dehydrogenase. These results suggest that changes in lipid metabolism resulting from endurance training are specific to skeletal muscle and may involve the peroxisome proliferator-activated receptor-α as a result of metabolic adaptations to training.[43]

C. MUSCLE TRIACYLGLYCEROL

1. IMTG Stores During Exercise

While plasma FFAs are the primary energy source utilized during exercise, intramuscular TGs stores may also be utilized. FFA availability from muscle TGs is challenging to determine because of the difficulty in distinguishing FFAs that are derived from lipid droplets in muscle fibers from those FFAs originating in adipocytes located between the fibers.[4] The adrenergic system, through β$_2$-adrenoreceptors, controls the release of FFAs from IMTGs by modulating the activity of a hormone-sensitive lipase similar to that found in adipocytes.[16,44] Utilization of IMTGs is seen primarily in Type IIa muscle fibers (fast-twitch) as opposed to Type I fibers (slow-twitch), which use FFAs from adipocytes.[45]

While generally accepted that both adipocyte- and muscle-derived TGs are used during exercise, some controversy exists regarding the utilization of IMTGs in untrained individuals.[46] Using skeletal muscle biopsy samples, several investigators have reported reduced IMTG following prolonged moderate-intensity exercise.[44,47] Other investigators, however, have not been able to replicate these findings using similar protocols.[48] Watt and coworkers[48] demonstrated that IMTG was reduced after 120 minutes of moderate-intensity exercise, but further reduction was not noted at 240 minutes. These results suggest that reduced utilization of IMTG during prolonged exercise may reflect greater plasma FFA delivery and oxidation.[48]

2.   Estimation of IMTG Use During Exercise

Oxidation of IMTG is well documented in endurance athletes.[49] For example, IMTG content in Type I fibers decreases following 2 hours of moderate-intensity exercise in endurance-trained athletes; however, the oxidation rate of IMTG decreases while plasma FFA oxidation rate increases over time.[49] In contrast, a short 2-week training period resulted in increased IMTG content and no change in IMTG utilization during exercise. These data support the theory that an increase in IMTG content may be an early adaptive response to exercise training, and this adaptation occurs prior to changes in fat oxidation.[50] While there appears to be a net utilization of IMTG following prolonged moderate intensity exercise, IMTG does not appear to contribute to enhanced lipid oxidation during recovery from exhaustive glycogen-depleting exercise.[51] Moreover, although IMTG is decreased in active muscle following moderate-intensity exercise, there is a concomitant increase in IMTG in non-exercising skeletal muscle that is associated with increases in plasma FFAs.[52]

Magnetic resonance spectroscopy has been frequently used to measure IMTGs. Johnson et al.[53] used magnetic resonance spectroscopy to assess IMTG content of vastus lateralis muscle before and after time trial cycling periods of 3-hour duration. In this investigation, six highly trained male cyclists completed a double-blind randomized crossover design of two experimental trials after a strenuous exercise bout and 48 hours of high- and low-carbohydrate diet. Resting IMTG content was significantly higher after low-carbohydrate versus high-carbohydrate diet and diminished during exercise by 64% and 57%, respectively. IMTG content was not different between conditions after exercise. The absolute degradation of IMTG content was greater during long-time low-carbohydrate diet when compared with the high-carbohydrate diet. Four of the six subjects had a reduction in IMTG content exceeding 70% during exercise. The results from this study suggest that IMTG stores may be exhausted by prolonged strenuous cycling exercise.[53]

D.   Lipid Ingestion Post Exercise: How Important Is It?

If IMTG is used during exercise, this short-chained fat must be replenished during a recovery period. However, repeated exercise periods without proper replenishment of IMTGs are thought to lead to decreased performance. Few studies have investigated replenishing IMTGs after endurance exercise, and the few that have been completed report that high levels of fat intake (35%–57% of total energy intake) will replenish IMTG stores more quickly than low levels of fat intake (10%–24%).[54] The amount of fat needed to completely replenish IMTG stores is estimated at approximately 2 g • kg^{-1} body mass per day.[55]

In a randomly assigned crossover design, Larson-Meyer et al.[56] investigated changes in IMTG stores from baseline after a 2-hour treadmill run at 67% $\dot{V}O_{2Max}$. During the recovery period, subjects consumed a low-fat (10% energy) and a moderate-fat (35%) diet. Utilizing nuclear magnetic resonance spectroscopic imaging before and 9 hours, ~22 hours, and 70 hours after the running period, Larson-Meyer et al.[56] showed IMTG content fell by approximately 25% during the endurance run. The consumption of a moderate fat diet allowed IMTG content to return to baseline within 22 hours and overshoot at 70 hours post-exercise. Unlike the high-fat diet, IMTG did not return to baseline with the low fat diet even after 70 hours post-exercise. These results suggest that a certain quantity of dietary fat is required to restore IMTG stores after running.[56]

High-fat diets are associated with increased lipid content in skeletal muscle and insulin resistance. Bachman and coworkers[57] examined the role of both high-fat and low-fat diets on IMTG storage and sensitivity to insulin in soleus and tibialis anterior muscle. While the low-fat diet did not alter IMTG storage or insulin sensitivity, the high-fat diet resulted in an increase in IMTG storage in the tibialis anterior but not the soleus muscle. Moreover, IMTG storage did not change with either diet in the soleus muscle. This study demonstrated that increases in circulating NEFA may result in increased IMTG storage as well as decreased insulin sensitivity.[57]

V. FUTURE DIRECTIONS

In the past 25 years a plethora of information has become available regarding fat consumption and physical performance. At the same time, information regarding the negative impact of high-fat diets and disease is overwhelming. Presently, more work is needed to assess the short term use of fat regarding exercise performance and its impact on negatively altering risk for disease. The recent USDA recommended diet of 30% fat, 15% protein, and 55% carbohydrates may be optimal for proper IMTG replenishment for individuals who exercise with at least one or more days of rest between exercise sessions,[54] but this is an area that still remains clouded. Another area where further work is needed concerns consuming a diet high in carbohydrates and low in fat during the initial 6 to 8 hours post-exercise in the replenishment of IMTG fat stores.[54] Additional work in these areas would not only give needed information on short-term dietary fat consumption and the improvement of exercise performance, but could also lead to improved treatment methods for diabetes, obesity, and other metabolically related disorders. Unfortunately, little information is known about whether starting an exercise session with less than normal IMTG will affect the performance of moderately intense exercise.

VI. SUMMARY

The abundant supply of fats and their high energy content per unit weight provides a vast potential for energy reserves. What is more important is the utilization of fats for a fuel source that will spare glucose and glycogen stores. The use of fats both from IMTG and adipose tissue during low to moderate intensity exercise (<25% to 65% $\dot{V}O_{2Max}$) can then allow for the use of carbohydrates as an energy substrate for times of sustained high-energy demand (>65% $\dot{V}O_{2Max}$). Of special interest is the fact that the capacity for fat utilization is enhanced after endurance exercise training. This enhanced fat utilization is characterized by increased adipocyte lipolysis resulting in increased plasma FFAs circulating to working tissue and the increased mitochondrial content found after exercise training. The increased availability of circulating FFAs and the increased number of muscle mitochondria augment superior endurance capacity found after endurance exercise training. One must remember that enhanced exercise performance as a result of enhanced fat oxidation is seen only at low- to moderate-exercise intensities, because at higher-exercise intensities (>65% $\dot{V}O_{2Max}$) carbohydrates and not fats are the primary fuel for exercise performance.

REFERENCES

1. Horowitz, J.F. and Klein, S. Lipid metabolism during endurance exercise. *Am J Clin Nutr* 72: 588S–63S, 2000.
2. Holloszy, J.O. and Kohrt, W.M. Regulation of carbohydrate and fat metabolism during and after exercise. *Ann Rev Nutr* 16: 121–38, 1996.
3. Despopoulos, A. and Silbernagl, S. *Color Atlas of Physiology.* 5th edition, Thieme Publishers, Stuttgart, 2003.
4. Ranallo, R.F. and Rhodes, E.C. Lipid metabolism during exercise. *Sports Med* 26: 29–42, 1998.
5. Raclot, T. Selective mobilization of fatty acids from adipose tissue triacylglycerols. *Prog Lipid Res* 42: 257–88, 2003.
6. Raclot, T. Selective mobilization of fatty acids from white fat cells: evidence for relationship to the polarity of triacylglycerols. *Biochem J* 322: 483–89, 1997.
7. Horowitz, J.F. Adipose tissue lipid mobilization during exercise. In: *Exercise Metabolism* Hargreaves, M. and Spriet, L., eds., Human Kinetics, 89–104, 2006.
8. Stich, V. and Berlan, M. Physiological regulation of NEFA availability: lipolysis pathway. *Proc Nutr Soc* 63: 369–74, 2004.
9. Horowitz, J.F., Coppack, S.W., Paramore, D., Cryer, P.E., Zhao, G., and Klein, S. Effect of short-term fasting on lipid kinetics in lean and obese women. *Am J Physiol* 276: E278–84, 1999.
10. Evans, K., Clark, M.L., and Frayn, K.N. Effects of an oral and intravenous fat load on adipose tissue and forearm lipid metabolism. *Am J Physiol* 276: E241–8, 1999.
11. Frayn, K.N., Summers, L.K.M., and Fielding, B.A. Regulation of plasma non-esterified fatty acid concentration in the postprandial state. *Proc Nutr Soc* 56: 713–21, 1997.
12. Brooks, G.A., Fahey, T.D., White, T.P., and Baldwin, K.M. *Exercise Physiology: Human Bioenergetics and Its Applications.* (3rd ed.) Mountain View: Mayfield, 2000.

13. Vukovich, M.D., Costill, D.L., and Fink, W.J. Carnitine supplementation: Effect on muscle carnitine and glycogen content during exercise. *Med Sci Sports Exer*, 26:1122–1129, 1994.

14. Decombaz, P., Deriaz, O., Acheson, K., Gmuender, B., and Jequier, E. Effect of L-carnitine on submaximal exercise metabolism after depletion of muscle glycogen. *Med Sci Sports Exer*, 25:733–740, 1993.

15. Lee, J.K., Lee, J.S., Park, H., Cha, Y-S, Yoon, C.S., and Kim, C.K. Effect of L-carnitine supplementation and aerobic training on FABP$_c$ content and beta-HAD activity in human skeletal muscle. *Eur J Appl Physiol* 2006. [e-pub ahead of print].

16. Turcotte, L.P. Role of fats in exercise. *Clinics in Sports Med* 18: 485–98, 1999.

17. Coyle, E.F., Jeukendrup, A.E., Wagenmakers, A.J.M., and Saris, W.H. Fatty acid oxidation is directly regulated by carbohydrate metabolism during exercise. *Am J Physiol* 273: E268–75, 1997.

18. Zderic, T.W., Davidson, C.J., Schenk, S., Byerley, L.O. and Coyle, E.F. High-fat diet elevated resting intramuscular triglyceride concentration and whole body lipolysis during exercise. *Am J Physiol Endocrinol Metab* 286: E217–25, 2004.

19. Schrauwen, P, Wagenmakers, A.J.M., van Marken Lichtenbelt, W.D., Saris, W.H.M., and Westerterp, K.R. Increase in fat oxidation on a high-fat diet is accompanied by an increase in triglyceride-derived fatty acid oxidation. *Diabetes* 49: 640–6, 2000.

20. Rowlands, D.S. and Hopkins, W.G. Effects of high-fat and high-carbohydrate diets on metabolism and performance in cycling. *Metabolism* 51: 678–90, 2002.

21. Coyle, E.F., Jeukendrup, A.E., Oseto, M.C., Hodgkinson, B.J., and Zderic, T.W. Low-fat diet alters intramuscular substrates and reduces lipolysis and fat oxidation during exercise. *Am J Physiol Endocrinol Metab* 280: E391–8, 2001.

22. Lambert, E.V., Hawley, J.A., Goedecke, J., Noakes, T.D., and Dennis, S.C. Nutritional strategies for promoting fat utilization and delaying the onset of fatigue during prolonged exercise. *J Sports Sci* 15: 315–24, 1997.

23. Helge, J.W., Watt, P.W., Richtor, E.A., Rennie, M.J., and Kiens, B. Fat utilization during exercise: Adaptation to a fat-rich diet increases utilization of plasma fatty acids and very low density lipoprotein-triacylgylcerol in humans. *J Physiol* 537: 1009–20, 2001.

24. Carey, A.L., Staudacher, H.M., Cummings, N.K., Stepto, N.K., Nikolopoulos, V., Burke, L.M., and Hawley, J.A. Effects of fat adaptation and carbohydrate restoration on prolonged endurance exercise. *J Appl Physiol* 91: 115–22, 2001.

25. Horowitz, J.F. Fatty acid mobilization from adipose tissue during exercise. *Trends Endocrinol Metab* 14: 386–92, 2003.

26. Weinberg, J.M. Lipotoxicity. *Kidney Intl* 70: 1560–66, 2006.

27. Wolins, N.E., Brasaemle, D.L., and Bickel, P.E. A proposed model of fat packaging by exchangeable lipid droplet proteins. *Fed Eur Biochem Soc* 580: 5484–91, 2006.

28. Russell, A.P. Lipotoxicity: The obese and endurance-trained paradox. *Intl J Obesity* 28: S66–S71, 2004.

29. Roy, H.J., Lovejoy, J.C., Keenan, M.J., Bray, G.A., Windhauser, M.M., and Wilson, J.K. Substrate oxidation and energy expenditure in athletes and nonathletes consuming isoenergetic high- and low-fat diets. *Am J Clin Nutr* 67: 405–11, 1998.

30. Jacobs, K.A., Krauss, R.M., Fattor, J.A., Horning, M.A., Friedlander, A.L., Bauer, T.A., Hagobian, T.A., Wolfel, E.E., and Brooks, G.A. Endurance training has little effect on active muscle free fatty acid, lipoprotein cholesterol, or triglyceride net balances. *Am J Physiol Endocrinol Metab*, 291: E656–E665, 2006.

31. Wolfe, R.R., Klein, S., Carraro, F., and Weber, J.M. Role of triglyceride–fatty acid cycle in controlling fat metabolism in humans during and after exercise. *Am J Physiol* 258: E382–9, 1990.

32. Klein, S., Coyle, E.F., and Wolfe, R.R. Fat metabolism during low-intensity exercise in endurance trained and untrained men. *Am J Physiol* 267:E934–40, 1994.

33. Romijn, J.A., Coyle, E.F., Sidossis, L.S., Gastaldelli, A., Horowitz, J.F., Endert, E., and Wolfe, R.R. Regulation of endogenous fat and carbohydrate metabolism in relation to exercise intensity and duration. *Am J Physiol* 265: E380–91, 1993.

34. Romijn, J.A., Klein, S., Coyle, E.F., Sidossis, L.S., and Wolfe, R.R. Strenuous endurance training increases lipolysis and triglyceride–fatty acid cycling at rest. *J Appl Physiol* 75(1): 108–13, 1993.

35. Phillips, S.M., Green, H.J., Tarnopolsky, M.A., Heigenhauser, G.J.F., Hill, R.E., and Grant, S.M. Effects of training duration on substrate turnover and oxidation during exercise. *J Appl Physiol* 81(5): 2182–91, 1996.

36. Schrauwen, P., van Aggel-Leijssen, D.P.C., Hul, G., Wagenmakers, A.J.M., Vidal, H., Saris, W.H.M., and van Baak, M.A. The effect of a 3-month low-intensity endurance training program on fat oxidation and acetyl-CoA carboxylase-2 expression. *Diabetes* 51: 2220–6, 2002.

37. Coggan, A.R., Raguso, C.A., Gastaldelli, A., Sidossis, L.S., and Yeckel, C.W. Fat metabolism during high-intensity exercise in endurance-trained and untrained men. *Metabolism* 49: 122–8, 2000.

38. Tremblay, A., Simoneau, J.A., and Bouchard, C. Impact of exercise intensity on body fatness and skeletal muscle metabolism. *Metabolism* 43: 814–8, 1994.

39. Wahrenberg, H, Engfeldt, P., Bolinder, J., and Arner, P. Acute adaptation in adrenergic control of lipolysis during physical exercise in humans. *Am J Physiol* 253: E382–9, 1987.

40. Klein, S., Coyle, E.F., and Wolfe, R.R. Effect of exercise on lipolytic sensitivity in endurance-trained athletes. *J Appl Physiol* 78: 2201–6, 1995.

41. Horowitz, J.F., Braudy, R.J., Martin, W.H., and Klein, S. Endurance exercise training does not alter lipolytic or adipose tissue blood flow sensitivity to epinephrine. *Am J Physiol* 277: E325–31, 1999.

42. Horton, T.J., Pagliassotti, M.J., Hobbs, K., and Hill, J.O. Fuel metabolism in men and women during and after long-duration exercise. *J Appl Physiol* 85: 1823–32, 1998.

43. Horowitz, J.F., Leone, T.C., Feng, W., Kelly, D.P., and Klein, S. Effect of endurance training on lipid metabolism in women: A potential role for PPARα in the metabolic response to training. *Am J Physiol Endocrinol Metab* 279: E348–55, 2000.

44. Cleroux, J., Van Nguyen, P., Taylor, A.W., and Leenen, F.H. Effects of β_2- vs β_1- + β_2-blockade on exercise endurance and muscle metabolism in humans. *J Appl Physiol* 66: 548–54, 1989.

45. Williams, R.S., Caron, M.G., and Daniel, K. Skeletal muscle β-adrenergic receptors: Variations due to fiber type and training. *Am J Physiol* 246: E160–7, 1984.

46. Watt, M.J., Heigenhauser, G.J.F., and Spriet, L.L. Intramuscular triacylglycerol utilization in human skeletal muscle during exercise: Is there a controversy? *J Appl Physiol* 93: 1185–95, 2002.

47. Phillips, S.M., Green, H.J., Tarnopolsky, M.A., Heigenhauser, G.J.F., and Grant, S.M. Progressive effect of endurance training on metabolic adaptations in working skeletal muscle. *Am J Physiol* 270: E265–72, 1996.

48. Watt, M.J., Heigenhauser, G.J.F., Dyck, D.J., and Spriet, L.L. Intramuscular triacylglycerol, glycogen and acetyl group metabolism during 4 h of moderate exercise in man. *J Physiol* 541: 969–78, 2002.

49. van Loon, L.J.C., Koopman, R., Stegen, J.H.C.H., Wagenmakers, A.J.M., Keizer, H.A., and Saris, W.H.M. Intramyocellular lipids form an important substrate source during moderate intensity exercise in endurance-trained males in a fasted state. *J Physiol* 553: 611–25, 2003.

50. Schrauwen-Hinderling, V.B., chrauwen, P., Hesselink, M.K.C., van Engelshoven, J.M.A., Nicolay, K., Saris, W.H., Kessels, A.G., and Kooi, M.E. The increase in intramyocellular lipid content is a very early response to training. *J Clin Endocrinol Metab* 88: 1610–6, 2003.

51. Kimber, N.E., Heigenhauser, G.J.F., Spriet, L.L., and Dyck, D.J. Skeletal muscle fat and carbohydrate metabolism during recovery from glycogen-depleting exercise in humans. *J Physiol* 548: 919–27, 2003.

52. Schrauwen-Hinderling, V.B., van Loon, L.J.C., Koopman, R., Nicolay, K., Saris, W.H.M., and Kooi, M.E. Intramyocellular lipid content is increased after exercise in nonexercising human skeletal muscle. *J Applied Physiol* 95: 2328–32, 2003.

53. Johnson, N.A., Stannard, S.R., Mehalski, K., Trenell, M.I., Sachinwall, T., Thompson, C.H., and Thompson, M.W. Intramyocellular triacylglycerol in prolonged cycling with high- and low-carbohydrate availability. *J Appl Physiol* 94: 1365–72, 2003.

54. Spriet, L.L. and Hargreaves, M. The metabolic system: Interaction of lipid and carbohydrate metabolism. In *ACSM's Advanced Exercise Physiology*, Lippincott, Williams and Wilkins: 410–420, 2006.

55. Decombaz, J. Nutrition and recovery of muscle energy stores after exercise. *Sportmedizin Sporttraumatologie* 51: 31–38. 2003.

56. Larson-Meyer, D.E., Newcomer, B.R., and Hunter, G.R. Influence of endurance running and recovery diet on intramyocellular lipid content in women: a ^{1}H NMR study. *Am J Physiol Endocrinol Metab* 282: E95–E106, 2002.

57. Bachman, O.P., Dahl, D.B., Brechtel, K., Machann, J., Haap, M., Maier, T., Loviscach, M., Stumvoll, M., Claussen, C.D., Schick, F., Haring, H.U., and Jacob, S. Effects of intravenous and dietary lipid challenge on intramyocellular lipid content and the relation with insulin sensitivity in humans. *Diabetes* 50: 2579–84, 2001.

58. Jeukendrup, A.E. and Aldred S. Fat supplementation, health, and endurance performance. *Nutrition* 20:678–688, 2004.

4 Utilization of Proteins in Energy Metabolism

Mauro G. Di Pasquale

CONTENTS

I. INTRODUCTION

Of the three macronutrients — carbohydrates, fats and protein — that compose our food, protein is the most important and versatile. Not only do proteins make up three quarters of body solids[1] (including structural and contractile proteins, enzymes, nucleoproteins, and proteins that transport oxygen) but protein and amino acids have potent biological effects that involve all tissues in the body and extend to almost all metabolic processes.

There is a vast body of research on the effects of protein and the individual amino acids on athletic performance. The results of this research have shown that not only do athletes need more protein than their sedentary counterparts, but has also described the profound effects that protein and amino acids have on athletic performance, primarily on muscle size and strength, energy metabolism, and immune function.

Since all cells in the body require energy for maintenance, repair, growth, and to maintain function, procuring this energy from food is the foundation for life. All three of the macronutrients are sources of energy. However, the focus in this chapter is on the utilization of proteins and amino acids in energy production. In following this thread we'll see that amino acids are involved in every aspect of energy metabolism and under certain conditions can be the main players. In fact, theoretically, amino acids can replace carbohydrates completely and replace fats as an energy source, leaving only the need for essential fatty acids for life. The major drawback to using protein to replace carbohydrates and fat is the problem of nitrogen elimination, which under certain circumstances can be toxic.[2]

A discussion of the role of proteins in energy production of necessity involves at least touching on other aspects of protein metabolism, including the dietary intake of proteins and the metabolic processes of which protein and amino acids are an integral part.

II. THE STRUCTURE AND PROPERTIES OF PROTEIN

A. STRUCTURAL, CONTRACTILE, ENZYMES AND OTHER PROTEINS

The word protein comes from the Greek word "proteios" which means "of the first rank" or "importance." Protein is indeed important for life, being involved in every biological process within the body. The average human body is approximately 18% protein. Proteins are essential components of muscle, skin, cell membranes, blood, hormones, antibodies, enzymes and genetic material, and almost all other body tissues and components. They serve as structural components, biocatalysts (enzymes), antibodies, lubricants, messengers (hormones), and carriers.

B. FREE AMINO ACID POOL

Of the body's vast content of amino acids, only a small amount is not bound up in protein structures of one sort or another. Only 0.5 to 1% of the amino acids in the body is present as free amino acids and make up the body's free amino acid pool.

The free amino acid pool represents the most bioactive part of the body's proteins and amino acid content. This pool is made up of free amino acids in plasma and in the intracellular and extracellular space, with the concentration of amino acids being higher in the intracellular pool. The relatively small amounts of free amino acids in the free amino acid pool, in equilibrium with the body's much larger amounts of proteins and amino acids, are responsible for all the metabolic and substrate protein and amino acid interactions that take place in the body, including muscle protein balance.[3]

Various amino acids are represented in this pool, with the non-essential or conditionally essential amino acids glutamine, glycine, and alanine making up the highest concentrations. Of the essential amino acids, lysine, threonine, and the branched-chain amino acids (BCAA), valine, leucine, and isoleucine are present in the highest concentrations.

The amino acids present in the plasma portion and extracellular portions of the pool are in a sort of equilibrium with the amino acids in the intracellular portion. Since this equilibrium between the intracellular and extracellular portions of the amino acid pool is due in most cases to active transport of the amino acids, it is not a true equilibrium but in fact a sort of steady state based on both concentrations of amino acids and the existing metabolic state. As such, the levels of free and protein-bound amino acids vary considerably. Measuring one portion of the pool without the other can give a false impression of the movement or flux of amino acids through the free pool.

The small free amino acid pool, while highly regulated and active, is relatively stable in size and content. However, some relatively small but important changes take place in amino acid concentrations in response to various stimuli such as exercise, food intake, and various diseases.

C. PROTEIN BALANCE

Protein balance is a function of intake relative to output (utilization and loss). Intake comes from dietary sources and the recycling of proteins, especially of cellular protein sloughed off in the intestinal lumen, while losses occur due to the use of the carbon skeletons of amino acids with the excretion of nitrogenous compounds, as well as protein losses in feces, urine, sweat, and the integumentary system.[4]

Body proteins are in a constant state of flux, with both protein degradation and protein synthesis constantly going on. Normally, these two processes are equal with neither net loss nor net gain of protein taking place. Protein intake usually equals protein lost.

However, if protein synthesis (anabolism) is greater than protein degradation (catabolism), then the overall result is anabolic with a net increase in body protein. If protein degradation is greater than protein synthesis, the overall result is catabolic with a net decrease in body protein.

Nitrogen balance, when nitrogen intake equals nitrogen loss, is essentially synonymous with protein balance since amino acids are involved in forming other important nitrogen-containing compounds such as ammonia and urea as well as creatine, peptide hormones, and some neurotransmitters. However, nitrogen balance is at times a more useful concept as it allows us to make some determination about protein and energy metabolism. For example, if urinary nitrogen increases in respect to a constant intake then we can suspect that amino acids are being deaminated and used as energy. However, with the limited information on hand we can't say for certain what's going on.

Although the end result may be the same, protein balance and protein turnover are not synonymous. Protein turnover, which is a measure of the rate of protein metabolism, involves both protein synthesis and catabolism.

1. Factors Affecting Protein Synthesis and Catabolism

Accelerated protein breakdown and a net protein loss occur secondary to exhaustive exercise and in injury and various diseases. The negative nitrogen balance observed in such cases represents the net result of breakdown and synthesis; with breakdown increased and synthesis either increased or diminished. Under certain conditions protein catabolism can also be decreased. As well, protein synthesis can be increased or decreased under certain conditions. The net result depends on the conditions present and the effects on both synthesis and catabolism.

For example, to have a net increase in protein synthesis so that there is an increase in the concentration of a protein in a cell, its rate of synthesis would have to increase or its breakdown decrease, or both. There are several ways in which the concentration of protein in a cell could be increased, including the four outlined below:

1. The rate of synthesis of the mRNA that codes for the particular protein(s) could be increased (known as transcriptional control).
2. The rate of synthesis of the polypeptide chain by the ribosomal-mRNA complex could be increased (known as translational control).
3. The rate of degradation of the mRNA could be decreased (also translational control).
4. The rate of degradation of the protein could be decreased.

Table 4.1 outlines some of the conditions or factors affecting protein synthesis. Many of these conditions and factors are interrelated. Keep in mind that protein

---

TABLE 4.1
Some Conditions and Factors Affecting Protein Synthesis

Conditions or Factors	Effect on Rate of Protein Synthesis
Decreased protein intake	decreased
Increased protein intake	increased
Decreased energy intake	decreased
Increased cellular hydration[a]	increased
Decreased cellular hydration	decreased
Increased intake of leucine in presence of sufficiency of other amino acids	increased
Increased intake of glutamine in presence of sufficiency of other amino acids	increased
Lack of nervous stimulation	decreased
Muscle stretch, or exercise	increased
Overtraining	decreased
Testosterone (and anabolic steroids)	increased
Growth hormone	increased
Insulin-like growth factor one (IGF-I)	increased
Normal thyroid hormone[b]	increased
Excess thyroid hormone	decreased
Catecholamines (including synthetic β-adrenergic agonist such as clenbuterol)	increased
Glucocorticoids	decreased
Physical trauma, infection	decreased

[a] It is important to understand that cellular hydration refers to an intracellular state and as such is different from extracellular hydration that is manifested either as water retention or volume depletion (extracellular dehydration) as measured by the degree of peripheral edema, overall blood volume, blood pressure, and serum concentrations of electrolytes.

[b] Thyroid hormone (thyroxine and triiodothyronine) stimulate both protein synthesis and degradation, depending on their levels in the body. Not enough or too much can be detrimental to protein synthesis. Higher than normal levels of thyroid hormone lead to the catabolism of protein.

From: Di Pasquale, Mauro G., *Amino Acids and Proteins for the Athlete: The Anabolic Edge*. CRC Press, Boca Raton, FL (1997).

---

synthesis is increased as the result of a net positive change secondary to changes in both (or less commonly one of) synthesis and catabolism.

III. DIETARY PROTEIN

Every cell in the body is partly composed of proteins, which are subject to continuous wear and replacement. Carbohydrates and fats contain no nitrogen or sulfur, two essential elements in all proteins. Whereas the fat in the body can be derived from dietary carbohydrates and the carbohydrates from proteins, the proteins of the body are inevitably dependant for their formation and maintenance on the proteins in food. Protein from food is digested and the resultant amino acids and peptides are absorbed and used to synthesize body proteins.

Proteins consist of large molecules with molecular weights ranging from 1000 to over 1,000,000. In their native state some are soluble and some insoluble in water. Although a great variety of proteins can be subdivided into various categories, they are all are made up of the same building blocks called amino acids.

Every species of animal has its characteristic proteins — the proteins of beef muscle, for instance, differ from those of pork muscle. It is the proteins that give each species its specific immunological characters and uniqueness.

Plants can synthesize all the amino acids they need from simple inorganic chemical compounds, but animals are unable to do this because they cannot synthesize the amino (NH_2) group; so to obtain the amino acids necessary for building protein they must eat plants — or other animals that have in their turn lived on plants.

The human body has certain limited powers of converting one amino acid into another. This is achieved in the liver, at least partly by the process of transamination, whereby an amino group is shifted from one molecule across to another under the influence of aminotransferase, the coenzyme of which is pyridoxal phosphate. However, the ability of the body to convert one amino acid into another is restricted. There are several amino acids which the body cannot make for itself and that must be obtained from the diet. These are termed essential amino acids.

Under normal circumstances, the adult human body can maintain nitrogenous equilibrium on a mixture of eight pure amino acids as its sole source of nitrogen. These eight are: isoleucine, leucine, lysine, methionine, phenylalanine, threonine, tryptophan, and valine. Several amino acids, including arginine, histidine, and glutamine, are believed by some to be conditionally essential. That is, under certain conditions such as growth, these amino acids are not able to be synthesized in adequate amounts and thus need to be supplied in the diet.

Synthesis of the conditionally essential and nonessential amino acids depends mainly on first forming appropriate alpha-keto acids, the precursors of the respective amino acids. For instance, pyruvic acid, which is formed in large quantities during the glycolytic breakdown of glucose, is the keto acid precursor of the amino acid alanine. Then, by the process of transamination, an amino radical is transferred from certain amino acids to the alpha-keto acid, while the keto oxygen is transferred to the donor of the amino radical. In the formation of alanine, for example, the amino radical is transferred to the pyruvic acid from one of several possible amino acid donors including asparagine, glutamine, glutamic acid, and aspartic acid.

Transamination is promoted by several enzymes, among which are the aminotransferases, which are derivatives of pyridoxine (B_6), one of the B vitamins. Without this vitamin, the nonessential amino acids are synthesized only poorly and, therefore, protein formation cannot proceed normally. The formation of protein can also be affected by other vitamins, minerals and nutrients.

A. QUALITY OF PROTEINS

All proteins are made up of varying numbers of amino acids attached together in a specific sequence and having a specific architecture. The sequence of the amino acids and form of the protein differentiate one protein from another and give the protein special physiological and biological properties.

The quantity and quality of protein in the diet is important in determining the effects on protein metabolism. Increasing protein intake leads to increased amino acid levels systemically, which in turn leads to increased protein synthesis, decreased endogenous protein breakdown, and increased amino acid oxidation.[5]

The quality of dietary protein is also important in determining changes in protein metabolism. Certain proteins are considered to be biologically more effective. An example would be the difference between soy and milk proteins. Consumption of a soy protein meal, as compared with casein, results in lower protein synthesis and higher oxidation of amino acids, as seen by the greater urea production than consumption of a casein protein meal.[6]

In a recent review, milk proteins were found to be more effective in stimulating amino acid uptake and net protein deposition in skeletal muscle after resistance exercise than hydrolyzed soy proteins.[8]

The findings revealed that even when balanced quantities of total protein and energy are consumed, milk proteins are more effective in stimulating amino acid uptake and net protein deposition in skeletal muscle after resistance exercise than are hydrolyzed soy proteins. Importantly, the finding of increased amino acid uptake was independent of the differences in amino acid composition of the two proteins. The authors of this review proposed that the improved net protein deposition with milk protein consumption is also not due to differences in amino acid composition, but to a different pattern of amino acid delivery associated with milk versus hydrolyzed soy proteins. These findings suggest that, in healthy human subjects, casein has a higher biological value than soy protein.

In addition, it has been shown that proteins found in whole foods may impact on protein metabolism differently because of the presence of other macronutrients. In a recent study, milk ingestion was found to stimulate net uptake of phenylalanine and threonine, representing net muscle protein synthesis following resistance exercise.[9] The results of this study suggest that whole milk may have increased utilization of available amino acids for protein synthesis. That is likely because carbohydrates and fats alter the rate of absorption of the amino acids and the hormonal response, and subsequently the fate of the amino acids absorbed. For example, the addition of sucrose to milk proteins increased whole-body nitrogen retention, but primarily in splanchnic tissues, whereas the addition of fat to milk proteins resulted in greater dietary N retention in peripheral tissues.[10]

B. Slow and Fast Dietary Proteins

We know that there are differences in carbohydrate — high glycemic, low glycemic, simple sugars, starches, etc. And we know that different carbohydrates are absorbed in the gut and appear in the blood at different rates depending on various factors — for example, simple sugars are absorbed quickly, and more complex ones, depending on how quickly they can be broken down, are absorbed more slowly. This makes up the basis for the glycemic index (GI) of not only foods but whole meals, since the presence of protein and fat with the carbohydrates usually slows down the absorption over the whole digestive process. Fast and slow carbohydrates have different metabolic effects on the hormones and on various metabolic processes.

There are also slow and fast dietary proteins. The speed of absorption of dietary amino acids by the gut varies according to the type of ingested dietary protein and the presence of other macronutrients. The speed of absorption can affect postprandial (after-meal) protein synthesis, breakdown, and deposition.[11,12]

It has been shown that the postprandial amino acid levels differ significantly depending on the mode of administration of a dietary protein; a single-protein meal results in an acute but transient peak of amino acids, whereas the same amount of the same protein given in a continuous manner, which mimics a slow absorption, induces a smaller but prolonged increase.

Since amino acids are potent modulators of protein synthesis, breakdown, and oxidation, different patterns of postprandial amino acidemia (the level of amino acids in the blood) might well result in different postprandial protein kinetics and gain. Therefore, the speed of absorption by the gut of amino acids derived from dietary proteins will have different effects on whole-body protein synthesis, breakdown, and oxidation, which in turn control protein deposition.

For example, one study looked at both casein and whey protein absorption and the subsequent metabolic effects.[13] In this study, two labeled milk proteins, casein (CAS) and whey protein (WP), of different physicochemical properties were ingested as one single meal by healthy adults, and postprandial whole-body leucine kinetics were assessed. WP induced a dramatic but short increase of plasma amino acids. CAS induced a prolonged plateau of moderate hyperaminoacidemia, probably because of a slow gastric emptying. Whole-body protein breakdown was inhibited by 34% after CAS ingestion but not after WP ingestion. Postprandial protein synthesis was stimulated by 68% with the WP meal and to a lesser extent (+31%) with the CAS meal.

Under the conditions of this study, i.e., a single protein meal with no energy added, two dietary proteins were shown to have different metabolic fates and uses. After WP ingestion, the plasma appearance of dietary amino acids is fast, high, and transient. This amino acid pattern is associated with an increased protein synthesis and oxidation and no change in protein breakdown. By contrast, the plasma appearance of dietary amino acids after a CAS meal is slower, lower, and prolonged, with a different whole-body metabolic response: protein synthesis slightly increases and oxidation is moderately stimulated, but protein breakdown is markedly inhibited.[13]

This study demonstrates that dietary amino acid absorption is faster with WP than with CAS. It is very likely that a slower gastric emptying was mostly responsible for the slower appearance of amino acids in the plasma. Indeed, CAS clots in the stomach, whereas WP is rapidly emptied from the stomach into the duodenum. The results of the study demonstrate that amino acids derived from casein are indeed slowly released from the gut and that slow and fast proteins differently modulate postprandial changes of whole-body protein synthesis, breakdown, oxidation, and deposition.[13]

After WP ingestion, large amounts of dietary amino acids flood the small body pool in a short time, resulting in a dramatic increase in amino acid concentrations. This is probably responsible for the stimulation of protein synthesis. This dramatic stimulation of protein synthesis and absence of protein breakdown inhibition is quite different from the pattern observed with classic feeding studies and with the use of only one protein source.

In conclusion, the study demonstrated that the speed of amino acid absorption after protein ingestion has a major impact on the postprandial metabolic response to a single protein meal. The slowly absorbed CAS promotes postprandial protein deposition by an inhibition of protein breakdown without excessive increase in amino acid concentration. By contrast, a fast dietary protein stimulates protein synthesis but also oxidation. This impact of amino acid absorption speed on protein metabolism is true when proteins are given alone, but as for carbohydrate, this might be blunted in more complex meals that could affect gastric emptying (lipids) or insulin response (carbohydrate).

C. Effects of Dietary Protein on Protein Metabolism

Protein metabolism is affected by several factors including energy, protein and macronutrient intake, and exercise.[14,15] An increase in dietary protein results in an increase in nitrogen retention[16] and an increase in amino acid oxidation, as well as increases in the rate of protein turnover.[17,18]

As mentioned elsewhere, the speed of absorption can also modulate protein metabolism by modulating protein synthesis, protein catabolism, and amino acid oxidation. The speed of absorption is a function of the state of the gastrointestinal system (previous dietary intake and presence or absence of any pathology), the type of dietary protein (free amino acids, hydrolysates and whey protein are rapidly absorbed in comparison to, for example, casein; see discussion under fast and slow dietary proteins),[19] and the presence of other dietary macronutrients.[20]

Both a high-protein diet and the rapid absorption of amino acids tends to increase amino acid oxidation[21] as well as gluconeogenesis.[22] Both processes underlie the importance of dietary protein and amino acids to overall energy metabolism.

D. Dietary Reference Intakes and Recommended Daily Allowances

The Recommended Dietary Allowances (RDAs, 1941–1989) were established to try to cover the nutritional needs of all normal, healthy persons living in the United States without the necessity of determining individual nutrient requirements. Canada had a similar system called the Recommended Nutrient Intake (RNI). Several foreign countries each have their own RDAs.

In the past, RDAs were established for protein (there was no RDA for fat or carbohydrate), vitamins A, D, E, K, thiamin, riboflavin, niacin, B_{12}, folacin, C, calcium, magnesium, iron, iodine, phosphorus, selenium, and zinc. The RDAs were set to allow for the vast majority of all normal healthy persons in the U.S. but did not cover people with illness or chronic disease. To cover some of the outliers, there is a margin of safety built into the RDAs so that the average healthy person can consume one third less than the RDA and still not run into any deficiencies. The Food and Nutrition Board of National Academy of Sciences (FNBNAS) set the values for the RDAs based on human and animal research. The Board meets about every 5 years to review current research on nutrients. As research accumulated for each of the many essential nutrients, its associated RDA was revised. The last revision for the RDAs was in 1989.[23]

In the past decade, some significant changes have taken place in the detail and scope of official dietary recommendations. In 1997, the FNBNAS introduced dietary reference intakes (DRIs), changing the way nutritionists and nutrition scientists evaluate the diets of healthy people. There are four types of DRI reference values: the estimated average requirement (EAR), the RDA, the adequate intake (AI) and the tolerable upper intake level (UL). The primary goal of having new dietary reference values was to not only prevent nutrient deficiencies, but also to reduce the risk of chronic diseases such as osteoporosis, cancer, and cardiovascular disease. 10 DRI reports have been completed since 1997 as well as several articles and hundreds of papers discussing them.[24-26] Definitions of DRIs are as follows:

- Recommended Dietary Allowance (RDA): the average daily dietary intake level that is sufficient to meet the nutrient requirement of nearly all (97% to 98%) healthy individuals in a particular life stage and gender group.
- Adequate Intake: a recommended intake value based on observed or experimentally determined approximations or estimates of nutrient intake by a group (or groups) of healthy people, that are assumed to be adequate — used when an RDA cannot be determined.
- Tolerable Upper Intake Level: the highest level of daily nutrient intake that is likely to pose no risk of adverse health effects for almost all individuals in the general population. As intake increase above the UL, the potential risk of adverse effects increases.
- Estimated Average Requirement: a daily nutrient intake value that is estimated to meet the requirement of half of the healthy individuals in a life stage and gender group — used to assess dietary adequacy and as the basis for the RDA.
- Acceptable Macronutrient Distribution Range (AMDR): a range of intakes for a particular energy source that is associated with reduced risk of chronic diseases while providing adequate intakes of essential nutrients.
- Estimated Energy Requirement (EER): the average dietary energy intake that is predicted to maintain energy balance in a healthy adult of a defined age, gender, weight, height, and level of physical activity consistent with good health.

In 2000 an expert nutrition review panel, consisting of both American and Canadian scientists selected by the National Academy of Sciences (NAS), was formed to establish the DRIs for macronutrients and energy. The panel's mission was, based on the current scientific literature, to update, replace, and expand upon the old RDAs in the United States (NRC 1989) and RNIs in Canada (Health and Welfare Canada 1990). In 2002, the DRI report was released with new recommendations for healthy individuals for energy, dietary carbohydrates and fiber, dietary fats (which include fatty acids and cholesterol), dietary protein, and the indispensable amino acids.[27]

Although the panel was instructed to consider increased physical activity as a factor affecting requirements, the DRIs for protein that applied to most healthy individuals were thought to be adequate for those who were physically active. After reviewing the scientific literature investigating the protein needs of athletes, the panel stated: "In view of the lack of compelling evidence to the contrary, no additional dietary protein is suggested for healthy adults undertaking resistance or endurance exercise."[28]

The general criterion used to establish the EAR for protein in the adult, and subsequently the RDA, was to determine the point at which the body is able to maintain body protein content at its current level (i.e., maintenance of nitrogen balance). This daily value was 0.66 g kg of body mass per day for adults (men and women 19 years of age and older), which resulted in an RDA of 0.80 g kg. This is the same daily value as the 1989 RDA and slightly lower than the 1990 RNI of 0.86 g kg (Health and Welfare Canada 1990).[29]

In the case of protein and amino acid requirements, the RDA is age- and gender-dependent and is set at twice the minimum value of the subject who required the most protein or amino acid in all the studies conducted. By greatly increasing the recommended intake figure over that experimentally determined, it was hoped that the protein and amino acid needs of the majority of the U.S. population would be met.

The RDA for protein was originally quite high. For many years, it was set at 1 g/kg body weight for the average adult male, who was assumed to weigh 70 kg (about 155 pounds), so the RDA was 70 g/day. In the last three decades, however, until 1989, the RDA for protein has been adjusted steadily downward.

1. How was the RDA Established?

Ideally, sufficient research is conducted to show (1) that a given nutrient is needed by the human, (2) that certain deficiency signs can be produced, (3) that these signs can be avoided or reversed if the missing nutrient is administered, and (4) that no further improvement is observed if the nutrient is administered at levels above that which reversed the deficiency symptoms.

Next, studies are conducted on a variety of subjects to determine their minimal need. Since humans vary so much, it is not possible to measure the requirements over a broad range of human variability. To allow for this variability, a safety factor is added on to the determined minimum needs of the group of subjects studied. As more subjects are studied and more data accumulated, the added safety factor becomes smaller.

For the purposes of determining protein needs, some shortcuts are taken. For example, since proper nitrogen balance studies are laborious and are performed over a period of several days, a shortcut is often taken and an estimate of nitrogen balance is made by collecting and measuring nitrogen in the urine — since the end products of protein metabolism leave the body mainly via this route — and estimating other losses. Estimations are made of the nitrogen lost in the feces and the small losses of protein from skin, hair, fingernails, perspiration, and other secretions.

About 90% of the nitrogen in urine is urea and ammonia salts — the end products of protein metabolism. The remaining nitrogen is accounted for by creatinine (from creatine), uric acid (products of the metabolism of purines and pyrimidines), porphyrins, and other nitrogen-containing compounds.

Urinary nitrogen excretion is related to the basal metabolic rate (BMR). The larger the muscle mass in the body, the more calories are needed to maintain the BMR. Also, the rate of transamination is greater as amino acids and carbohydrates are interconverted to fulfill energy needs in the muscle. One to 1.3 mg of urinary nitrogen is excreted for each kilocalorie required for basal metabolism. Nitrogen excretion also increases during exercise and heavy work.

Fecal and skin losses account for a significant amount of nitrogen loss from the body in normal conditions, and these may vary widely in disease states. Thus, measurement of urinary nitrogen loss alone may not provide a predictable assessment of daily nitrogen requirement when it is most needed. Fecal losses are due to the inefficiency of digestion and absorption of protein (93% efficiency). In addition, the intestinal tract secretes proteins in the lumen from saliva, gastric juice, bile, pancreatic enzymes, and enterocyte sloughing.

Taking all these losses into consideration and using nitrogen balance as a tool, the minimum daily dietary allowance for protein can be derived on the following bases:

1. Obligatory urinary nitrogen losses of young adults amount to about 37 mg/kg of body weight.
2. Fecal nitrogen losses average 12 mg/kg of body weight.
3. Amounts of nitrogen lost in the perspiration, hair, fingernails, and sloughed skin are estimated at 3 mg/kg of body weight.
4. Minor routes of nitrogen loss such as saliva, menstruation, and seminal ejaculation are estimated at 2 mg/kg of body weight.
5. The total obligatory nitrogen lost — that which must be replaced daily — amounts to 54 mg/kg, or in terms of protein lost this is 0.34 g/kg ($0.054 \cdot 6.25$ — 1 gram of nitrogen = 6.25 grams of protein).
6. To account for individual variation the daily loss is increased by 30%, or 70 mg/kg. In terms of protein, this is 0.45 g/kg of body weight.
7. This protein loss is further increased by 30%, to 0.6 g/kg of body weight, to account for the loss of efficiency when consuming even a high-quality protein such as egg.
8. The final adjustment is to correct for the 75% efficiency of utilization of protein in the mixed diet of North Americans. Thus, the RDA for protein becomes 0.8 g/kg of body weight for normal healthy adult males and females, or 63 g of protein per day for a 174 lb (79 kg) man and 50 g per day for a 138 lb (63 kg) woman.

The need for dietary protein is influenced by age, environmental temperature, energy intake, gender, micronutrient intake, infection, activity, previous diet, trauma, pregnancy, and lactation.

The minimum daily requirement, that is, the minimum amount of dietary protein that will provide the needed amounts of amino acids to optimally maintain the body, is impossible to determine for each individual without expending a good deal of time and effort for each person.

At present, the normal amount of protein recommended for sedentary people is 0.8 grams of protein per kilogram (0.36 grams per pound) of body weight per day. This RDA for protein presumes that the dietary protein is coming from a mixed diet containing a reasonable amount of good-quality proteins. For the average person subsisting on mixtures of poor-quality proteins, this RDA may not be adequate.

E.   RECOMMENDED DIETARY ALLOWANCES (RDA) FOR ATHLETES

The Recommended Dietary Allowances make little provision for changes in nutrient requirements for those who exercise. Energy requirements increase with exercise as the lean (muscle) mass increases and as resting metabolic energy expenditure increases. Increased physical activity at all ages promotes the retention of lean muscle mass and requires increased protein and energy intake.

In athletes, several factors can increase the amount of protein needed, including duration and intensity of exercise, degree of training and current energy, and protein intake of the diet. Athletes who train hard need more protein than the average individual. This holds true for both endurance and power sports.

1.   Historical Overview

The history of protein requirements for athletes is both interesting and circular. In the mid-1800's the popular opinion was that protein was the primary fuel for working muscle.[30] This was an incentive for athletes to consume large amounts of dietary protein.

In 1866 a paper based on urinary nitrogen excretion measures (for protein to provide energy, its nitrogen must be removed and subsequently excreted primarily in the urine), suggested that protein was not an important fuel, and contributed about 6% of the fuel used during a 1,956 m climb in the Swiss Alps.[31] This paper and others led to the perception that exercise does not increase one's need for dietary protein. This view has persisted to the present.

Recently, however, there is some evidence to show that protein contributes more than is generally believed today. The data in the 1866 study likely underestimated the actual protein use for several methodological reasons. For example, the subjects consumed a protein-free diet before the climb, post-climb excretion measures were not made, and other routes of nitrogen excretion may have been substantial.

However, based largely on these data, this belief has persisted throughout most of the 20th century. This is somewhat surprising because Cathcart[32] in an extensive review of the literature prior to 1925 concluded "the accumulated evidence seems to me to point in no unmistakable fashion to the opposite conclusion that muscle activity does increase, if only in small degree, the metabolism of protein." Based on results from a number of separate experimental approaches, the conclusions of several more recent investigators support Cathcart's conclusion.[33]

Several studies have shown that the current RDA for protein is not enough for many people, including athletes and the elderly.

The current dietary protein recommendations for protein (0.8 grams per kilogram) may be insufficient for athletes and those wishing to maximize lean body mass and strength. These athletes may well benefit from protein supplementation. With exercise and under certain conditions, the use of protein and amino acid supplements may have significant anabolic and anticatabolic effects.

Athletes who train hard, because of the increased use of amino acids for energy metabolism and protein synthesis, need more protein than the average individual.

Over a decade ago, Peter Lemon, of the Applied Physiology Research Laboratory, Kent State University, addressed the issue of the protein requirements of athletes.[34] Lemon remarked that current recommendations concerning dietary protein are based primarily on data obtained from sedentary subjects. However, both endurance and strength athletes, he says, will likely benefit from diets containing more protein than the current RDA of 0.8 g/kg/day, though the roles played by protein in excess of the RDA will likely be quite different between the two sets of athletes.

For strength athletes, Lemon states that protein requirements will probably be in the range of 1.4–1.8 g/kg/day, whereas endurance athletes need about 1.2–1.4 g/kg/day. There is no indication that these intakes will cause any adverse side effects in healthy humans. On the other hand, there is essentially no valid scientific evidence that protein intakes exceeding about 1.8–2.0 k/kg day will provide an additional advantage.

F. Effects of Exercise on Dietary Protein Requirements

High protein intake has been the mainstay of most athlete's diets. Athletes in general and strength athletes and bodybuilders in particular, consume large amounts of protein.[35] One reason for their increased protein consumption is their increased caloric intake. Another is that most athletes deliberately increase their intake of protein-rich foods and often use protein supplements.

As we've seen, many scientific and medical sources believe that protein supplementation and high-protein diets are unnecessary and that the RDA supplies more than adequate amounts of protein for the athlete.[36] In fact, overloading on protein is felt to be detrimental because of the increased load to the kidneys of the metabolic breakdown products formed when the excess protein is used as an energy source.

The results of a number of investigations involving both strength and endurance athletes indicate that, in fact, exercise does increase protein/amino acid needs.[37–41] In Lemon's review, the consensus was that all athletes need more protein than sedentary people, and that strength athletes need the most.[42]

Over a decade ago, a group of researchers at McMaster University in Hamilton, Ontario concluded that the current Canadian Recommended Nutrient Intake for protein of 0.86 g/kg/day is inadequate for those engaged in endurance exercise.[43] Moreover, their results indicated that male athletes may have an even higher protein requirement than females. A recent study found that endurance athletes need a protein intake of at least 1.2 g/kg to achieve a positive nitrogen balance.[44]

Butterfield[45] performed a review of the literature and recommended high protein intakes (up to 2–3 g/kg) for physically active individuals. She found evidence for the existence of an intricate relationship between protein and energy utilization with exercise:

When energy intake is in excess of need, the utilization of even a marginal intake of protein will be improved, giving the appearance that protein intake is adequate. When energy intake and output are balanced, the improvement in nitrogen retention accomplished by exercise seems to be fairly constant at protein intakes greater than 0.8 g/kg/d, but falls off rapidly at protein intakes below this. When energy balance is negative, the magnitude of the effect of exercise on protein retention may be decreased as the activity increases, and protein requirements may be higher than when energy balance is maintained.

Somewhat in agreement with Butterfield's conclusions are the results of another study by Piatti et al.[46] They investigated the effects of two hypocaloric diets (800 kcalories) on body weight reduction and composition, insulin sensitivity and proteolysis in 25 normal obese women. The two diets had the following composition: 45% protein, 35% carbohydrate, and 20% fat (high-protein diet); and 60% carbohydrate, 20% protein, and 20% fat (high-carbohydrate diet). The results, said the authors, suggest that (1) a hypocaloric diet providing a high percentage of natural protein can improve insulin sensitivity; and (2) conversely, a hypocaloric high-carbohydrate diet decreases insulin sensitivity and is unable to spare muscle tissue.

In another study it was shown that a protein intake as high as four times the recommended RDA (3.3 grams per kilogram of bodyweight per day vs. RDA of 0.8 grams per kilogram per day) resulted in significantly increased protein synthesis even when compared with a protein intake that was almost twice the RDA.[47] This observation that a protein intake of approximately four times the RDA, in combination with weight training, can promote greater muscle size gains than the same training with a diet containing what is considered by many to be more than adequate protein, is in tune with what many bodybuilders and other weight training athletes believe.

The effects of two levels of protein intake (1.5 g/kg/day or 2.5 g/kg/day) on muscle performance and energy metabolism were studied in humans submitted to repeated daily sessions of prolonged exercise at moderate altitude.[48] The study showed that the higher level of protein intake greatly minimized the exercise-induced decrease in serum branched chain amino acids.

Several studies and papers in the last decade have championed the need for protein above the RDA for athletes and those involved in physical exercise. The reasons are many and involve those athletes in strength and endurance sports and those wanting to increase muscle mass.

Many support the idea that the protein needs of athletes are substantially higher than those of sedentary subjects because of the oxidation of amino acids during exercise and gluconeogenesis, as well as the retention of nitrogen during periods of muscle building.[49–51] Intense muscular activity increases both protein catabolism and protein utilization as an energy source.[52,53] Thus, a high-protein diet may decrease the catabolic effects of exercise by several means — including the use of dietary protein as an energy substrate, thereby decreasing the catabolism of endogenous protein during exercise.

Athletes have for years maintained that a high-protein diet is essential for maximizing lean body mass. And even though there have been attempts to discourage them, the popularity of high-protein diets has not waned. Athletes seem to feel intuitively that they need higher levels of protein than the average sedentary person. This intuitive feeling is backed up by their claims of the ergogenic effects of high-protein diets.

Are these effects simply psychological? Not according to studies that have shown the anabolic effects of increased dietary protein intake. For example, in one study done in rats,[54] dietary energy had no identifiable influence on muscle growth. In contrast, increased dietary protein appeared to stimulate muscle growth *directly* by increasing muscle RNA content and inhibiting proteolysis, as well as increasing insulin and free T3 levels.

Although perhaps popular for a while, supplements that may work through a placebo effect but have no intrinsic effects eventually fall by the wayside and are abandoned by the majority. High-protein diets are used because they work. As well, the use of protein supplements is popular because of their effectiveness above and beyond a whole-food high-protein diet.

Although there has been some concern about the effects of a high dietary protein intake on the kidneys, there seems to be no basis for these concerns in healthy individuals.[55,56] In fact, some animal studies have pointed to a beneficial effect of high-protein diets on kidney function.[57]

A recent review of some of the issues of high dietary protein intake in humans suggested that the maximum protein intake based on bodily needs, weight control evidence, and avoiding protein toxicity would be about 25% of energy requirements at approximately 2 to 2.5 g per kg of weight corresponding to 176 g protein per day for an 80-kg individual on a 12,000 kJ/d or 3000 cal/d diet.[58] The authors also stated that this is well below the theoretical maximum safe intake range for an 80-kg person (285 to 365 g/d).

There has also been some concern about the adverse effects of high-protein diets on the serum lipid profile and on blood pressure. However, it would seem that these concerns also have little basis in fact.

In one study, a diet higher in lean animal protein, including beef, was found to result in more favorable HDL ("good" cholesterol) and LDL ("bad" cholesterol) levels.[59] The study involved ten moderately hypercholesterolemic subjects (six women, four men). They were randomly allocated to isocaloric high- or low-protein diets for 4 to 5 weeks, after which they switched over to the other. Protein provided either 23% or 11% of energy intake; carbohydrate provided 65% or 53%; and fats accounted for 24%. During the high-protein diet, mean fasting plasma total cholesterol, LDL, and triglycerides were significantly lower, HDL was raised by 12%, and the ratio of LDL to HDL consistently decreased. Other studies by the same group of researchers found that increased levels of dietary proteins resulted in beneficial changes in blood lipids in both normolipemic and dyslipemic humans.[60,61] As well, recent studies have found that increasing dietary plant and animal protein lowers blood pressure in hypertensive persons.[62,63]

Intense muscular activity increases protein catabolism (breakdown) and protein use as an energy source. The less protein available, the less muscle you're going to be able to build. A high-protein diet protects the protein to be turned into muscle by, among other things, providing another energy source for use during exercise. The body will burn this protein instead of the protein inside the muscle cells.

In fact, studies have shown that the anabolic effects of intense training are increased by a high-protein diet. When intensity of effort is at its maximum and stimulates an adaptive, muscle-producing response, protein needs accelerate to provide for that increased muscle mass. It's also well known that a high-protein diet is necessary for anabolic steroids to have full effect.

Once a certain threshold of work intensity is crossed, dietary protein becomes essential in maximizing the anabolic effects of exercise. Exercise performed under that threshold, however, may have little anabolic effect and may not require increased protein. As a result, while serious athletes can benefit from increased protein, other athletes who do not undergo similar rigorous training may not.

Whether you need to supplement your diet with extra protein depends on your goals. For those who don't have to worry about gaining some fat along with the muscle (traditionally athletes in sports without weight classes or those in the heavyweight classes, where mass is an advantage — for example in the shotput and in weightlifting), high-caloric diets will usually supply all the protein necessary, provided plenty of meat, fish, eggs, and dairy products are provided. With the increased caloric intake and including high-quality protein foods, extra protein will be obtained at the dinner table without specific planning.

Most athletes, however, need the economy of maximizing lean body mass and minimizing body fat. These athletes, both competitive and recreational, are on a moderate- or at times a low-caloric intake. To increase their protein intake, they need to plan their diets carefully and in many cases use protein supplements, since they can't calorically afford to eat food in the volume necessary to get enough protein.

On the average, I recommend a minimum of 1 gram of high-quality protein per pound of bodyweight (2.2 grams per kg) every day for anyone involved in competitive or intense recreational sports who wants to maximize lean body mass but does not wish to gain weight or have excessive muscle hypertrophy. This would apply to athletes who wish to stay in a certain competitive weight class or those involved in endurance events.

However, athletes involved in strength events such as the Olympic field and sprint events, those in football or hockey, weightlifters, powerlifters, and bodybuilders, may need even more than my recommendation to maximize body composition and athletic performance. In those attempting to minimize body fat and thus maximize body composition, for example in sports with weight classes and in bodybuilding, it's possible that protein may well make up over 50% of their daily caloric intake.

Such an increase is important if one is trying to lose weight and/or body fat it is important to keep dietary protein levels high. The body transforms and oxidizes more protein on a calorie-deficient diet than it would in a diet that has adequate calories. The larger the body muscle mass, the more transamination of amino acids occurs to fulfill energy needs. Thus, for those wishing to lose weight but maintain or even increase lean body mass in specific skeletal muscles, I recommend at least 1.5 grams of high-quality protein per pound of bodyweight. The reduction in calories needed to lose weight should be at the expense of the fats and carbohydrates, not protein.

G. Essential, Conditionally Essential, and Nonessential Amino Acids

The requirement for dietary protein consists of two components:

1. The requirement for the nutritionally essential amino acids (isoleucine, leucine, lysine, methionine, phenylalanine, threonine, tryptophan, and valine) under all conditions and for conditionally essential amino acids (arginine, cysteine, glutamine, glycine, histidine, proline, taurine and tyrosine) under specific physiological and pathological conditions.
2. The requirement for nonspecific nitrogen for the synthesis of the nutritionally dispensable amino acids (aspartic acid, asparagine, glutamic acid, alanine, serine) and other physiologically important nitrogen-containing compounds such as nucleic acids, creatine, and porphyrins.

With respect to the first component, it is usually accepted that the nutritive values of various food protein sources are to a large extent determined by the concentration and availability of the individual indispensable amino acids. Hence, the efficiency with which a given source of food protein is utilized in support of an adequate state of nutritional health depends on both the physiological requirements for the indispensable amino acids and total nitrogen and on the concentration of specific amino acids in the source of interest.

1. Essential Amino Acids

Essential amino acids, also called indispensable amino acids, must be supplied in the diet either as free amino acids or as constituents of dietary proteins. By this criterion, the following eight amino acids are essential in man (Table 4.2).

TABLE 4.2
Essential Amino Acids

*Isoleucine
*Leucine
Lysine
Methionine
Phenylalanine
Threonine
Tryptophan
*Valine

* Branched Chain Amino Acids —
Leucine, Isoleucine, Valine

---

2. Conditionally Dispensable Amino Acids

Several amino acids are considered conditionally essential (dispensable) as they are rate limiting for protein synthesis under certain conditions. Individual amino acids are often described as conditionally essential, based on requirements for optimal growth and maintenance of positive nitrogen balance. While in extreme circumstances, such as in the absence of certain nonessential amino acids from the diet and the presence of limited amounts of essential amino acids from which to synthesize the nonessential amino acids, any of the amino acids might be considered conditionally essential, including arginine, citrulline, ornithine, proline, cysteine, tyrosine, histidine, taurine etc.[64-68] However, practically, only seven other amino acids can be considered essential under certain conditions.

The following amino acids can be considered to be conditionally essential based on the body's inability to actually synthesize them from other amino acids under certain conditions. By this criterion, the following seven amino acids are conditionally essential in man (Table 4.3).

3. Nonessential or Dispensable Amino Acids

Dispensable amino acids, also called nonessential amino acids, can be synthesized by the body from other amino acids. The following eight amino acids can be considered to be nonessential in man based on the body's ability to actually synthesize them from other amino acids under almost all conditions, although, as discussed above, there is likely no amino acid that is nonessential since limiting amounts of the precursors of these amino acids in a diet that does not contain adequate amounts of these amino acids will limit the body's ability to synthesize them (Table 4.4).

4. The Distinction is Blurred

Although I've made the distinction among the three amino acid groups as far as essentiality, there is a blurring of the lines among the three groups and there is still much controversy regarding the determination of amino acid requirements in humans.[69] The blurring can be minor, for example, the amino acid histidine. Some consider histidine an indispensable amino acid rather than a conditionally indispensable

---

**TABLE 4.3
Conditionally Essential
Amino Acids**

Arginine
Cysteine, Cystine
Glutamine
Histidine
Proline
Taurine
Tyrosine

TABLE 4.4
Nonessential Amino Acids

Alanine
Asparagine
Aspartic Acid
Citrulline
Glutamic Acid
Glycine
Serine

---

one. In the neonate, the only truly dispensable amino acids are alanine, aspartic acid, glutamic acid, serine and asparagine.[70]

The blurring, however, can also be major and further research is needed before we can make a decision as to which amino acids are truly dispensable. For example, some believe that no amino acid is dispensable since, among other issues, there is some doubt as to whether we can actually synthesize amino acids, and that in fact we may need to obtain almost all — if not all — amino acids from dietary sources.[71,72]

IV. EXERCISE AND PROTEIN METABOLISM

Exercise has profound effects on skeletal muscle. Skeletal muscle increases its contractile protein content, resulting in muscular hypertrophy as it successfully adapts to increasing work loads. Studies have shown that certain stimuli produce muscle hypertrophy.

In a review on the effects of exercise on protein turnover in man, Rennie et al.[73] concluded the following:

1. Exercise causes a substantial rise in amino acid catabolism.
2. Amino acids catabolized during exercise appear to become available through a fall in whole-body protein synthesis and a rise in whole-body protein breakdown.
3. After exercise, protein balance becomes positive through a rise in the rate of whole-body synthesis in excess of breakdown.
4. Studies of free 3-methylhistidine in muscle, plasma, and urine samples suggest that exercise decreases the fractional rate of myofibrillar protein breakdown, in contrast with the apparent rise in whole-body breakdown.

In contrast to exercise, most of the increased proteolysis during fasting is due to the degradation of myofibrillar proteins (contractile proteins) in skeletal muscle.[74,75]

A number of studies have examined the influence of exercise on protein synthesis and protein degradation. In general, it seems that exercise suppresses protein synthesis and stimulates protein degradation in skeletal muscle proportional to the level of exertion. In one early study using rats, mild exercise decreased protein synthesis by 17%. More intense treadmill running reduced synthesis by 30% and an exhaustive 3-hour run inhibited synthesis by 70%.[76]

Another study by the same author examined the effects of exhaustive running on protein degradation and found that exhaustive running stimulates protein degradation in skeletal muscle.[77] Other studies have also shown that exercise produces a catabolic condition. In one study looking at aerobic exercise in humans, six male subjects were exercised on a treadmill for 3.75 hours at 50% VO_2 max and the rates of protein synthesis and degradation were measured.[78] During exercise there was a 14% decrease in protein synthesis and a 54% increase in the rate of degradation.

This study is one of the few to make measurements during recovery after exercise. Its authors found that, after exercise, protein synthesis increased above the initial resting levels while protein degradation decreased, returning eventually to pre-exercise levels. Any gains in the recovery phase seem therefore to be due to increases in protein synthesis rather than to decreases in protein catabolism.

In another study, multiple amino acid tracers were used to further elucidate the changes in protein synthesis and degradation that occur during prolonged aerobic exercise.[79,80] In these studies, male subjects were exercised on a bicycle ergometer at 30% VO_2 max for 105 minutes. The results of the study showed that, while exercise inhibited protein synthesis, the degree of inhibition varied depending on the amino acid tracer used. For example, the authors found decreases in protein synthesis of 48% using labeled leucine and 17% using lysine. With the relatively light workloads used in these studies, there were no changes in protein degradation or increases in urea production.

Even though the acute effect of exercise on protein turnover is catabolic, the long-term effects are an overall increase in protein synthesis and lean body mass. Routine exercise produces maintenance or hypertrophy of muscle mass. Few studies have looked at the postexercise recovery of protein turnover. The above report and a later report by Devlin et al.[81] suggest that recovery occurs through stimulation of protein synthesis.

Preliminary studies by Layman et al. reported in the second edition of *Nutrition in Exercise and Sport* provide additional support for this recovery pattern.[82] The authors found that after a 2-hour bout of running on a motor-driven treadmill at 26 m per minute, protein synthesis in the gastrocnemius muscle was suppressed by 26 to 30% in fasted male rats. Recovery of protein synthesis occurred during the next 4 to 8 hours even if the animals were withheld from eating. These data suggest that muscles have a very high capacity for recovery even during conditions of food restriction. Several recent studies have shown that exercise training and protein intakes before and after exercise are important for maximizing the effects of exercise on muscle protein synthesis and on subsequent recovery.[83-89]

Just what factors control protein synthesis during exercise are being worked out, although some general trends and associations have been recognized. For example, high-intensity exhaustive bouts of exercise produce a transient catabolic effect on protein synthesis. This effect is controlled presumably at the translation level of protein synthesis. Transcription is depressed but RNA concentrations are unchanged during the relatively brief period of the exercise bout. At the level of translation, potential regulatory controls include (1) availability of substrates, (2) hormones, (3) energy states, and (4) initiation factors.[90]

Recent studies have shown that, in part, the decline in protein synthesis is a result of repressed signaling through a protein kinase referred to as the mammalian target of rapamycin (mTOR), which in turn affects translation initiation and elongation phases of mRNA translation.[91-93]

A. Exercise-Induced Amino Acid Flux

The changes that occur in the BCAAs, alanine, and glutamine in the liver, plasma, and muscle during exercise suggest that individual amino acids may be limiting as substrates for protein synthesis and that they may be an important source of energy for various tissues and organs in the body. In general, decreases in protein synthesis and increases in protein degradation produce a net release of amino acids into the intracellular free pool that may or may not be reflected by increased plasma levels.

Exercise is accompanied by changes in anabolic and catabolic hormones. It would appear that the molecular mechanism for the action of these hormones on translation remains equivocal, but most evidence points to changes in the initiation phase of translation.

The availability of energy may also be a limiting factor for muscle protein synthesis. Studies have found that decreases in protein synthesis that occur in proportion to the number of contractions induced by electrical stimulation were in proportion to the decline in the level of ATP in muscle cells.[94]

V. ENERGY METABOLISM

A. Introduction

The production of a steady supply of energy is crucial in maintaining life. Energy is needed to form and repair cellular materials, to maintain the integrity of the body's cells and tissues, and for movement. Mammals derive energy from the carbon skeleton of macronutrients such as proteins, carbohydrates, and lipids.

The ultimate fate of any nutrient, if not used structurally in the body — for example as skeletal muscle — as readily available substrates in tissues and circulation (this "reservoir" of glucose, amino acids, glycerol, ketones, and fatty acids is very small in comparison with total body macronutrient availability), or immediately for energy, is to be transformed into glucose and deposited as glycogen, or into lipids and deposited mainly as triglycerides in fat cells.

Energy is released when carbon–carbon and carbon–hydrogen bonds of the macronutrients that come from our diets and are part of our bodies are broken and either used directly or stored in other chemical bonds such as the high-phosphate bonds of adenosine triphosphate (ATP). When the high-phosphate body is broken, energy is released and made available to do work.

Energy production in the human body revolves around the rebuilding of ATP and to a lesser extent other nucleoside triphosphates such as guanosine triphosphate (GTP), cytidine triphosphate (CTP), thymidine triphosphate (TTP), and uridine triphosphate (UTP). ATP generation is normally accomplished mostly under aerobic conditions by shuttling different proportions of all three micronutrients through the citric acid cycle and oxidative phosphorylation, ending up with ATP, CO_2 and water.

The mechanisms regulating energy production are complex, involving interactions on many levels, including control of protein synthesis and breakdown, under resting and exercising conditions. For example, increased energy demands, reflected by several changes including increased levels of adenosine monophosphate (AMP) and decreased levels of ATP and creatine phosphate, leads to adenosine monophosphate kinase (AMPK) activation, inhibiting the mammalian target of rapamycin (mTOR) which in turn decreases protein synthesis and increases protein breakdown.[95–97] Another example is the need for energy during exercise leading to increases in AMPK activity and reduced the translation repressor protein elf-4E-binding-protein (4E-BP1) phosphorylation, which in turn leads to decreases in protein synthesis.[98]

B. METABOLIC PATHWAYS PRODUCING ATP

Energy, mainly in the form of ATP, can be produced by both aerobic and anaerobic pathways. Overall, the aerobic pathways produce most of the ATP while the anaerobic pathways are crucial for maintaining energy production under general or tissue hypoxic conditions, such as intense exercise and ischemia. During strenuous exercise, regeneration of ATP, on which muscle contraction is dependent, is based on both aerobic and anaerobic processes in varying degrees depending on oxygen availability.

1. Anaerobic Energy Production

There are at least four anaerobic pathways. Three of these involve substrate-level phosphorylation from phosphocreatine during anaerobic glycolysis, and in one of the steps in the tricarboxylic acid (TCA) cycle. The fourth is less well known and also involves the TCA cycle. The former two reactions occur in the cytoplasm while the latter occur in the mitochondria.

a. Cytoplasmic Anaerobic Substrate Level Phosphorylation

1. Phosphagen mobilization is the simplest mechanism for generating ATP. The best known example is creatine phosphate (PCr), catalyzed by creatine phosphokinase (CPK), can readily transfer its phosphoryl group to ADP to form ATP.

$$PCr + ADP + H+ \rightarrow ATP + creatine$$

Phosphagen mobilization also occurs between ATP, ADP and AMP. This recoupling allows the formation of more ATP from shuffling high-phosphate groups, for example, 2 ADP recouple to form 1 ATP and 1 AMP.[99,100]

Phosphocreatine levels can be influenced by creatine levels in the diet, levels of amino acid precursors in the diet, and by supplementation with creatine and to a lesser extent from the amino acids methionine, arginine, and glycine.

2. Anaerobic substrate-level glycolysis, the partial catabolism of glucose to lactate, is the second cytoplasmic anaerobic means of forming ATP. If glycogen is the substrate instead of glucose, an extra mole of ATP is generated. The overall reaction is:

$$glucose + 2\ Pi + 2ADP \Longleftrightarrow 2\ lactate + 2\ H_2O + 2\ ATP$$

and this can be broken down to the two specific ATP-producing steps, which are offset somewhat by the ATP-requiring step early on in glycolysis:

$$1,3\text{-BPG} + ADP \rightarrow 3\text{-PG} + ATP$$

$$PEP + ADP \rightarrow Pyruvate + ATP$$

Several factors involved in anaerobic glycolysis influence the amount of ATP generated. For example, the formation of lactate by lactate dehydrogenase generates nicotinamide adenine dinucleotide (NAD^+), which allows glycolysis to continue. If NAD^+ is not being regenerated by the lactate dehydrogenase reaction there is an inhibition of glyceraldehyde-3-phosphate dehydrogenase, which in turn blocks ATP generation by substrate level phosphorylation.

b. Anaerobic Mitochondrial Phosphorylation

Anaerobic mitochondrial metabolism can generate ATP via two pathways. The first is by substrate-level phosphorylation during the conversion of succinyl-CoA to succinate. In this reaction succinyl-CoA synthetase drives the reaction in which succinyl-CoA + GDP + Pi forms succinate + GTP + CoA. GTP is then coupled with ADP to produce ATP. The GTP and ATP formed in this way are generally considered to contribute to the overall mitochondrial ATP generation, most of which is formed by oxidative phosphorylation. However, there is some speculation that the products of mitochondrial substrate level phosphorylation may be qualitatively different.[101]

In the second pathway, ATP is formed via electron transport in complexes I and II driven by reduction of fumarate to succinate coupled to the oxidation of reduced ubiquinone that is generated via NADH (the reduced form of NAD^+) from TCA cycle reducing equivalents.[102–106]

Both pathways contribute to elevations of succinate and are operative to some extent in all vertebrates, with the extent being dependent on adaptive responses. For example, it has been shown that in diving vertebrates there is an accumulation of succinate in the blood during breath-hold dives.[107] This production is thought to result from amino acid catabolism leading to TCA cycle intermediates such as fumarate, malate, succinyl-CoA, and alpha-ketoglutarate, which in turn are fermented with succinate.

Amino acids can contribute to both aerobic and anaerobic energy metabolism in several ways, both directly and indirectly — directly by providing the carbon skeletons that contribute to TCA cycle anaplerosis and indirectly by being used as substrates for gluconeogenesis.

2. Aerobic Energy Production

The TCA cycle, also called the Krebs cycle and the citric acid cycle, is a mitochondrial metabolic pathway that underlies most of the metabolic processes in the body and is essential for aerobic energy production. For example, this pathway is an important source of biosynthetic building blocks used in gluconeogenesis, amino acid biosynthesis, and fatty acid biosynthesis.

The basic energy process of the TCA cycle is the energy-producing oxidation of acetyl-CoA through a series of intra-mitochondrial reactions. The acetyl-CoA that enters the Krebs cycle comes from several sources, including the conversion of pyruvate from glycolysis to acetyl-CoA by pyruvate dehydrogenase, the oxidation of fatty acids, ketone bodies, and the carbon skeletons of some amino acids. The energy released is trapped primarily as the reduced high-energy electron carriers NADH and FADH2, which transfer their chemical energy via oxidative phosphorylation to the electron transport chain to produce ATP.

During the nine steps of the TCA cycle, an acetyl-CoA molecule (2 carbons) enters the cycle and condenses it with oxaloacetate (4 carbons) to create citrate (6 carbons). The citrate is subsequently decarboxylated twice (forming 2 molecules of CO_2, which, along with the CO_2 released by pyruvate dehydrogenase when acetyl-CoA is formed from pyruvate, is the source of CO_2 released into the atmosphere when you breathe) through a series of steps until it reaches oxaloacetate again, leaving the net carbons the same with each turn of the cycle. The TCA cycle can be summarized as follows:

$$\text{Acetyl-CoA} + 3\ NAD^+ + FAD + GDP + P_i + 2\ H_2O + 1\ \text{CoA-SH} \rightarrow 2\ \text{CoA-SH}$$

$$+ 3\ NADH + 3\ H^+ + FADH_2 + GTP + 2\ CO_2 + 1\ H_2O$$

While none of the steps in the pathway directly use oxygen, the activity of the TCA cycle is linked to oxygen consumption to regenerate NAD+. If the oxygen supply is low, the TCA cycle cannot continue even though some steps may proceed forward anaerobically to provide a limited amount of energy in the form of GPT. As well as oxygen, some TCA cycle enzymes need specific co-factors to function. For example, thiamine deficiency may lead to decreased activity of pyruvate dehydrogenase and alpha-ketoglutarate dehydrogenase, and a decrease in the ability of the TCA cycle to meet metabolic demands.

3. TCA Cycle

The TCA cycle is more than just a catabolic pathway generating ATP. It is also a metabolic hub where the intermediates are used to produce other biological compounds. For example, a transamination reaction converts interconverts glutamate and alpha-ketoglutarate. Glutamate is a precursor for the synthesis of other amino acids and purine nucleotides. Succinyl-CoA is a precursor for porphyrins. Oxaloacetate can be transaminated to form aspartate. Aspartate itself is a precursor for other amino acids and pyrimidine nucleotides. Oxaloacetate and malate are substrates for gluconeogenesis and they in turn can be produced by the increase in other TCA cycle intermediates (TCAI).

Cytoplasmic and mitochondrial pathways are intertwined by the transfer of TCA cycle intermediates back and forth. For example, citrate can be exported out of the mitochondria into the cytostol where is broken down by ATPcitrate lyase to yield oxaloacetate and acetyl-CoA. Under certain circumstances, the acetyl-CoA produced can be used as a precursor for fatty acids. The oxaloacetate produced in this reaction is reduced to malate, which can either be transported back into the matrix of the mitochondria where it is reoxidized into oxaloacetate, or be oxidatively decarboxylated to pyruvate by malic enzyme, which can then be transported back to the mitochondria. All of these reactions and interchanges serve to optimize metabolic processes involved in anabolic and catabolic functions, as well as contributing to anaplerotic and cataplerotic pathways.

The level of TCA cycle intermediates (TCAI) and the flux rate of the TCA cycle are both important determinants in TCA cycle function and energy production. While the amount of TCAI is relatively small and constant, varying in size by three or four times, the turnover and throughput of the cycle can vary dramatically depending on demand. To sustain flux through the TCA cycle and thus regenerate ATP, it is important that TCAI be maintained within certain ranges, which requires that leakage of TCAI and their use in various metabolic pathways, termed as cataplerosis, must be balanced by anaplerosis, supplying TCAI to the cycle from various sources.

The main anaplerotic sources are pyruvate, certain amino acids, and 3 to 5 carbon derivatives of fatty acid metabolism. Amino acids are involved not only in supplying anaplerotic substrates directly into the TCA cycle, but also in supplying oxaloacetate and malate either by supplying glucose for glycolysis via gluconeogenesis or by supplying pyruvate and phosphoenolpyruvate, which in turn are carboxylated to form oxaloacetate and malate.

C. ROLE OF PROTEIN AND AMINO ACIDS IN ENERGY METABOLISM

Amino acids have three possible fates in the body. They can be used for and influence protein synthesis, used to produce pyruvate and/or TCA cycle intermediates (and thus be used for gluconeogenesis, glyconeogenesis, and fatty acid synthesis), or their carbon skeletons can be used for energy production. All three processes are ongoing to some extent — the degree that each is active depends on the nutritional environment. For example, in times of dietary surplus, the potentially toxic nitrogen of amino acids is eliminated via transaminations, deamination, and urea formation; the carbon skeletons, while used to some extent for energy production, are mostly conserved as carbohydrate via gluconeogenesis, or as fatty acid via fatty acid synthesis pathways.

However, even though amino acids have traditionally been relegated to a minor role in energy production, with fats and carbohydrates considered the major substrates, they nonetheless under some circumstances have a substantial and crucially important role in energy metabolism. In extreme cases, by providing substrates for direct energy production, and indirectly by providing carbon skeletons for the formation of TCAI, glucose, glycogen, acetyl units, and fatty acids, amino acids can provide up to half or more of energy requirements.

As we have seen, the history of protein requirements for athletes and protein's energy contribution has had its up and downs. In the mid-1800s, popular opinion was that protein was the primary fuel for working muscle. The consensus lately is that proteins are not major contributors to energy metabolism. However, we are now starting to reexamine the role of protein in energy metabolism and are finding that, while it may not be the primary fuel, it is at times a major source of energy.

Under normal conditions it is generally accepted today that the contribution made by proteins to the energy value of most well-balanced diets is usually between 10 and 15% of the total and seldom exceeds 20%. For example, at rest and with a diet that contains significant amounts of carbohydrates, fats, and proteins, carbohydrates and fats are the preferred substrates for energy production. At that time the oxidation of amino acids accounts for less than 10% of the total energy needs. However, under certain conditions, for example very low-carbohydrate diets, because of the role that protein has in gluconeogenesis and TCA cycle anaplerosis, proteins make a much larger contribution to energy metabolism.

An example would be when energy consumption in the form of carbohydrates and fats is low. In these cases, whether due to a lack of fat and carbohydrates availability even in diets containing adequate energy in the form of protein, or due to a hypocaloric diet, the energy needs of the body take priority and dietary and tissue proteins will be utilized at the expense of the building or repair processes of the body.

However, the amount of protein involved in energy metabolism can be substantial, and in some cases, overshadow the roles of both fats and carbohydrates, at least as far as the ultimate source of energy. As such, in people on high-protein, low-carbohydrate diets, and especially in bodybuilders and elite endurance and power athletes who may be on very high-protein isocaloric and hypocaloric diets, the contribution can be as high as 50%, and in selective cases even more. As well, protein oxidation rises in various other situations such as trauma and sepsis.

In my view, the contribution that protein makes to energy metabolism, including both the complete oxidation of the carbon skeletons, directly or indirectly by the various transformations (gluconeogenesis and glycolytic-TCA cycle interactions) is underappreciated and more studies need to be done to determine the amount of protein carbon that actually contributes to energy metabolism both at rest and during exercise. As it stands, even in studies where the contribution of protein is obvious,[108] that contribution is often glossed over.

D. Fate of Dietary Protein

Unlike the fats and carbohydrates that can be stored in the form of triglycerides and glycogen, there is no storage form of protein or amino acids. All of the protein and amino acids (except for a very small but important amount of free amino acids that make up the plasma and intracellular amino acid pool) serve either a structural or metabolic function. Recently, however, there is some evidence to show that, under some circumstances, protein plays a prominent role in energy metabolism.

Excess amino acids from dietary protein are normally deaminated or transaminated by the liver, while the non-nitrogenous portion of the molecule is transformed into glucose and used directly, or into fat or glycogen. The unneeded nitrogen is converted to urea and excreted in the urine. Endogenous protein goes through anabolic and catabolic phases, usually in time with absorptive and postabsorptive states, and under various stressors including exercise. Part of this protein is also used for energy metabolism.

In general, the more protein that is ingested and the larger the body muscle mass, the more deamination and transamination of amino acids occurs to fulfill energy needs. Each kilocalorie needed for basal metabolism leads to the excretion of 1 to 1.3 mg of urinary nitrogen. Because of the increased use of amino acids for energy production, nitrogen excretion increases during exercise and heavy work, although this increase in not always in proportion to the amount of energy generated.

Protein requirements and the use of amino acids for energy production are raised if other energy sources are not ingested in adequate amounts — as is sometimes seen in persons and athletes on either low-fat or low-carbohydrate diets to decrease their weight and body fat levels.

Amino acids ingested without other energy sources makes for a less than ideal diet. This inefficiency is partly because of the energy lost during amino acid metabolism and the energy cost of protein synthesis — incorporation of each amino acid molecule into peptides requires three high-energy phosphate bonds. Consequently, excess of dietary energy over basal needs, whether as fats, carbohydrates, or proteins, improves the efficiency of nitrogen utilization.

E. PROTEIN CONTRIBUTION TO ENERGY METABOLISM

In the body, amino acids may be used for primarily protein synthesis or energy production, depending upon (1) protein quality, (2) caloric level of the diet, (3) stage of development, including growth, pregnancy, and lactation, (4) prior nutritional status, and (5) stress factors such as exercise, fever, injury, and immobilization. Protein oxidation is a term used to describe the release of energy from the carbon skeleton of amino acids after deamination.

Four ways that proteins provide energy are through (1) direct oxidation of the carbon skeletons; (2) gluconeogeneis via alanine, glutamine, and lactate; (3) storage as fat or glycogen; and (4) anapleurotic contributions that cycle through the mitochondria and cytoplasm and result in the oxidation of resulting 2 carbon units in the TCA cycle.

F. AMINO ACID CATABOLISM

The catabolism of amino acids yields energy, about 4 Calories (kcal) per gram of protein, notwithstanding the higher energy costs of processing dietary protein. To allow amino acids to be used for energy, the amino group (NH_2) must first be removed by a process known as deamination, where the amino group is removed; or transamination, where the amino group is transferred to another structure to form a new amino acid (see below).

The deaminated carbon skeletons — alpha keto acid residues — that are not used for forming new amino acids enter the glycolytic and TCA cycle, intertwining between mitochondrial and cytoplasm pathways involving 2, 3, and 4 carbon intermediates (see below) are either converted to glucose and glycogen (glucogenic, gycogenic pathways) or metabolized in fat pathways (ketogenic pathway) either to be fully oxidized via the TCA cycle, or used for fatty acid formation. For more information see section 4.5.2.3.

When energy consumption in the form of carbohydrates and fats is low, the energy needs of the body take priority and dietary and tissue proteins will be utilized at the expense of the building or repair processes of the body.

1. Oxidation of Amino Acids

Once the needed proteins are synthesized and the amino acid pools replenished, additional amino acids are degraded and used for energy or stored mainly as fat and, to a lesser extent, as glycogen. The primary site for degradation of most amino acids is the liver. The liver is unique because of its capacity to degrade amino acids and synthesize urea for elimination of the amino nitrogen.

A number of mechanisms are brought into play to both conserve nitrogen when fed a low-protein diet, and to oxidize the surplus when presented with an immediate excess. For example, the nitrogen catabolic enzymes and those involved in the first step in the catabolism of the essential amino acids are up- and down-regulated in response to an increase or decrease in dietary protein.

The first step in the degradation of amino acids begins with deamination — the removal of the alpha-amino group from the amino acid to produce an oxoacid, which may be a simple metabolic intermediate itself (e.g., pyruvate) or be converted to a simple metabolic intermediate via a specific metabolic pathway. The intermediates are either oxidized via the citric acid cycle or converted to glucose via gluconeogenesis. For instance, deaminated alanine is pyruvic acid. This can be converted into glucose or glycogen. Or it can be converted into acetyl-CoA, which can then be polymerized into fatty acids. Also, two molecules of acetyl-CoA can condense to form acetoacetic acid, which is one of the ketone bodies.

The larger the body muscle mass, the more transamination of amino acids occurs to fulfill energy needs. Each kcal needed for basal metabolism leads to the excretion of 1 to 1.3 mg of urinary nitrogen. For the same reason, nitrogen excretion increases during exercise and heavy work.

The human body, through metabolic and hormonal controls, has evolved to meet its continuous metabolic and energy needs even though eating, and thus provision of essential nutrients, is intermittent. Nutrients in the absorptive state (the time during and right after a meal, usually lasting about 4–8 hours depending on the composition of the meal and the state of the organism) are filtered through the liver (with the liver modifying or simply conveying glucose, amino acids, and fatty acids to the systemic circulation and thus to the rest of the body). Such nutrients, coming from the food ingested, are used preferentially for energy production and energy storage.

In the postabsorptive period (after a meal has been completely digested and the resulting nutrients absorbed into the body — again, usually 4–8 hours after a meal during which the transition from the postprandial to the fasting state occurs, and even under fasting conditions (as long as the fasting state is not extensive), the body tends to keep a constant energy output by mobilizing internal substrates (glycogen, cellular and body fat, cellular protein) that can be used as energy sources.

Postabsorptive energy sources include both circulating and stored macronutrients. Those that are readily available include circulating glucose, fatty acids, and triglycerides, liver and muscle glycogen, muscle triglycerides, the branched chain amino acids (used by skeletal muscle) and the amino acids alanine and glutamine, which are released from skeletal muscle and used for gluconeogenesis — in the case of glutamine, directly as fuel by the immune system and gastrointestinal tract).[109,110]

Circulating glucose is replenished mainly through hepatic glycogenolysis (breakdown of glycogen) and gluconeogenic (formation of glucose from other compounds such as lactate, glycerol, alanine, and glutamine) processes mainly in the liver, but also involving skeletal muscle, kidney and GI tract.

In a normal 70-kg man these postabsorptive energy sources provide up to 1200 kcal (800 calories from carbohydrate sources). These sources are exhausted in less than 24 hours if no other food is consumed.

In an individual who is dieting to lose weight or in an athlete who is limiting both caloric and fat intake to maximize lean body mass and minimize body fat, these sources may amount to less than 500 kcal, since liver and muscle glycogen levels as well as circulating triglycerides and fatty acids are often limited, and, in the case of the athlete, would easily be exhausted during a training session. In cases where the available energy is used up while training, other energy sources are called upon to supply the energy needed both during and after training until nutrients are able to be absorbed from a post-training meal.

Fatty acids and ketones formed by the catabolism of body fat (triglycerides) can be used by most tissues in the body. However, in the short term, certain tissues such as the brain can only use glucose for energy. Thus, glucose or substances that can be converted to glucose are vital to survival. The lack of glucose in the short term results in the formation of glucose through gluconeogenesis, a process by which glucose is formed from other substrates, mainly lactate, pyruvate, glycerol and amino acids.[111-113] Amino acids, a major substrate for glucose production, come from skeletal muscle, leading to a loss of both contractile and non-contractile protein.

Short-term extreme adaptations to energy needs beyond the immediate available energy are varied. Certain tissues, such as the heart, kidney, and skeletal muscle, change their primary fuel substrate from glucose to fatty acids and ketone bodies rather readily. Others, such as the brain, take longer and use only glucose (from gluconeogenesis) and ketones as energy sources.[114]

Although fatty acids cannot be directly converted to glucose, the energy produced from the oxidation of free fatty acids (FFAs) can be used to fuel the conversion of certain other substrates into glucose (gluconeogenesis being an energy-requiring process), thus sparing somewhat the use of structural and contractile protein for glucose formation. For example, lactate and pyruvate are formed from anaerobic glycolysis and released systemically. In the liver they are converted to glucose, which is then released for other tissues to use. This shuttle is called the Cori cycle.[115,116] As well, the energy garnered through fatty acid oxidation is used for transforming glycerol into glucose.

With ongoing energy deprivation or low-carbohydrate intake, other adaptations appear. The brain, which ordinarily obtains energy only by glucose oxidation, acquires the ability to use keto acids for its fuel requirements, and this further contributes to protein conservation.

G. GLUCONEOGENESIS

As we have seen, certain processes such as glycogenolysis, gluconeogenesis, increasing fatty acid oxidation, utilization of ketones, proteolysis, and others ensure that the body has a continuous supply of available energy and substrates for its metabolic needs. Endogenous glucose production depends on glycogenolysis (glucose from glycogen) and gluconeogenesis (glucose from amino acids, lactate, and glycerol).

The rise in blood glucose and the subsequent rise in insulin that occur after a meal promote glycogen storage in liver and muscle, and fat deposition in adipose tissue, skeletal muscle, and liver. After a meal, both glucose and insulin levels fall and liver glycogen through the process of glycogenolysis becomes the primary source of available glucose.

Maintenance of plasma glucose concentrations within a narrow range despite wide fluctuations in the demand (e.g., vigorous exercise) and supply (e.g., large carbohydrate meals) of glucose results from coordination of factors that regulate glucose release into and removal from the circulation.[117]

The degree of contribution to glucose production from glycogenolysis vs. gluconeogenesis varies with the metabolic environment, macronutrient intake, and body composition.[118] For example, due to limited endogenous carbohydrate stores, dietary restriction of carbohydrate results in an increase in gluconeogenesis to both supply glucose directly and to increase hepatic glycogen levels, thus supporting glycogenolysis.[119]

Muscle glycogen levels cannot contribute to blood glucose levels directly although it can contribute to glycolysis providing anaerobic ATP for skeletal muscle contractions, and contribute to the formation of lactate, glycerol, alanine, and glutamine, substrates for hepatic gluconeogenesis.

It is often believed that gluconeogenesis from amino acids is a process that occurs only under physical stress and starvation in order to provide glucose, and that the need to provide glucose is a driving factor in the increased gluconeogenesis taking place at these times. It is also generally believed that gluconeogenesis from amino acids is a minor process in the fed state. In fact, conversion of the glucogenic moieties of the degraded amino acids to glucose occurs even in the fed state.

A detailed quantitative analysis of the energy exchanges associated with the degradation of amino acids in man demonstrates that gluconeogenesis and export of glucose is essential, because complete oxidation of the amino acid mixture by the liver would provide much more ATP than needed by the liver and the oxygen consumption greater than that available to the liver.[120] Gluconeogenesis from amino acids must thus be regarded as a normal process associated with amino acid degradation, occurring at higher rates under conditions of normal food intake than during fasting.

1. Amino Acids and Gluconeogenesis

Lactate, pyruvate, glycerol, and certain amino acids are used by the liver, kidney, and intestinal tract to form glucose. Under normal conditions, amino acids, especially alanine and glutamine, serve as major substrates for gluconeogenesis.[121]

It has been shown that, even under normal conditions, a major fate of dietary amino acids is for hepatic gluconeogenesis. Interestingly enough, dietary carbohydrate content only minimally affects hepatic gluconeogenesis from dietary amino acids, with only a slight increase seen during severe carbohydrate restriction.[122] As well, an increase in free fatty acids has been shown to increase gluconeogenesis but only at high plasma FFA concentrations.[123]

In one study, the contribution under various nutritional regimens of several amino acids and lactate to gluconeogenesis was estimated by measuring the glucose formation from 14C-labeled substrates.[124] Isolated rat hepatocytes were incubated for

60 minutes in a Krebs-Ringer bicarbonate buffer pH 7.4 containing lactate, pyruvate, and all the amino acids at concentrations similar to their physiological levels found in rat plasma, with one precursor labeled in each flask. In all conditions, lactate was the major glucose precursor, providing over 60% of the glucose formed. Glutamine and alanine were the major amino acid precursors of glucose, contributing 9.8 and 10.6% of the glucose formed, respectively, in hepatocytes isolated from starved rats. Serine, glycine, and threonine also contributed to gluconeogenesis in the starved liver cells at 2.6, 2.1, and 3.8%, respectively, of the glucose formed.

In this study it was shown that the availability of dietary carbohydrates varies the gluconeogenic response. The rate of glucose formation from the isolated hepatocytes of the starved rats and those fed either high protein or high fat was higher than from rats fed a nonpurified diet.[124]

The low-insulin and high-glucagon output that characterizes the post-absorptive phase and fasting (the lower the glucose level the lower the insulin and higher the glucagon output) stimulates both glycogenolysis and gluconeogenesis. Initially, approximately 70 to 75% of the hepatic glucose output is derived from glycogenolysis and the remainder from gluconeogenesis.

Starvation is associated initially with an increased release of the gluconeogenic amino acids from muscles and an increase in gluconeogenesis.[125] In one study looking at amino acid balance across forearm muscles in post-absorptive (overnight fasted) subjects, fasting significantly reduced basal insulin and increased glucagon, and increased muscle release of the principal glycogenic amino acids (alanine, glutamine, glycine, threonine, serine, methionine, tyrosine, and lysine).[126] In this study, alanine release increased 59.4%. The increase in release for all amino acids averaged 69.4% and was statistically significant for threonine, serine, glycine, alanine, alpha-aminobutyrate, methionine, tyrosine, and lysine. In the same study, seven subjects were also fasted for 60 hours. In these subjects there was a reduction of amino acid release as the fasting continued.

Since these changes reproduce those observed after a few days of total fasting, it has been suggested that it is the carbohydrate restriction itself, and the subsequent decrease in insulin and increase in glucagon, that is responsible for the metabolic and hormonal adaptations of brief fasting.[127] A reduction in the release of substrate amino acids from skeletal muscle largely explains the decrease in gluconeogenesis characterizing prolonged starvation.

A similar response, an initial increase in gluconeogenesis followed in time by a decrease, is seen in trauma such as burn injury[128] and in prolonged exercise.[129]

During prolonged mild exercise that increases the hepatic glucose output two-fold, the relative contribution of gluconeogenesis to the overall hepatic output increases from 25 to 45%, indicating a three-fold rise in the absolute rate of gluconeogenesis. After 12 to 13 hours of fasting, hepatic gluconeogenesis replaces glycogenolysis as the main source of glucose.[130] In one study on six subjects the contribution of gluconeogenesis to glucose production was 41, 71, and 92% at 12, 20 and 40 hours, respectively.[131]

As well, there is an increase in gluconeogenesis with type II diabetes[132] and obesity. A recent study found that the fractional and absolute contribution of gluconeogenesis to glucose production is higher in obesity and is associated with increased rates of protein turnover and insulin resistance of glucose, lipid, and protein metabolism.[133] The study also found a lower contribution to glucose production from hepatic glycogenolysis.

Insulin resistance, by mechanisms that involve suppression of PI3K/Akt signaling leading to activation of caspase-3 and the ubiquitin-proteasome proteolytic pathway, leads to an increase in muscle protein degradation,[134] and a subsequent increase in gluconeogenesis.

2. Hormonal Control of Gluconeogenesis

Among the hormones responsible for a rise in gluconeogenesis one must take into account adrenaline, glucagon, glucocorticoids, growth hormone, and insulin. These hormones can act either directly on the gluconeogenic enzymes or on the mobilization of precursors necessary for gluconeogenesis (the 3-carbon precursors, including lactate, alanine, and glycerol). On a moment-to-moment basis, however, these processes are controlled mainly by the glucocorticoids insulin and glucagon, whose secretions are reciprocally influenced by the plasma glucose concentration. The glucocorticoids increase the activity of the glucose-alanine cycle. Insulin decreases the supply of gluconeogenic substrates and inhibits the glucose-alanine cycle. Thus, the exercise-induced hypoinsulinemia is a promoting factor in gluconeogenesis. In the resting postabsorptive state, release of glucose from the liver (usually equally via glycogenolysis and gluconeogenesis) is the key regulated process.

Glycogenolysis depends on the relative activities of glycogen synthase and phosphorylase, the latter being the more important. The activities of fructose-1,6-diphosphatase, phosphoenolpyruvate carboxylkinase, and pyruvate dehydrogenase, whose main precursors are lactate, alanine, and glutamine, regulate gluconeogenesis.

In the immediate postprandial state, due to the availability of substrates coming from the GI tract, suppression of liver glucose output and stimulation of skeletal muscle glucose uptake are the most important factors. Glucose disposal by insulin-sensitive tissues is regulated initially at the transport step and then mainly by glycogen synthase, phosphofructokinase, and pyruvate dehydrogenase. Hormonally induced changes in intracellular fructose 2,6-bisphosphate concentrations play a key role in muscle glycolytic flux and both glycolytic and gluconeogenic flux in the liver.

Under stressful conditions (e.g., hypoglycemia, trauma, vigorous exercise), increased secretion of other hormones such as adrenaline, cortisol, and growth hormone, and increased activity of the sympathetic nervous system, come into play. Their actions to increase hepatic glucose output and to suppress tissue glucose uptake are partly mediated by increases in tissue fatty acid oxidation.

In diabetes, the most common disorder of glucose homeostasis, fasting hyperglycemia results primarily from excessive release of glucose by the liver due to increased gluconeogenesis; postprandial hyperglycemia results from both impaired suppression of hepatic glucose release and impaired skeletal muscle glucose uptake. These abnormalities are usually due to the combination of impaired insulin secretion and tissue resistance to insulin.

As noted above, under normal conditions the amount of readily available energy coming from carbohydrate sources is only about 800 kcal — and includes the 120 grams or so of glycogen from the body's skeletal muscle, 70 g of glycogen in the liver and 10 grams of glucose in the blood. Adipose tissue, on the other hand, provides an almost limitless supply of available energy, about 100,000 calories from the average person's 15 kg of fat.

Muscle glycogen and FFAs from adipose tissue and intramuscular stores provide energy both at rest and during low-intensity exercise. At these levels, substrate availability does not limit activity since there is so much potential energy available from body fat. FFA mobilization from adipose tissue (catecholamines stimulate adipose lipase, which breaks each triglyceride molecule down to form 1 glycerol and 3 fatty acid molecules) starts with any kind of activity. FFAs are metabolized in muscle cells to acetyl-CoA that subsequently enters the citric acid cycle, forming ATP as it is oxidatively metabolized.

While FFA mobilization may lag at first, it soon results in high FFA blood levels of up to six times the normal level. These levels of FFA are so high that it can't all be utilized by muscle. Perhaps one of the reasons for the overproduction of FFA is to release glycerol, a substrate for gluconeogenesis.

3. Effects of Amino Acids on Hepatic Glucose Metabolism

Amino acids have direct (substrate mediated) and indirect (hormone mediated) effects on hepatic glucose metabolism. The hormonal effects include the simultaneous increase in endogenous levels of insulin and glucagon.[135,136] This simultaneous increase leads to an increase in endogenous glucose production mainly by gluconeogenesis, since higher insulin concentrations are needed to suppress gluconeogenesis as compared with glycogenolysis.[137]

One study found that conditions creating postprandial amino acid elevation stimulate secretion of insulin and glucagon, but do not affect glycaemia despite markedly increased gluconeogenesis.[138] The rise in endogenous glucose production was counterbalanced by an insulin-stimulated increase in glucose disposal, which thereby served to maintain fasting plasma glucose concentrations.

H. Use of Amino Acids for Energy — Catabolic Effects of Exercise

Typical responses to acute exercise are suppressed protein synthesis and elevated protein degradation. Comparison of these responses in muscle containing various types of fibers indicated that the rate of protein synthesis was suppressed and the rate of protein degradation was elevated mainly in muscles less active during exercise. Thus, the less active muscles, but not those that fulfill the main task during exercise performance, are used as a reservoir for mobilization of protein resources. The exercise-induced catabolism is not extended to contractile proteins. During exercise, the catabolic response is extended to the smooth muscle of the gastrointestinal tract, lymphoid tissue, liver, and kidney.

Both the anti-anabolic and catabolic effects have to be considered as tools for mobilization of protein resources during a stressful situation. As a result, an increased pool of available free amino acids is created. Due to the suppressed protein synthesis, the free amino acids pool is used for supplying the necessary protein synthesis by "building materials" only to a minor extent. The amino acids are mainly used for additional energy supply to contracting muscles.

There are at least three pathways connecting free amino acids with energy processes. One of these consists in the oxidation of branched-chain amino acids. The main site of this pathway is the contracting muscle. An increased oxidation of leucine during exercise was established in human as well as in animal studies. The metabolism of several amino acids leads to the formation of metabolites of the citric cycle, which also has a beneficial effect on muscle metabolism by increasing the capacity of the citric cycle for oxidizing the acetyl-CoA units generated from pyruvate and FFAs.

1. Amino Acid Metabolism in Muscle

There are three principal sources of amino acids for energy metabolism: dietary protein, plasma and tissue free amino acid pools, and endogenous tissue protein.

All three sources are in equilibrium. Dietary protein is a relatively minor source of amino acids during normal exercise since ingesting a large protein meal prior to exercise is rarely done. The plasma pool of free amino acids is much smaller than the free amino acid pool of human skeletal muscle largely because skeletal muscle makes up about 40% of bodyweight and contains about 75% of the whole-body free amino acids.

The free amino acid pools, however, are much smaller than the amount of amino acids available from endogenous protein breakdown. It has been estimated that the intramuscular amino acid pool contains less that 1% of the metabolically active amino acids. It has also been estimated that the amount of leucine oxidized during a prolonged exercise bout is approximately 25 times greater than the free leucine concentration in muscle, liver, and plasma. Therefore, the free amino acid pool is only a minor source of amino acids during exercise, whereas the most important source is endogenous protein breakdown.

2. Pathways of Amino Acid Metabolism in Muscle

Many of the amino acids can be oxidized by skeletal muscle including alanine, arginine, aspartate, cysteine, glutamate, glycine, phenylalanine, threonine, tyrosine, and the three BCAA. Not all of these amino acids, however, have the same metabolic potential in muscle and it appears that the BCAA are the dominant amino acids oxidized by skeletal muscle. The catabolism of amino acids involves the removal of the alpha-amino group by transamination or oxidative deamination, followed by conversion of the carbon skeleton to metabolites that are common to the pathways of carbohydrate and fat metabolism. It should be noted that the avenues available for amino acid catabolism and conversion are extensive, and the final products, their fates, and the pathways available to them are all quite complex.

3. Skeletal Muscle Catabolism

Significant gaps remain in our knowledge of the pathways of amino acid catabolism in humans. Sufficient information, however, does exist to allow a broad picture of the overall process of amino acid oxidation to be developed along with approximate quantitative assessments of the role played by liver, muscle, kidney, and small intestine. For example, one study found that amino acids are the major fuel of liver, i.e., their oxidative conversion to glucose accounts for about one-half of the daily oxygen consumption of the liver, and no other fuel contributes nearly so importantly.[139]

The daily supply of amino acids provided in the diet cannot be totally oxidized to CO_2 in the liver because such a process would provide far more ATP than the liver could utilize and not enough ATP would be generated in other tissues. Instead, most amino acids are oxidatively converted to glucose. This results in an overall ATP production during amino acid oxidation very nearly equal to the ATP required to convert amino acid carbon to glucose.

ATP is thus produced in the muscle cells both by anaerobic glycolysis and oxidation of amino acids, while ATP is used up in liver cells to produce glucose from the carbon skeletons. Thus the glucose-alanine cycle in an indirect way transfers ATP from the liver to the peripheral tissues.

It is commonly thought that only ATP, phosphocreatine, and glycolysis (the conversion of glucose into pyruvic acid) provides cellular energy under anaerobic conditions. Such is not the case, however, because, as we have seen, amino acid catabolism coupled with the TCA cycle can also provide a source of anaerobic energy production.

In a study on anoxic heart muscle, glutamate and aspartate catabolized at a higher rate as compared with oxygenation.[140] The data obtained from this study suggests that the constant influx of intermediates into the cycle from amino acids is supported by coupled transamination of glutamate and aspartate. This leads to the formation of ATP and GTP in the citric acid or tricarboxylic acid cycle during blocking of aerobic energy production. Succinate, a component of the citric acid cycle, is thought to result from amino acid catabolism.

In another study on cat heart papillary muscle, supplying hypoxic contracting muscles with aspartate resulted in maintenance of muscular function to some extent and led to augmented release of succinate and lactate.[141] The data from this study indicate that anaerobic succinate formation is correlated to the energy-requiring processes of the myocardium. Maintenance of myocardial function by the supply of amino acids may be related to their conversion into succinate. In some studies, it has been shown that in the human heart glutamate may be used as an anaerobic fuel through conversion to succinate coupled with GTP formation.[142]

Since amino acids can be used as fuel in both aerobic and anaerobic states, muscle catabolism occurs under both conditions to provide the needed substrates. The use of parenteral or enteral amino acid mixtures and combinations of specific amino acids can attenuate this catabolic and counterproductive response to exercise.

4. Oxidation of Amino Acids

The contribution made by proteins to the energy value of most well-balanced diets is usually between 10 and 15% of the total and seldom exceeds 20%. In some athletes in power sports and in bodybuilders who may be on very high-protein diets, the contribution can be as high as 50%, and in selective cases even more.

Once the needed proteins are synthesized and the amino acid pools replenished, additional amino acids are degraded and used for energy or stored mainly as fat and to a lesser extent as glycogen. The primary site for degradation of most amino acids is the liver, which is unique because of its capacity to degrade amino acids and to synthesize urea for elimination of the amino nitrogen.

The first step in the degradation of amino acids begins with deamination — the removal of the alpha-amino group from the amino acid to produce an oxoacid, which may be a simple metabolic intermediate itself (e.g., pyruvate) or be converted to a simple metabolic intermediate via a specific metabolic pathway. The intermediates are either oxidized via the citric acid cycle or converted to glucose via gluconeogenesis. For instance, deaminated alanine is pyruvic acid. This can be converted into glucose or glycogen, or it can be converted into acetyl-CoA, which can then be polymerized into fatty acids. Also, 2 molecules of acetyl-CoA can condense to form acetoacetic acid, which is one of the ketone bodies.

Deamination occurs mainly by transamination, the transfer of the amino group to some other acceptor compound. Deamination generally occurs by the following transamination pathway:

$$\text{alpha-ketoglutaric acid} + \text{amino acid} \rightarrow \text{glutamic acid} + \text{alpha-keto acid}$$

$$\text{glutamic acid} + \text{NAD+} + \text{H2O} \rightarrow \text{NADH} + \text{H+} + \text{NH3} + \text{alpha-ketoglutaric acid}$$

Note from this schema that the amino group from the amino acid is transferred to alpha-ketoglutaric acid, which then becomes glutamic acid. The glutamic acid can then transfer the amino group to still other substances or can release it in the form of NH_3. In the process of losing the amino group the glutamic acid once again becomes alpha-ketoglutaric acid, so that the cycle can be repeated again and again.

To initiate this process, the excess amino acids in the cells, especially in the liver, induce the activation of large quantities of aminotransferases, the enzymes responsible for initiating most deamination. Hepatic tissue contains high concentrations of the degradative enzymes, including the aminotransferases (with the exception of the branched-chain aminotransferase), which remove the alpha-amino groups during the first step in amino acid degradation. Branched chain aminotransferase results in the release of BCAA into circulation and is exclusively a mitochondrial enzyme in skeletal muscles.[143]

For example, degradation of the BCAAs is initiated by the reversible transamination of the BCAA to the alpha-keto acid with transfer of the alpha-amino group to alpha-ketoglutarate, forming glutamate. This step appears to be nearly at equilibrium with little physiological control. The second and rate-limiting step is decarboxylation of the branched-chain keto acids by branched-chain keto acid dehydrogenase (BCKAD). BCKAD activity is highly regulated by phosphorylation and dephosphorylation to the inactive and active forms, respectively. This step is stimulated by increases in the concentration of the leucine keto acid, alpha-ketoisocaproate (KIC).

During periods of increased energy needs, such as starvation, trauma, and exercise, increased levels of BCAAs stimulate BCKAD and the BCAAs are degraded to energy in skeletal muscle. During absorption periods when muscles are using glucose as a primary fuel, muscle transaminates the BCAA and releases the keto acids into circulation for complete oxidation by the liver or kidney. In the liver, these intermediates, formed either in the liver or from other tissues, are either oxidized via the citric acid cycle or converted to glucose via gluconeogenesis. A deaminated amino acid can enter the citric acid cycle at different levels, including acetyl-CoA, pyruvate, oxaloacetate, alpha-ketoglutarate, succinyl-CoA, or fumarate.[144] Both isoleucine and valine form succinyl-CoA, whereas leucine forms acetyl-CoA. Of these, only the carbons of acetyl-CoA from leucine can be oxidized directly in the citric acid cycle; the other intermediates must first be converted to pyruvate via phosphoenolpyruvate before their carbons are available for oxidation in the citric acid cycle as acetyl-CoA.

Within skeletal muscle, BCAA degradation involves transfer of the alpha-amino group to ketoglutarate to form glutamate. Glutamate serves as an important intermediate in nitrogen metabolism. While glutamate is formed *de novo* in skeletal muscle, there is no net release. Once the amino group is transferred to glutamate, there are three primary fates. The amino group can be transferred either to pyruvate in synthesis of alanine or onto oxaloacetate for the synthesis of aspartate, or the glutamate can release the amino group in the form of NH_3 and reform ketogluterate, at the same time releasing 2 hydrogen atoms, which are oxidized to form ATP.

Alanine is released from muscle into circulation and is ultimately removed by the liver for gluconeogenesis. Aspartate is an important component of the purine nucleotide cycle, which is central to maintaining the pool of ATP in muscle. The purine nucleotide cycle serves to regenerate IMP and also produces fumarate and free NH_3. The ammonia can be combined with glutamate via glutamine synthetase to form glutamine (glutamate + ammonia + ATP → glutamine + ADP).[145] Glutamine is ultimately released from muscle, with the majority of glutamine being used by the gut and the immune system as a primary energy source.

Together, alanine and glutamine represent 60 to 80% of the amino acids released from skeletal muscle while they account for only 18% of the amino acids in muscle protein. During exercise, glutamine synthesis and glutamine levels in muscle decline due to inhibition of glutamine synthetase.

The net effect of oxidation of amino acids to glucose in the liver is to make nearly two-thirds of the total energy available from the oxidation of amino acids available to peripheral tissues, without necessitating that peripheral tissues synthesize the complex array of enzymes needed to support direct amino acid oxidation.

As a balanced mixture of amino acids is oxidized in the liver, nearly all carbon from glucogenic amino acids flows into the mitochondrial aspartate pool and is actively transported out of the mitochondria via the aspartate-glutamate antiport linked to proton entry. In the cytoplasm the aspartate is converted to fumarate utilizing urea cycle enzymes; the fumarate flows via oxaloacetate to phosphoenolpyruvate and on to glucose.

Thus carbon flow through the urea cycle is normally interlinked with gluconeogenic carbon flow because these metabolic pathways share a common step. Liver mitochondria experience a severe nonvolatile acid load during amino acid oxidation.

It is suggested that this acid load is alleviated mainly by the respiratory chain proton pump in a form of uncoupled respiration.

I. GLUCOGENIC AND KETOGENIC AMINO ACIDS

All tissues have some capability for synthesis of the non-essential amino acids, amino acid remodeling, and conversion of non-amino acid carbon skeletons into amino acids and other derivatives that contain nitrogen. However, the liver is the major site of nitrogen metabolism in the body. In times of dietary surplus, the potentially toxic nitrogen of amino acids is eliminated via transaminations, deamination, and urea formation; the carbon skeletons are generally conserved as carbohydrate, via gluconeogenesis, or as fatty acid via fatty acid synthesis pathways.

In this respect, amino acids fall into three categories: glucogenic, ketogenic, or glucogenic and ketogenic. Glucogenic amino acids are those that give rise to a net production of pyruvate or TCA cycle intermediates, such as a-ketoglutarate or oxaloacetate, all of which are precursors to glucose via gluconeogenesis. All amino acids except lysine and leucine are at least partly glucogenic. Lysine and leucine are the only amino acids that are solely ketogenic, giving rise only to acetylCoA or acetoacetylCoA, neither of which can bring about net glucose production. See Figure 4.1 to see the entry of amino acids into the pathway of gluconeogenesis.

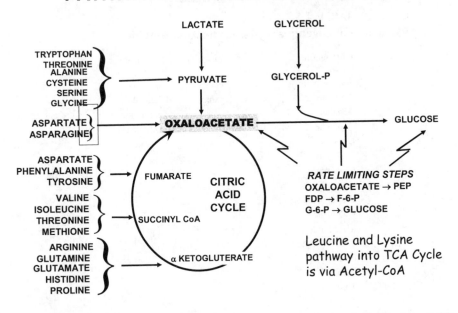

ENTRY OF PRECURSORS INTO THE PATHWAYS OF GLUCONEOGENESIS

FIGURE 4.1 Abbreviations: PEP, phosphoenolpyruvate; FDP, fructose-1, 6-phosphate; F-6-P, fructose 6-phosphate; G-6-P, glucose 6-phosphate.

A small group of amino acids comprising isoleucine, phenylalanine, threonine, tryptophan, and tyrosine give rise to both glucose and fatty acid precursors and are thus characterized as being glucogenic and ketogenic. Finally, it should be recognized that amino acids have a third possible fate. During times of stress and starvation there is an increase in the use of the reduced carbon skeleton, through the transformation to acetylCoA either directly or indirectly via the TCA cycle, for energy production, with the result that it is oxidized to CO_2 and H_2O.

1. Glucogenic Amino Acids

For a list of the glucogenic amino acids that are metabolized to alpha-ketoglutarate, pyruvate, oxaloacetate, fumarate, or succinyl CoA, see Table 4.5.

2. Ketogenic Amino Acids

The ketogenic amino acids are metabolized to acetylCoA or acetoacetate. Leucine and Lysine are the only amino acids that are solely ketogenic giving rise only to acetylCoA or acetoacetylCoA, neither of which can bring about net glucose production. For lists of the ketogenic amino acids and the five amino acids that are both glucogenic and ketogenic, see Table 4.5.

3. Alanine and Glutamine

Intense exercise has dramatic effects on amino acid metabolism. After an exhausting load a significant rise and concurrent drop of serum isoleucine, threonine, ornithine,

TABLE 4.5
Glucogenic and Ketogenic Amino Acids

Glucogenic	Ketogenic	Both
Alanine	Leucine	Isoleucine
Arginine	Lysine	Phenylalanine
Asparagine		Threonine
Aspartate		Tryptophan
Cysteine		Tyrosine
Glutamate		
Glutamine		
Glycine		
Histidine Hydroxyproline		
Isoleucine		
Methionine		
Phenylalanine		
Proline		
Serine		
Threonine		
Tryptophan		
Tyrosine		
Valine		

leucine, serine, glycine, asparagine and glutamine occurs with a rise in serum alanine.[146] The rise of alanine suggests the existence of a glucose-alanine cycle. The drop of branched amino acids is probably due to their enhanced entry into muscles. The drop of glutamine reflects increased use by the gut and immune system, even though the release of glutamine by muscle cells increases secondary to proteolysis.

Similarly, under stress, glucose consumption increases and the efflux of lactate, alanine, glutamine, and total amino acid nitrogen (i.e., net muscle protein catabolism) increases.

In a series of studies, Brown et al. have shown that catabolic hormones alone fail to reproduce the stress-induced efflux of amino acids.[147] In this study the net balance of amino acids was determined in five healthy volunteers prior to and following a 2-hour infusion of the catabolic hormones epinephrine, cortisol, and glucagon into the femoral artery. This hormonal simulation of stress in normal volunteers increased glutamine efflux from the leg to an extent similar to that of burn patients.

Alanine efflux, however, was not affected by the hormonal infusion. Because alanine efflux constituted a major proportion of the total peripheral amino acid catabolism in the burn patients, there was significantly less total amino acid nitrogen loss from the healthy volunteers receiving the stress hormones. Thus catabolic hormones alone fail to reproduce the stress-induced pattern and quantity of amino acid efflux from human skeletal muscle. This discrepancy is largely due to an unresponsiveness of alanine to hormonally induced muscle protein catabolism.

In states of stress, alanine becomes increasingly important to sustain increases in gluconeogenesis. Alanine, via deamination to pyruvate, is a principal precursor for hepatic gluconeogenesis and is normally produced secondary to insulin resistance — important since insulin is known to inhibit muscle protein breakdown especially in severely stressed states.

In another study, Brown et al. showed that alanine efflux may depend on pyruvate availability during stress and the rate of glycolysis within peripheral tissues may be a major factor in regulating the quantity of alanine efflux.[148]

Several studies have hypothesized that alanine decreases plasma ketone body levels by increasing availability of oxaloacetate, thus allowing acetyl groups to enter the citric acid cycle and releasing coenzyme A (CoA). The significant elevation in plasma free carnitine concentration found after alanine ingestion is consistent with the hypothesis that alanine increases the oxidation of acetylCoA by providing oxaloacetate for the citric acid cycle.[149]

Glutamine also becomes increasingly important during stress due to both its role as a major precursor for ammoniagenesis by the kidney and its avid consumption by visceral organs, fibroblasts, and lymphoid tissue.[150]

The authors of this study suggest that "any attempt to minimize muscle protein catabolism should be accompanied by amino acid supplementation, especially of glutamine and alanine." Thus the provision of exogenous alanine may decrease insulin resistance, and the provision of exogenous alanine and glutamine may decrease the need to obtain these amino acids from endogenous protein and therefore decrease muscle protein breakdown.

4.   Interorgan Exchange of Amino Acids

Many of the alterations in the hormonal ensemble during exercise favor (or even constitute the main cause of) protein and amino acid mobilization. As a result of exercise, there is an interorgan exchange of amino acids, particularly the BCAAs, alanine, and glutamine. The main features of this interorgan exchange include:

- The movement of the branched-chain amino acids (leucine, valine, and isoleucine) from the splanchnic bed (liver and gut) to skeletal muscles.
- The movement of alanine from muscle to the liver
- The movement of glutamine from muscle to the gut.

The interorgan exchange of these amino acids has several functions including:

- Maintaining amino acid precursors for protein synthesis
- Assisting in the elimination of nitrogen wastes
- Providing substrates for gluconeogenesis
- Providing glutamine for gut and immune system function
- Maintaining the purine nucleotide cycle.

Early studies by Felig et al. provided evidence about amino acid movement among tissues.[151] By examining arterial-venous differences in substrate concentrations across tissues, they observed that skeletal muscle had a net uptake of BCAAs with a subsequent release of alanine greater than the amount present in muscle protein. The released alanine was removed by the splanchnic bed. On the basis of these observations, the study's authors proposed the existence of a glucose-alanine cycle for maintenance of blood glucose and the shuttling of nitrogen and gluconeogenic substrate from muscle to liver.

Another study by Ahlborg et al. using six untrained adult males examined the arterial-venous differences across the splanchnic bed and across the leg during 4 hours of cycling at 30% of VO_2max.[152] They observed decreases in plasma glucose and insulin, and increases in glucagon and FFAs. Plasma glucose declined from a pre-exercise level of 90 mg/dl but stabilized at 60 mg/dl as release of glucose by the liver continued throughout the exercise period. Glucose remained an important fuel throughout exercise, but there was a significant increase in use of FFAs.

There was also a significant increase in amino acid flux, including a fourfold increase in the release of branched-chain amino acids from the splanchnic area and a corresponding increase in the uptake by exercising muscles. In return, muscles released alanine, which was removed by the liver for gluconeogenesis. This study demonstrated a change in amino acid flux during exercise with movement of branched-chain amino acids from visceral tissues to skeletal muscles and the return of alanine as a precursor for hepatic synthesis of glucose.

Lemon and Mullin further established the relationship of amino acid metabolism to glucose homeostasis.[153] In this study they demonstrated a dramatic increase in sweat urea nitrogen in men previously depleted of glycogen stores and exercised for 1 hour at 61% VO_2 max, but no change in urinary urea nitrogen. The authors found that amino acid catabolism provided 10.4% of total energy for the exercise in carbohydrate-depleted individuals, while in the carbohydrate-loaded group protein provided 4.4% of the energy needs. These results suggest that production of nitrogen wastes during exercise is related to carbohydrate status and that sweating may be an important mechanism for elimination of nitrogen wastes. Other studies also support the relationship of increased amino acid degradation with maintenance of hepatic glucose production.[154,155]

Exercise and periods of food restriction or fasting share many similarities in amino acid metabolism. In both there is a net release of amino acids from protein due to suppression of protein synthesis and an increase in protein breakdown. This change in protein turnover results in an increase in tissue levels of free amino acids and net release of amino acids from most tissues. Tissues with high rates of protein turnover are most affected, with the liver and gastrointestinal tract incurring the largest losses during short-term fasts. Skeletal muscle, which has lower rates of protein turnover, responds somewhat less dramatically, but because of its total mass, muscle is the predominant source of free amino acids during prolonged periods of food restriction.

Amino acids have been shown to play important roles in energy homeostasis during periods of high energy need or low energy intake. While the qualitative role is becoming clear, the quantitative level of this role remains uncertain. Most of the studies examining this role have been designed using leucine and alanine as metabolic tracers. These studies establish changes in protein turnover, increases in amino acid flux, and increase in leucine oxidation. However, questions remain about the potential to generalize from these findings to other amino acids or to dietary protein requirements. Endurance exercise causes a reduction in muscle protein synthesis and net protein breakdown, but is there a real loss of amino acids; are there increases in urea production during exercise; are the effects unique to leucine or do they relate to other amino acids? These questions remain to be fully answered.

Using multiple isotope tracers, Wolfe et al.[156] examined amino acid metabolism during aerobic exercise. They found inhibition of protein synthesis, increased leucine oxidation, and increased flux of alanine. These findings are consistent with most earlier reports. However, using direct isotopic measures, they failed to find any increase in urea synthesis. Further, using lysine, a second indispensable amino acid, they demonstrated that the inhibition of protein synthesis was less than half that estimated by leucine (17 vs. 48%) and that there was no increase in lysine oxidation.

J. PROTEIN METABOLISM AND AMMONIA

1. Metabolism of Ammonia

Ammonia is formed in a number of reactions in the body during the degradation of amines, purines, and pyrimidines,[157-159] and the metabolism of amino acids. It seems, however, that the quantitatively important source of ammonia during exercise is the metabolism of amino acids.[160]

Skeletal muscle produces a large quantity of ammonia during prolonged submaximal (i.e., endurance) exercise, the source of which is the subject of some controversy.

Ammonia production in skeletal muscle involves the purine nucleotide cycle and the amino acids glutamate, glutamine, and alanine and probably also includes the branched chain amino acids as well as aspartate.[161]

Several authors have proposed that the degradation of amino acids, specifically, the branched-chain amino acids leucine, valine, and isoleucine, may be a source of ammonia during this type of activity. The ammonia response can be suppressed by increasing the carbohydrate availability and this may be mediated by decreasing the oxidation of the branched chain amino acids.[162]

MacLean et al. performed a study in which the purpose was to examine the effects of oral BCAA supplementation on amino acid and ammonia metabolism in exercising humans.[163] Five men exercised the knee extensors of one leg for 60 minutes with and without (control) an oral supplement of BCAA. The subjects consumed 77 mg/kg of the supplement administered in two equal doses of 38.5 kg/mg at 45 and 20 minutes before the onset of exercise. According to the authors of the study, the 500-mg capsules of the commercially available BCAA supplement were reported to contain only the three BCAAs in the following proportions: 220, 150, and 130 mg L-leucine, L-valine, and L-isoleucine, respectively. This was confirmed by dilution of the capsules in water and with analysis by high-performance liquid chromatography.

The researchers concluded that their study clearly shows that BCAA supplementation results in significantly greater muscle ammonia production during exercise. Also, BCAA supplementation imposes a substantial ammonia load on muscle, as indicated by the consistently larger total alanine and glutamine releases observed during exercise. The elevated BCAA levels also suppress the degree of net protein degradation that normally occurs during exercise of this magnitude and duration.

Also of importance in this was the finding that the degree of contractile protein degradation was not increased during exercise for either trial. The authors noted that previous studies have reported that muscle protein catabolism occurs primarily in noncontractile protein while contractile protein catabolism is spared or even decreased. MacLean et al. found no significant elevations in the release of 3-methylhistidine (a marker of contractile protein catabolism — 3-methylhistidine is a muscle-specific amino acid that is produced and lost in the urine only when muscle protein is broken down) from muscle for either trial.

Since it is produced in degradation reactions, ammonia is usually considered an end product of metabolism that must be converted to urea, a non-toxic compound, for excretion. In most mammals, including man, urea is produced in the liver by a cyclical series of reactions known as the urea cycle. The urea cycle, because of the intricacy of amino acid metabolism, and in particular the contribution of different tissues, is more complex than is generally thought.

In addition to its role in the urea cycle, ammonia can play a number of other roles in metabolism including:

- Acting as a substrate for the glutamate dehydrogenase reaction in the formation of non-essential amino acids; as a substrate for glutamine synthetase in the formation of glutamine in muscle

- Acting as an important regulator of the rate of glycolysis in muscle, brain, and possibly other tissues
- The regulation of acid/base balance by the kidney.

Ammonia, generated from glutamine within the tubule cells, acts as a third renal system to help the body cope with large acid loads. Once formed, ammonia diffuses into the tubule to combine with the protons as follows:

$$NH3 + H+ \; NH4+$$

Through the activity of the glutaminase enzyme, the hydrolysis of glutamine to glutamate in the distal tubules of the kidney is the primary pathway for renal ammonia production, although additional ammonia can also be produced by the further conversion of glutamate to a-ketoglutarate through the activity of the enzyme glutamate dehydrogenase. Furthermore, oxidation of glutamine carbons by the kidney gives rise to bicarbonate ($HCO3-$) ion production for release into the blood stream to further buffer hydrogen ion production. These processes allow the kidneys to effectively excrete excess protons and protect the body from acidosis.

Consequently, during acidosis, major changes in renal glutamine metabolism occur to support ammoniagenesis. Renal uptake of glutamine has been shown to be accelerated by activation of the Na+-dependent membrane transport system. The rate of glutamine hydrolysis and the maximal activity of the glutaminase enzyme were also increased, such that renal glutamine consumption was increased 6- to 10-fold, making the kidney the major organ of glutamine utilization during acidosis.

The glutamine is produced in muscle (although brain and liver may contribute small amounts) and transported to the kidney, where the two nitrogen atoms are released as ammonia. Since the glutamine release by muscle may be at the expense of alanine, the excretion of the nitrogen from amino acid metabolism in muscle is effectively switched from urea, which is produced from the metabolism of alanine in the liver, to ammonia, which is produced from glutamine metabolism in the kidney. In this way, the end product of nitrogen metabolism is put to good use by the body in achieving control of acidosis.

2. Urea Formation by the Liver

The ammonia released during deamination is removed from the blood almost entirely by conversion into urea; 2 molecules of ammonia and 1 molecule of carbon dioxide combine in accordance with the following net reaction:

$$2NH_3 + CO_2 \rightarrow H_2N\text{-}CO\text{-}NH_2 + H_2O$$

Practically all urea formed in the human body is synthesized in the liver. In pathological states such as serious liver dysfunction, ammonia can accumulate in the blood and become toxic. For example, high levels of ammonia can disrupt the functioning of the central nervous system, sometimes leading to a state called hepatic coma.

The stages in the formation of urea involve ornithine, citrulline, and arginine. Ornithine plus CO_2 and NH_3 forms citrulline, which combines with another molecule of NH_3 to form arginine. Arginine plus water produces urea and reforms ornithine through the action of arinase. Once formed, urea diffuses from the liver cells into the body fluids and is excreted by the kidneys.

3. High Levels of Protein Intake and Ammonia

With increasing protein intake there is an increased oxidation of amino acids and subsequently an increased production of ammonia. Animals can adapt to a high-protein diet by upregulating urea synthesis and excretion, and also by upregulating amino acid metabolizing enzymes such as alanine and aspartate aminotransferases, glutamate dehydrogenase, and argininosuccinate synthetase,[164] and can increase mitochondrial glutamine hydrolysis in hepatocytes.[165] As well, the metabolism of increased dietary protein can be modulated at the gastrointestinal level, for example, with decreased gastric emptying to decrease the rate of absorption, thus allowing the liver to better deal with the amino acid load.[166–168]

Even with all of these mechanisms in play it is possible that high dietary protein can lead to toxic effects and hyperammonemia, perhaps secondary to the liver's limited capacity to form urea. Unfortunately there is very little documentation on the effects of the chronic intake of large amounts of dietary protein on normal people. One phenomenon, known as "rabbit starvation," seems to occur in diets that are very high in protein and very low in fat and carbohydrates, such as the consumption of very lean rabbit meat.[169] I believe the basis behind the toxicity associated with eating just lean meat is hyperammonemia, which occurs secondary to the large amount of protein needed in an attempt to derive all of one's energy from protein alone.

This is accentuated by the fact that the amount of useable energy derived from protein is less than that derived from carbs and fats. Using amino acids as a primary energy source is less efficient than using either carbs or fats. That is because the deamination and formation of urea, as well as the oxidation of amino acids and conversion into glucose, require energy and this decreases the net amount of energy obtainable from amino acids. As such, more protein needs to be metabolized to meet the energy requirements of the body and this potentially leads to even higher levels of systemic ammonia.

It has been shown that, as the protein content of meals is increased, the rate of urea synthesis maxes out and beyond this point ammonia levels increase. In one study, the maximum rate corresponded to a protein intake of just over 3 grams per kg of bodyweight or approximately 40% of dietary energy.[170] However, anecdotally, higher levels than this have not caused any adverse effects — for example, the Inuit's ancestral diet consisted of fat and protein with protein levels approximating 50% of the energy intake. It is possible that with time an upregulation of hepatic enzymes would make it possible to subsist without adverse effects on a diet in which protein makes up more than 50% of total energy intake.

It has been demonstrated that when protein intake is either decreased or increased urinary nitrogen output is adjusted to match protein intake.[171] As well, in one study, measurements were made at 6-hour intervals, of urinary nitrogen output and of the activity of some hepatic enzymes in the rat during adaptation from one level of dietary protein to another. The enzymes measured were arginase, argininosuccinate lyase, argininosuccinate synthetase, glutamate dehydrogenase, and alanine and aspartate aminotransferases.[172]

When the dietary protein content was reduced from 135 to 45 g casein/kg, the urinary N output and the activities of the hepatic enzymes reached their new steady-state levels in 30 hours. The reverse adaptation, from 45 to 135 g casein/kg, was also complete in 30 hours. The rate of change of enzyme activity and the final activity as percentage of initial activity were very similar for all six enzymes, suggesting a common control mechanism. There was no simple relationship between the activity of the urea cycle enzymes and the amount of N excreted. When an equal amount of gelatin was substituted for casein, the N output was doubled but there was no change in the activity of the liver enzymes. The authors concluded that the results suggest that the activity of the urea cycle enzymes depends in part on the amount of N available for excretion after the demands for synthesis have been met. The enzymes, however, appear to be present in excess so that an increased N load was not necessarily accompanied by an increase in enzyme activity.

K. LOW-CARBOHYDRATE, HIGH-PROTEIN DIETS AND ENERGY METABOLISM

The macronutrient mix of low-carbohydrate diets takes the body along energy metabolic pathways that differ from the more traditional higher carbohydrate diets. Following a low-carb diet shifts the body energy metabolism to the use of more fat and protein, both as immediate substrates and for the formation of ketones (in the case of both fats and amino acids) and glucose (in the case of amino acids). This shift changes the dynamics of energy metabolism to the extent where dietary carbohydrates no longer make up an important energy substrate. Instead, fat oxidation is increased, glycogen spared, and amino acids are used to provide carbon skeletons for gluconeogenesis, which in turn is used to supply baseline glucose and glycogen levels, which are used for glycolysis as needed.

Two pivotal enzymes in energy metabolism are pyruvate dehydrogenase (PDH), which decarboxylates pyruvate to form the two carbon unit acetyl CoA, and pyruvate carboxylase (PC) that carboxylates pyruvate to form oxaloacetate. Both enzymes are intimately involved in carbohydrate oxidation and help to control the degree of involvement of fatty acids and amino acids in energy metabolism. With low dietary carbs PDH is downregulated so that less pyruvate is converted to acetyl CoA, and subsequently the formation of acetyl CoA from fatty acid oxidation increases proportionally. At the same time, because glucose cannot be formed from fat (except for the case of odd chain fatty acids where the remaining 3 carbon units can enter the TCA cycle and be used for gluconeogenesis) more amino acid carbon skeletons are involved in the formation of glucose, pyruvate, and TCA cycle intermediates.

1. Metabolic Advantage of a High Protein, Low-carbohydrate Diet

The metabolic advantage in low-carbohydrate diets — greater weight loss than isocaloric diets of different composition.

a. Dietary Calories from Macronutrients

It is widely held that a calorie is a calorie and by this it is usually meant that two isocaloric diets lead to the same weight loss. A calorie is a measure of heat energy and when food is being referenced, it represents the total amount of energy stored in food. Used in this way, all calories are equal, whether from fat, protein, or carbohydrates. However, the idea that a dietary calorie is a calorie as far as how it influences useable and storable energy, body weight, and composition under all conditions is simplistic at best.

Many factors influence how much energy is actually derived from dietary macronutrient intake. Calories can be "wasted" in many ways. Decreased absorption from the GI tract and increased excretion are two obvious ways. An increase in thermogenesis and energy expenditure will also waste calories. In the case of thermogenesis (thermic effect of feeding), or the heat generated in processing food, the thermic effect of nutrients is approximately 2–3% for lipids, 6–8% for carbohydrates, and 25–30% for proteins.[173] This in itself is almost enough to explain the metabolic advantage of low-carb, high-protein diets. But there's more involved. For example it has been shown that increasing dietary protein increases fat oxidation. As well, the calorie cost in the use of the various macronutrients for energy also differs, with protein being the least efficient.

Through the interaction of both cytoplasmic and mitochondrial pathways it is possible to store both carbohydrates and protein as body fat. In the case of protein, it involves both the glucogenic and ketogenic amino acids. The ketogenic influence on body fat is obvious, since ketones are readily metabolized to two carbon units and can be directly used for lipogenesis. The glucogenic amino acids can enter the TCA cycle as intermediates and either through a short or long pathway end up as 2 carbon units that can be exported to the cytoplasm for lipogenesis.

Low-carbohydrate and higher-protein diets do more than increase weight loss. It's also been shown that low-carbohydrate, high-protein diets favorably affect body mass and composition[174] and that these changes are independent of energy intake.[175]

But this is nothing new. Prior research also found that a low-carbohydrate diet results in a significant fat loss and an increased retention of muscle mass, either alone or in comparison with a high-carbohydrate diet.

For example, in 1971 a group of researchers looked at the effects of three diets that had the same calorie and protein levels, but varying fat and carbohydrate content.[176] They found that, as the carbohydrates in the diets went down, there was an increased weight and fat loss. In other words, the men who were on the lower-carbohydrate diets lost the most weight and body fat.

In 1998, another study, this time involving obese teenagers, came up with similar results.[177] After 8 weeks on a low-carbohydrate diet, the teens not only lost significant amounts of weight and body fat, but even managed to increase their lean body mass.

In the study, a 6-week carbohydrate-restricted diet resulted in a favorable response in body composition (decreased fat mass and increased lean body mass) in normal-weight men. The results of this study indicate that a low-carbohydrate diet mobilizes and burns up body fat more than a high-carbohydrate diet, while at the same time preserving muscle mass.

Insulin, by varying the amount of fat and carbohydrate storage, can also make the body more efficient in the use of dietary calories. For example, decreased insulin levels, increased insulin sensitivity and even lack of an insulin receptor in fat tissue leads to increases in energy expenditure and helps to protect against obesity even in obesiogenic environments.[178]

Calories from different macronutrient mixes can affect appetite, satiety, compliance, short- and long-term compensatory responses, and changes in the oxidation of other substrates and thus make a difference as far as weight loss and body composition are concerned. For example, one study found that fat mass status and the macronutrient composition of an acute dietary intake influence substrate oxidation rates.[179] This study found that the intake of a high-protein, lower-carbohydrate single meal improved postprandial lipid oxidation in obese women and produced an increased thermic response. These responses were due to elevated insulin levels that occurs with higher-carbohydrate meals as well as the increased energy needs associated with the higher-protein meal.

The enhanced weight loss on protein-enriched diets as compared with balanced diets has been often assigned to a greater food-derived thermogenesis, an effect generally attributed to the metabolic costs of peptide-bond synthesis and breakdown, urogenesis, and gluconeogenesis.[180]

2. Low-Carbohydrate Controversy

There has been much controversy about both the effectiveness and safety of lower-carbohydrate diets. New studies from leading institutions including Duke and Harvard Universities have shown that low-carbohydrate diets are safe, healthy, lead to more permanent fat and weight loss, and have shown improvements in the dieters' blood lipid and cholesterol levels.

Several studies have shown that low-carbohydrate diets are more effective for weight and fat loss than the high-carbohydrate diets. The results of a study published in 2002 showed that the long-term use of a low-carbohydrate diet resulted in increased weight and fat loss, and a dramatic improvement in the lipid profile (decreased cholesterol, triglycerides and LDL, and increased HDL levels).[181]

Two studies published in 2003 in the *New England Journal of Medicine* found that people on the high-protein, high-fat, low-carbohydrate diet lost twice as much weight over 6 months as those on the standard low-fat diet recommended by most major health organizations.[182,183] In both studies, the low-carbohydrate dieters generally had better levels of "good" cholesterol and triglycerides, or fats in the blood. There was no difference in "bad" cholesterol or blood pressure.

The 132 men and women in the study conducted by the Veterans Affairs Department[182] started out weighing an average of 286 pounds. After 6 months, those on the low-carbohydrate diet had lost an average of 12.8 pounds (5.7 kg); those on the low-fat diet 4.2 pounds (1.8 kg).

The other study involved 63 participants who weighed an average of 217 pounds (98.4 kg) at the start. After 6 months, the low-carbohydrate group lost 15.4 pounds (7 kg), the group on the standard diet 7 pounds (3.2 kg). In a follow-up to this study, the authors found that after 1 year there were several favorable metabolic responses to the low-carbohydrate diet.[184]

Another scientific study published in the same year compared the effects of a low-carbohydrate diet with a low-fat control diet on weight loss and commonly studied cardiovascular risk factors.[185] In this study, healthy obese women on the low-carbohydrate diet lost 8.5 kg, more than twice the amount of weight lost by women on the control diet, over a 6-month period. Loss of fat mass was also significantly greater in the low-carbohydrate group.

In a follow-up study the authors concluded that short-term weight loss is greater in obese women on a low-carbohydrate diet than in those on a low-fat diet even when reported food intake is similar.[186] The authors did not find an explanation for these results since there were no measurable changes between the dieters.

Another study published in 2004 found that not only was weight loss greater but serum triglyceride levels decreased more and high-density lipoprotein cholesterol level increased more with the low-carbohydrate diet than with the low-fat diet.[187]

In the latest study, researchers from the Harvard School of Public Health, after analyzing data collected over 20 years from more than 82,000 women participating in the Nurses' Health Study, concluded that low-carbohydrate diets do not seem be linked to a higher risk of heart disease in women.[188]

VI. CONCLUSIONS AND RECOMMENDATIONS

Both endurance and power athletes need more protein than the RDAs to maximize body composition and performance. How much more is still under debate, as is the upper tolerable level. From the available research, and from my clinical and personal experience, athletes will benefit by taking in a minimum of twice the present RDA for protein, and for those wishing to gain significant muscle mass, up to four times the RDAs.

The contribution that protein makes to energy metabolism depends on several variables, including the state of the organism, the energy and macronutrient content of the diet, and level of physical activity. For those following a low-carbohydrate diet or on an energy-restricted diet, it is important to keep dietary protein levels relatively high as this will increase weight loss as well as help minimize the loss of muscle mass and increase the loss of body fat.

In my view, the contribution protein makes to energy metabolism, including both the complete oxidation of the carbon skeletons, directly or indirectly by the various transformations (gluconeogenesis and glycolytic-TCA cycle interactions) is underappreciated.

Obviously, more research needs to be done in humans in several areas including determining:

- The amount of protein carbon that actually contributes to energy metabolism both at rest and during exercise
- The adaptive responses to acute and chronic increased dietary protein intake
- The response to protein intake when taken alone and with other macro and micronutrients

- The response to dose and timing of protein intake during the day, and in and around training
- Tolerable upper intake levels both for proteins as a whole and for individual amino acids
- If and how the high intake of protein from whole foods presents any risks, including investigating "rabbit starvation" where the primary food eaten is lean meat
- If and how the use of protein (both high- and low-quality) and amino acid supplements presents any risks, including the effects of fast (for example individual amino acids, hydrolysates, and whey protein) and slow proteins (for example casein) on protein dynamics (oxidation, gluconeogenesis, ammonia excretion, etc.) in the body.
- The effects of exercise on substrate utilization and the roles of various energy depots (liver glycogen, muscle glycogen, adipose triacylglycerol, intramuscular triacylglycerol) in exercise and recovery.
- The effects of high-protein diets, with or without restrictions on the other two macronutrients, on health, body composition, and athletic performance.
- Alternating a low-carb, high-protein phase, with a higher-carb phase (phase shift diet) will result in increased performance for both strength and endurance athletes secondary to an improvement in protein and energy metabolism and also to the increased availability of both intramyocellular lipids and glycogen
- The effects of specific amino acids on energy metabolism, for example, their anaplerotic usefulness and subsequently their effects on both aerobic and anaerobic energy systems, including their contribution to and their effects on carbohydrate and fat metabolism.
- The mechanisms by which acute and chronic physical activity alter substrate utilization and subsequently affect athletic performance and body composition.

REFERENCES

1. Guyton, A.C. and Hall, J.E., *Textbook of Medical Physiology*, 9th ed., W.B. Saunders Co., Amsterdam, The Netherlands, 1996, 877.
2. Lieb, C., The effect on human beings of a twelve month exclusive meat diet, *JAMA*, 93, 20–22, 1929.
3. Pitkanen, H.T., Nykanen, T., Knuutinen, J., Lahti, K., Keinanen, O., Alen, M., Komi, P.V., and Mero, A.A., Free amino acid pool and muscle protein balance after resistance exercise, *Med. Sci. Sports Exerc.*, 35(5), 784–792, 2003.
4. Tomé, D. and Bos, C., Dietary protein and nitrogen utilization, *J. Nutr.*, 130, 1868S–1873S, 2000.
5. Pacy, P.J., Price, G.M., Halliday, D., Quevedo, M.R., and Millward, D.J., Nitrogen homeostasis in man: The diurnal responses of protein synthesis and degradation and amino acid oxidation to diets with increasing protein intakes. *Clin. Sci.* (Lond.), 86, 103–116, 1994.

6. Luiking, Y.C., Deutz, N.E., Jakel, M., and Soeters, P.B., Casein and soy protein meals differentially affect whole-body and splanchnic protein metabolism in healthy humans, *J. Nutr.*, 135(5),1080–1087, 2005.

7. Elliot, T.A., Cree, M.G, Sanford, A.P., Wolfe, R.R., and Tipton, K.D., Milk ingestion stimulates net muscle protein synthesis following resistance exercise, *Med. Sci. Sports Exerc.*, 38(4), 667–674, 2006.

8. Phillips, S.M., Hartman, J.W., and Wilkinson, S.B., Dietary protein to support anabolism with resistance exercise in young men, *J. Am. Coll. Nutr.*, 24(2), 134S–139S, 2005.

9. Elliot, T.A., Cree, M.G., Sanford, A.P., Wolfe, R.R., and Tipton, K.D, Milk ingestion stimulates net muscle protein synthesis following resistance exercise. *Med. Sci Sports Exerc.*, 38(4), 667–674, 2006.

10. Fouillet, H., Gaudichon, C., Mariotti, F., Bos, C., Huneau ,J.F., and Tome, D., Energy nutrients modulate the splanchnic sequestration of dietary nitrogen in humans: A compartmental analysis, *Am. J. Physiol. Endocrinol. Metab.*, 281(2), E248–E260, 2001.

11. Dangin, M., Boirie, Y., Garcia-Rodenas, C., Gachon, P., Fauquant, J., Callier, P., Ballevre, O., and Beaufrere, B., The digestion rate of protein is an independent regulating factor of postprandial protein retention, *Am. J. Physiol. Endocrinol. Metab.*, 280, E340–E348, 2001.

12. Dangin, M., Boirie, Y., Guillet, C., and Beaufrere, B., Influence of the protein digestion rate on protein turnover in young and elderly subjects, *J. Nutr.*, 132(10), 3228S–3233S, 2002.

13. Boirie, Y., Dangin, M., Gachon, P., Vasson, M.P., Maubois, J.L., and Beaufrere, B., Slow and fast dietary proteins differently modulate postprandial protein accretion, *Proc. Natl. Acad. Sci. USA*, 94, 14930–14935, 1997.

14. Todd, K.S., Butterfield, G.E., and Calloway, D.H., Nitrogen balance in men with adequate and deficient energy intake at three levels of work, *J. Nutr.*, 114, 2107–2118, 1984.

15. Bowtell, J.L., Leese, G.P., Smith, K., Watt, P.W. Nevill, A., Rooyackers, O., Wagenmakers, A.J.M., and Rennie, M.J., Modulation of whole body protein metabolism, during and after exercise, by variation of dietary protein, *J. Appl. Physiol.*, 85, 1744–1752, 1998.

16. Friedman, J.E. and Lemon, P.W., Effect of chronic endurance exercise on retention of dietary protein, *Int. J .Sports Med.*, 10, 118–123, 1989.

17. Pannemans, D.L., Halliday ,D., Westerterp, K.R., and Kester, A.D., Effect of variable protein intake on Whole body protein turnover in young men and women, *Am. J. Clin. Nutr.*, 61, 69–74, 1995.

18. Gaine, P.C., Pikosky, M.A., Martin, W.F., Bolster, D.R., Maresh ,C.M., and Rodriguez, N.R., Level of dietary protein impacts whole body protein turnover in trained males at rest, *Metabolism*, 55(4), 501–507, 2006.

19. Mahe, S., Roos, N., Benamouzig, R., Davin, L., Luengo, C., Gagnon, L., Gausserges, N., Rautureau, J., and Tome, D., Gastrojejunal kinetics and the digestion of [15N]ß-lactoglobulin and casein in humans: The influence of the nature and quantity of the protein, *Am. J. Clin. Nutr.*, 63, 546–552, 1996.

20. Fouillet, H., Bos, C., Gaudichon, C., and Tome, D., Approaches to quantifying protein metabolism in response to nutrient ingestion, *J. Nutr.*, 132, 3208S–3218S, 2002.

21. Dangin, M., Boirie, Y., Guillet, C., and Beaufrere, B., Influence of protein digestion rate on protein turnover in young and elderly subjects, *J. Nutr.*, 132, 3228S–3233S, 2002.

22. Jungas, R.L., Halperin, M.L., and Brosnan, J.T., Qualitative analysis of amino acid oxidation and related gluconeogenesis in humans, *Physiol. Rev.*, 72, 419–448, 1992.

23. National Research Council, *Recommended Dietary Allowances*, 10th ed., National Academy of Sciences, Washington, DC, 1989.
24. Zello, G.A., Related Dietary Reference Intakes for the macronutrients and energy: Considerations for physical activity, *Appl. Physiol. Nutr. Metab.*, 31(1), 74–79, 2006.
25. Barr, S.I., Applications of Dietary Reference Intakes in dietary assessment and planning, *Appl. Physiol. Nutr. Metab.*, 31(1), 66–73, 2006.
26. Barr, S.I., Introduction to dietary reference intakes, *Appl. Physiol. Nutr. Metab.*, 31(1), 61–65, 2006.
27. Institute of Medicine, National Academy of Sciences, *Dietary Reference Intakes for Energy, Carbohydrate, Fiber, Fat, Fatty Acids, Cholesterol, Protein, and Amino Acids (Macronutrients)*, National Academy Press, Washington, DC, 2002.
28. Whiting, S.J., Symposium overview. Dietary Reference Intakes: Considerations for physical activity, *Appl. Physiol. Nutr. Metab.*, 31(1), 59–60, 2006.
29. Health and Welfare Canada, *Nutrition Recommendations. The Report of the Scientific Review Committee*, Canadian Government Publishing Center, Ottawa, Canada, 1990.
30. von Liebig, J., *Animal Chemistry or Organic Chemistry and Its Application to Physicology and Pathology* (translated by Gregory, W.), Taylor and Walton, London, 1842, 144.
31. Fick, A. and Wislicenus, J., On the origin of muscular power, *Phil. Mag.J. Sci.*, 41, 485–503, 1866.
32. Cathcart, E.P., Influence of muscle work on protein metabolism, *Physiol. Rev.*, 5, 225–243, 1925.
33. Astrand, P.O. and Rodahl, K., *Textbook of Work Physiology*, 3rd ed., McGraw-Hill Book Co, New York, 1986.
34. Lemon, P.W.R., Do athletes need more dietary protein and amino acids?, *Int. J. Sport. Nutr.*, 5, S39–S61, 1995.
35. Kleiner, S.M., Bazzarre, T.L., and Ainsworth, B.E., Nutritional status of nationally ranked elite bodybuilders, *Int. J. Sport Nutr.*, 4(1), 54–69, 1994.
36. Darden, E., Protein, *Nautilus magazine*, 3(1), 12–17, 1981.
37. Dohm, G.L., Protein nutrition for the athlete, *Clin. Sports Med.*, 3(3), 595–604, 1984.
38. Lemon, P.W., Maximizing performance with nutrition: Protein and exercise: update 1987, *Med. Sci. Sports Exerc.*, 19(5), S179–S190, 1987.
39. Burke, L.M. and Read, R.S., Sports nutrition: Approaching the nineties, *Sports Med.*, 8(2), 80–100, 1989.
40. Lemon, P.W., Protein requirements of soccer, *J. Sports Sci.*, 12, S17–S22, 1994.
41. Lemon, P.W., Do athletes need more dietary protein and amino acids?, *Int. J. Sports Med.*, 5, S39–S61, 1995.
42. Phillips, S.M., Atkinson, S.A., Tarnopolsky, M.A., and MacDougall, J.D. Gender differences in leucine kinetics and nitrogen balance in endurance athletes, *J. Appl. Physiol.*, 75, 2134–2141, 1993.
43. Gaine, P.C., Pikosky, M.A., Martin, W.F., Bolster, D.R., Maresh, C.M., and Rodriguez, N.R., Level of dietary protein impacts whole body protein turnover in trained males at rest, *Metabolism*, 55(4), 501–507, 2006.
44. Butterfield, G.E., Whole body protein utilization in humans, *Med. Sci. Sports Exerc.*, 19, S157–S165, 1987.
45. Piatti, P.M., Monti, L.D., and Magni, F., Hypocaloric high-protein diet improves glucose oxidation and spares lean body mass: Comparison to hypocaloric high-carbohydrate diet, *Metabolism*, 43, 1481–1487, 1994.
46. Fern, E.B., Bielinski, R.N., and Schutz, Y., Effects of exaggerated amino acid and protein supply in man, *Experientia*, 47(2), 168–172, 1991.

47. Bigard, A.X., Satabin, P., Lavier, P., Bigard, A.X., Satabin, P., and Lavier, P., Effects of protein supplementation during prolonged exercise at moderate altitude on performance and plasma amino acid pattern, *Eur. J. Appl. Physiol. Occup. Physiol.*, 66(1), 5–10, 1993.

48. Phillips, S.M., Protein requirements and supplementation in strength sports, *Nutrition*, 20(7–8), 689–695, 2004.

49. Volek, J.S., Forsythe, C.E., and Kraemer, W.J., Nutritional aspects of women strength athletes, *Br. J. Sports Med.*, 40(9):742–8, 2006.

50. Tarnopolsky, M., Protein requirements for endurance athletes, *Nutrition*, 20(7–8), 662–668, 2004.

51. Henriksson, J., Effect of exercise on amino acid concentrations in skeletal muscle and plasma, *J. Exp. Biol.*, 160, 149–165, 1991.

52. Dohm, G.L., Tapscott, E.B., and Kasperek, G.J., Protein degradation during endurance exercise and recovery, *Med. Sci. Sports Exerc.*, 19(5), S166–S171, 1987.

53. Millward, D.J., Bates, P.C., and Brown, J.G., Role of thyroid, insulin and corticosteroid hormones in the physiological regulation of proteolysis in muscle, *Prog. Clin. Biol. Res.*, 180, 531–542, 1985.

54. Lemon, P.W., Protein requirements of soccer, *J. Sports Sci.*, 12, S17–22, 1994.

55. Manz, F., Remer, T., Decher-Spliethoff, E., Hohler, M., Kersting, M., Kunz, C., and Lausen, B., Effects of a high protein intake on renal acid excretion in bodybuilders, *Zeit. Ernahrungswiss.*, 34(1), 10–15, 1995.

56. Sterck, J.G., Ritskes-Hoitinga,J., and Beynen, A.C., Inhibitory effect of high protein intake on nephrocalcinogenesis in female rats, *Br. J. Nutr.*, 67(2), 223–233, 1992.

57. Bilsborough, S. and Mann, N., A review of issues of dietary protein intake in humans, *Int. J .Sport Nutr. Exerc. Metab.*, 16(2), 129–152, 2006.

58. Wolfe, B.M. and Giovannetti, P.M., Short-term effects of substituting protein for carbohydrate in the diets of moderately hypercholesterolemic human subjects, *Metabolism: Clin.Exper.*, 40(4), 338–43, 1991.

59. Wolfe, B.M. and Giovannetti, P.M., High-protein diet complements resin therapy of familial hypercholesterolemia, *Clin Invest. Med.*, 15(4), 349–59, 1992.

60. Wolfe, B.M. and Piche, L.A., Replacement of carbohydrate by protein in a conventional-fat diet reduces cholesterol and triglyceride concentrations in healthy normolipidemic subjects, *Clin. Invest. Med.*, 22(4), 140–148, 1999.

61. Hodgson, J.M., Burke, V., Beilin, L.J., and Puddey, I.B., Partial substitution of carbohydrate intake with protein intake from lean red meat lowers blood pressure in hypertensive persons, *Am. J. Clin. Nutr.*, 83(4), 780–787, 2006.

62. He, J., Gu, D., Wu, X., Chen, J., Duan, X., Chen, J., and Whelton, P.K., Effect of soybean protein on blood pressure: A randomized, controlled trial, *Ann. Int. Med.*, 143(1), 1–9, 2005.

63. Hunnisett, A.G., Kars, A., Howard, J.M.H., and Davies, S., Changes in plasma amino acids during conditioning therapy prior to bone marrow transplantation: Their relevance to antioxidant status, *Amino Acids*, 4(1–2), 177–185, 1993.

64. Soon Cho, E., Krause, G.F., and Anderson, H.L., Effects of dietary histidine and arginine on plasma amino acid and urea concentrations of men fed a low nitrogen diet, *J. Nutr*, 107(11), 2078–2089, 1977.

65. Laidlaw, S.A. and Kopple, J.D., Newer concepts of the indispensable amino acids, *Am. J. Clin. Nutr.*, 46(4), 593–605, 1987.

66. Harper, A.E. and Yoshimura, N.N., Protein quality, amino acid balance, utilization, and evaluation of diets containing amino acids as therapeutic agents, *Nutrition*, 9(5):460–469, 1993.

67. Kihlberg, R., Bark, S., and Hallberg, D., An oral amino acid loading test before and after intestinal bypass operation for morbid obesity, *Acta Chir. Scand.*, 148(1), 73–86, 1982.

68. Furst, P. and Stehle, P., What are the essential elements needed for the determination of amino acid requirements in humans?, *J. Nutr.*, 134, 1558S–1565S, 2004.

69. Pencharz, P.B. and Azcue, M., Use of bioelectrical impedance analysis (BIA) measurements in the clinical management of malnutrition, *Am. J. Clin. Nutr.*, 64, S485–S488, 1996.

70. Katagiri, M. and Nakamura, M., Animals are dependent on preformed alpha-amino nitrogen as an essential nutrient, *IUBMB Life*, 53(2), 125–129, 2002.

71. Katagiri, M. and Nakamura, M., Reappraisal of the 20th-century version of amino acid metabolism, *Biochem. Biophys. Res. Comm.*, 312(1):205–208, 2003.

72. Rennie, M.J., Edwards, R.H., Krywawych, S., Davies ,C.T., Halliday, D., Waterlow, J.C., and Millward, D.J., Effect of exercise on protein turnover in man, *Clin. Sci.*, 61(5), 627–639, 1981.

73. Lowell, B.B., Ruderman, N.B., and Goodman, M.N., Regulation of myofibrillar protein degradation in rat skeletal muscle during brief and prolonged starvation, *Metabolism*, 35, 1121–1127, 1986.

74. Li, J.B. and Goldberg, A.L., Effects of food deprivation on protein synthesis and degradation in rat skeletal muscle, *Am. J. Physiol.*, 246, E32–E37, 1984.

75. Dohm, G.L., Tapscott, E.B., Barakat, H.A., and Kasperek, G.J., Measurement of *in vivo* protein synthesis in rats during an exercise bout, *Biochem. Med.*, 27, 367–372, 1982.

76. Dohm, G.L., Williams, R.T., and Kasperek, G.J., Increased excretion of urea and N tau-methylhistidine by rats and humans after a bout of exercise, *J. Appl. Physiol.*, 52(1), 27–33, 1982.

77. Millward, D.J., Davies, C.T., Halliday, D., Wolman,S.L., Matthews, D., and Rennie, M., Effect of exercise on protein metabolism in humans as explored with stable isotopes, *Fed. Proc.*, 41(10), 2686–2691, 1982.

78. Wolfe, R.R., Wolfe, M.H., Nadel, E.R., and Shaw, J.H.F., Isotopic determinations of amino acid–urea interactions in exercise, *J. Appl. Physiol.*, 56, 221–229, 1984.

79. Wolfe, R.R., Goodenough, R.D., Wolfe, M.H., Royle, G.T., and Nadel, E.R., Isotopic analysis of leucine and urea metabolism in exercising humans, *J. Appl. Physiol.*, 52, 458–466, 1982.

80. Devlin, J.T., Brodsky, I., Scrimgeour, A., Fuller, S., and Bier, D.M., Amino acid metabolism after intense exercise, *Am. J. Physiol.*, 258(2 Pt 1), E249–255, 1990.

81. Layman, D.K., Paul, G.L. and Olken, M.H., Amino Acid Metabolism during Exercise, in *Nutrition in Exercise and Sport*, Wolinsky, I. and Hickson, J.F. Jr., Eds., CRC Press, Boca Raton, FL, 1994, 127.

82. Flakoll, P.J., Judy, T., Flinn, K., Carr, C., and Flinn, S., Postexercise protein supplementation improves health and muscle soreness during basic military training in Marine recruits, *J. Appl. Physiol.*, 96(3), 943–950, 2004.

83. Levenhagen, D.K., Carr, C., Carlson, M.G., Maron, D.J., Borel, M.J., and Flakoll, P.J., Postexercise protein intake enhances whole-body and leg protein accretion in humans, *Med .Sci. Sports Exerc.*, 34(5), 828–837, 2002.

84. Esmarck, B., Andersen, J.L., Olsen, S., Richter, E.A., Mizuno, M., and Kjaer, M., Timing of postexercise protein intake is important for muscle hypertrophy with resistance training in elderly humans, *J. Physiol.*, 15(8), Pt 1, 301–311, 2001.

85. Levenhagen, D.K., Gresham, J.D., Carlson, M.G., Maron, D.J., Borel, M.J., and Flakoll, P.J., Postexercise nutrient intake timing in humans is critical to recovery of leg glucose and protein homeostasis, *Am. J. Physiol. Endocrinol. Metab.*, 280(6), E982–E993, 2001.

86. Willoughby, D.S., Stout ,J.R., and Wilborn, C.D., Effects of resistance training and protein plus amino acid supplementation on muscle anabolism, mass, and strength, *Amino Acids*, Sep 20, 2006 [Epub ahead of print].

87. Bird, S.P., Tarpenning, K.M., and Marino, F.E., Liquid carbohydrate/essential amino acid ingestion during a short-term bout of resistance exercise suppresses myofibrillar protein degradation, *Metabolism*, 55(5), 570–577, 2006.

88. Tipton, K.D., Elliott, T.A., Cree, M.G., Aarsland, A.A., Sanford, A.P., and Wolfe, R.R., Stimulation of net muscle protein synthesis by whey protein ingestion before and after exercise, *Am. J. Physiol. Endocrinol. Metab.*, Aug 8, 2006 [Epub ahead of print].

89. Layman, D.K., Paul, G.L., and Olken, M.H., Amino Acid Metabolism during Exercise, in *Nutrition in Exercise and Sport*, Wolinsky, I. and Hickson, J.F. Jr., Eds., CRC Press, Boca Raton, FL, 1994, 127.

90. Gautsch, T.A., Anthony, J.C., Kimball, S.R., Paul, G.L., Layman, D.K., and Jefferson, L.S., Availability of eIF-4E regulates skeletal muscle protein synthesis during recovery from exercise, *Am. J. Physiol.*, 274, C406–C414, 1998.

91. Williamson, D.L., Kubica, N., Kimball, S.R., and Jefferson, L.S., Exercise-induced alterations in extracellular signal-regulated kinase 1/2 and mammalian target of rapamycin (mTOR) signalling to regulatory mechanisms of mRNA translation in mouse muscle, *J. Physiol.*, 573(6) Pt 2, 497–510, 2006.

92. Atherton, P.J. and Rennie, M.J., Protein synthesis a low priority for exercising muscle, *J. Physiol.*, 573(6) Pt 2, 288–289, 2006.

93. Morgan, H.E., Earl, D.C.N., Broadus, A., Wolpert, E.B., Giger, K.E., and Jefferson, L.S., Regulation of protein synthesis in heart muscle: I. Effect of amino acid levels on protein synthesis, *J. Biol. Chem.*, 246, 2152–2162, 1971.

94. Hardie, D.G. and Hawley, S.A., AMP-activated protein kinase: the energy charge hypothesis revisited, *BioEssays*, 23,1112–1119, 2001.

95. Bolster, D.R., Crozier, S.J., Kimball, S.R., and Jefferson, L.S., AMP-activated protein kinase suppresses protein synthesis in rat skeletal muscle through a down-regulated mammalian target of rapamycin (mTOR) signaling, *J. Biol. Chem.*, 277, 23977–23980, 2002.

96. Meley, D., Bauvy, C., Houben-Weerts, J.H., Dubbelhuis, P.F., Helmond, M.T., Codogno, P., and Meijer, A.J., AMP-activated protein kinase and the regulation of autophagic proteolysis, *J. Biol. Chem.*, September 21, 2006 [Epub ahead of print].

97. Dreyer, H.C., Fujita, S., Cadenas, J.G., Chinkes, D.L., Volpi, E., and Rasmussen, B.B., Resistance exercise increases AMPK activity and reduces 4E-BP1 phosphorylation and protein synthesis in human skeletal muscle, *J. Physiol.*, 576(10) Pt 2, 613–624, 2006.

98. Noma, T., Dynamics of nucleotide metabolism as a supporter of life phenomena, *J. Med. Invest.*, 52(3–4):127–136, 2005.

99. Valero, E., Varon, R., and Garcia-Carmona, F., A kinetic study of a ternary cycle between adenine nucleotides, *FEBS J.*, 273(15), 3598–3613, 2006.

100. Lambeth, D.O., Reconsideration of the significance of substrate-level phosphorylation in the citric acid cycle, *Biochem. Educ.*, 34, 21–29, 2006.

101. Hochachka, P.W., Owen, T.G., Allen, J.F., and Whittow, G.C., Multiple end products of anaerobiosis in diving vertebrates, *Comp. Biochem. Physiol. Biochem. Mol. Biol.*, 50, 17–22, 1975.

102. Weinberg, J.M., Venkatachalam, M.A., Roeser, N.F., Saikumar, P., Dong, Z., Senter, R.A., and Nissim, I., Anaerobic and aerobic pathways for salvage of proximal tubules from hypoxia-induced mitochondrial injury, *Am. J. Physiol. Renal Physiol.*, 279, F927–F943, 2000.

103. Penney, D.G. and Cascarno, J., Anaerobic rat heart: Effects of glucose and tricarboxylic acid-cycle metabolites on metabolism and physiological performance, *Biochem. J.*, 118, 221–227, 1970.

104. Gronow, G.H.J. and Cohen, J.J., Substrate support for renal functions during hypoxia in the perfused rat kidney, *Am. J. Physiol. Renal Fluid Electrolyte Physiol.*, 247, F618–F631, 1984.

105. Weinberg, J.M., Venkatachalam, M.A., Roeser, N.F. and Nissim, I., Mitochondrial dysfunction during hypoxia/reoxygenation and its correction by anaerobic metabolism of citric acid cycle intermediates, *Proc. Natl. Acad. Sci. USA*, 97, 2826–2831, 2000.

106. Hochachka, P.W. and Dressendorfer, R.H., Succinate accumulation in man during exercise, *Eur. J. Appl. Physiol.*, 35, 235–242, 1976.

107. Degoutte, F., Jouanel, P., and Filaire, E., Energy demands during a judo match and recovery, *Br. J. Sports Med.*, 37(3), 245–249, 2003.

108. Piatti, P.M., Monti, L.D., Pacchioni, M., Pontiroli, A.E., and Pozza, G., Forearm insulin- and non-insulin-mediated glucose uptake and muscle metabolism in man: role of free fatty acids and blood glucose levels, *Metabolism*, 40(9), 926–933, 1991.

109. Felig, P., Wahren, J., Sherwin, R. and Palaiologos, G., Amino acid and protein metabolism in diabetes mellitus, *Arch. Internal Med.*, 137(4), 507–513, 1977.

110. Favier, R.J., Koubi, H.E., Mayet, M.H., Sempore, B., Simi, B., and Flandrois, R., Effects of gluconeogenic precursor flux alterations on glycogen resynthesis after prolonged exercise, *J. Appl. Physiol.*, 63(5), 1733–1738, 1987.

111. Azzout, B., Bois-Joyeux, B., Chanez, M., and Peret, J., Development of gluconeogenesis from various precursors in isolated rat hepatocytes during starvation or after feeding a high protein, carbohydrate-free diet, *J. Nutr.*, 117(1), 164–169, 1987.

112. Jahoor, F., Peters, E.J., and Wolfe, R.R., The relationship between gluconeogenic substrate supply and glucose production in humans, *Am. J. Physiol.*, 258(2) Pt 1, E288–E896, 1990.

113. Amiel, S.A., Archibald, H.R., Chusney, G., Williams, A.J., and Gale, E.A., Ketone infusion lowers hormonal responses to hypoglycaemia: evidence for acute cerebral utilization of a non-glucose fuel, *Clin. Sci.*, 81(2), 189–194, 1991.

114. Cori, C.F., Mammalian carbohydrate metabolism, *Physiol. Rev.*, 11, 143–275, 1931.

115. Reichard, G.A. Jr., Moury, F.N. Jr., Hochella, N.J., Patterson, A.L., and Weinhouse, S., Quantitative estimation of the Cori cycle in the human, *J. Biol. Chem.*, 238, 495–501, 1963.

116. Gerich, J.E., Control of glycaemia, *Baillieres Clin. Endocrinol. Metab.*, 7(3), 551–586, 1993.

117. Chevalier, S., Burgess, S.C., Malloy, C.R., Gougeon, R., Marliss, E.B., and Morais, J.A., The greater contribution of gluconeogenesis to glucose production in obesity is related to increased whole-body protein catabolism, *Diabetes*, 55(3), 675–681, 2006.

118. Harber, M.P., Schenk, S., Barkan, A.L., and Horowitz ,J.F., Alterations in carbohydrate metabolism in response to short-term dietary carbohydrate restriction, *Am. J. Physiol. Endocrinol. Metab.*, 289(2), E306–E312, 2005.

119. Jungas, R.L., Halperin, M.L., and Brosnan, J.T., Quantitative analysis of amino acid oxidation and related gluconeogenesis in humans, *Physiol. Rev.*, 72(2), 419–448, 1992.

120. Nurjhan, N., Bucci, A., Perriello, G., Stumvoll, M., Dailey, G., Bier, D.M., Toft, I., Jenssen, T.G., and Gerich, J.E., Glutamine: A major gluconeogenic precursor and vehicle for interorgan carbon transport in man, *J. Clin. Invest.*, 95(1), 272–277, 1995.

121. Bisschop, P.H., Pereira Arias, A.M., Ackermans, M.T., Endert, E., Pijl, H., Kuipers, F., Meijer, A.J., Sauerwein, H.P., and Romijn, J.A., The effects of carbohydrate variation in isocaloric diets on glycogenolysis and gluconeogenesis in healthy men, *J. Clin. Endocrinol. Metab.*, 85(5), 1963–1967, 2000.

122. Roden, M., Stingl, H., Chandramouli, V., Schumann, W.C., Hofer, A., Landau, B.R., Nowotny, P., Waldhausl, W., and Shulman, G.I., Effects of free fatty acid elevation on postabsorptive endogenous glucose production and gluconeogenesis in humans, *Diabetes*, 49(5), 701–707, 2000.

123. Kaloyianni, M. and Freedland, R.A., Contribution of several amino acids and lactate to gluconeogenesis in hepatocytes isolated from rats fed various diets, *J. Nutr.*, 120(1), 116–122, 1990.

124. Widhalm, K., Zwiauer, K., Hayde, M., and Roth, E., Plasma concentrations of free amino acids during 3 weeks treatment of massively obese children with a very low calorie diet, *Eur. J. Pediatr.*, 149(1), 43–47, 1989.

125. Pozefsky, T., Tancredi, R.G., Moxley, R.T., Dupre, J., and Tobin, J.D., Effects of brief starvation on muscle amino acid metabolism in nonobese man, *J. Clin. Invest.*, 57(2), 444–449, 1976.

126. Fery, F., Bourdoux, P., Christophe, J., and Balasse, E.O., Hormonal and metabolic changes induced by an isocaloric isoproteinic ketogenic diet in healthy subjects, *Diabete et Metabolisme*, 8(4), 299–305, 1982.

127. Cynober, L., Amino acid metabolism in thermal burns, *J. Parenter. Enteral Nutr.*, 13(2), 196–205, 1989.

128. Lemon, P.W. and Nagle, F.J., Effects of exercise on protein and amino acid metabolism, *Med. Sci. Sports Exerc.*, 13(3), 141–149, 1981.

129. Rothman, D.L., Magnusson, I., Katz, L.D., Shulman, R.G., and Shulman, G.I., Quantitation of hepatic glycogenolysis and gluconeogenesis in fasting humans with ^{13}C NMR, *Science*, 254:573–576, 1991.

130. Katz, J. and Tayek, J.A., Gluconeogenesis and the Cori cycle in 12-, 20-, and 40-h-fasted humans, *Am. J. Physiol. Endocrinol. Metab.*, 275(3), E537–542, 1998.

131. Boden, G., Chen, X., and Stein, T.P., Gluconeogenesis in moderately and severely hyperglycemic patients with type 2 diabetes mellitus, *Am. J. Physiol. Endocrinol. Metab.*, 280, E23–E30, 2001.

132. Chevalier, S., Burgess, S.C., Malloy, C.R., Gougeon, R., Marliss, E.B., and Morais, J,A., The greater contribution of gluconeogenesis to glucose production in obesity is related to increased whole-body protein catabolism, *Diabetes*, 55(3), 675–681, 2006.

133. Wang, X., Hu, Z., Hu, J., Du, J., and Mitch, W.E., Insulin resistance accelerates muscle protein degradation: Activation of the ubiquitin-proteasome pathway by defects in muscle cell signaling, *Endocrinology*, 147(9), 4160–4168, 2006.

134. Floyd, J., Fayans, S., Conn, J., Knopf, R., and Rull, J., Stimulation of insulin secretion by amino acids, *J. Clin. Invest.*, 45, 1487–1502, 1966.

135. Ohneda, A., Parada, E., Eisentraut, A., and Unger, R., Characterization of response of circulating glucagon to intraduodenal and intravenous administration of amino acids, *J. Clin. Invest.*, 47, 2305–2322, 1968.

136. Adkins, A., Basu, R., Persson, M., Dicke, B., Shah, P., Vella, A., Schwenk, W.F., and Rizza, R., Higher insulin concentrations are required to suppress gluconeogenesis than glycogenolysis in nondiabetic humans, *Diabetes*, 52, 2213–2220, 2003.

137. Krebs, M., Brehm, A., Krssak, M., Anderwald, C., Bernroider, E., Nowotny, P., Roth, E., Chandramouli, V., Landau, B.R., Waldhausl, W., and Roden, M., Direct and indirect effects of amino acids on hepatic glucose metabolism in humans, *Diabetologia*, 46(7), 917–925, 2003.

138. Jungas, R.L., Halperin, M.L., and Brosnan, J.T., Quantitative analysis of amino acid oxidation and related gluconeogenesis in humans, *Physiol. Rev.*, 72(2), 419–448, 1992.

139. Pisarenko, O.I., Solomatina, E.S., and Studneva, I.M., Formation of the intermediate products of the tricarboxylic acid cycle and ammonia from free amino acids in anoxic heart muscle, *Biokhimiia*, 51(8), 1276–1285, 1986.

140. Wiesner, R.J., Ruegg, J.C., and Grieshaber, M.K., The anaerobic heart: succinate formation and mechanical performance of cat papillary muscle, *Exper. Biol.*, 45(1), 55–64, 1986.

141. Camici, P., Marraccini, P., Lorenzoni, R., Ferrannini, E., Buzzigoli, G., Marzilli, M., and L'Abbate, A., Metabolic markers of stress-induced myocardial ischemia, *Circulation*, 83(5 Suppl), 1118–1113, 1991.

142. Hutson, S.M., Wallin, R., and Hall, T.R., Identification of mitochondrial branched chain aminotransferase and its isoforms in rat tissues, *J. Biol. Chem.*, 267(22), 15681–15686, 1992.

143. Fisher, A.G. and Jensen, C.R., *Scientific Basis of Athletic Conditioning*, Lea & Febiger, Philadelphia, 1991.

144. Kuhn, E., The effect of work load on amino acid metabolism, *Czech. Vnitrni Lekarstvi*, 40(7), 411–115, 1994.

145. Brown, J.A., Gore, D.C., and Jahoor, F., Catabolic hormones alone fail to reproduce the stress-induced efflux of amino acids, *Arch. Surg.*, 129(8), 819–824, 1994.

146. Brown, J., Gore, D.C., and Lee, R., Dichloroacetate inhibits peripheral efflux of pyruvate and alanine during hormonally simulated catabolic stress, *J. Surg. Res.*, 54(6), 592–596, 1993.

147. Carlin, J.I., Olson, E.B. Jr., Peters, H.A., and Reddan, W.G., The effects of post-exercise glucose and alanine ingestion on plasma carnitine and ketosis in humans, *J. Physiol.*, 390, 295–303, 1987.

148. Newsholme, E.A., Crabtree, B., and Ardawi, M.S., The role of high rates of glycolysis and glutamine utilization in rapidly dividing cells, *Biosci. Rep.*, 5(5), 393–400, 1985.

149. Felig, P., The glucose-alanine cycle, *Metabolism*, 22, 179–207, 1973.

150. Ahlborg, G., Hagenfeldt, L., and Wahren, J., Substrate turnover during prolonged exercise in man, *J. Clin. Invest.*, 53, 1080–1090, 1974.

151. Lemon, P.W.R. and Mullin, J.P., Effect of initial muscle glycogen levels on protein catabolism during exercise, *J. Appl. Physiol.*, 48, 624–629, 1980.

152. Lemon, P.W. and Nagle, F.J., Effects of exercise on protein and amino acid metabolism, *Med. Sci. Sports Exerc.*, 13(3), 141–149, 1981.

153. Brooks, G.A., Amino acid and protein metabolism during exercise and recovery, *Med. Sci. Sports Exerc.*, 19(5 Suppl), S150–S156, 1987.

154. Wolfe, R.R., Jahoor, F., Herndon, D.N., and Miyoshi, H., Isotopic evaluation of the metabolism of pyruvate and related substrates in normal adult volunteers and severely burned children: Effect of dichloroacetate and glucose infusion, *Surgery*, 110(1), 54–67, 1991.

155. Sewell, D.A. and Harris, R.C., Adenine nucleotide degradation in the thoroughbred horse with increasing exercise duration, *Eur. J. Appl. Physiol. Occup. Physiol.*, 65(3), 271–277, 1992.

156. Sewell, D.A., Gleeson, M., and Blannin, A.K., Hyperammonaemia in relation to high-intensity exercise duration in man, *Eu.r J. Appl. Physiol. Occup. Physiol.*, 69(4), 350–354, 1994.

157. Sahlin, B.S., Adenine nucleotide depletion in human muscle during exercise: causality and significance of AMP deamination, *Int. J. Sports Med.*, 11 Suppl 2, S62–S67, 1990.

158. van Hall, G., van der Vusse, G.J., Soderlund, K., and Wagenmakers, A.J., Deamination of amino acids as a source for ammonia production in human skeletal muscle during prolonged exercise, *J. Physiol.*, 489(Pt 1), 251–261, 1995.

159. Graham, T.E. and MacLean, D.A., Ammonia and amino acid metabolism in human skeletal muscle during exercise, *Can. J. Physiol. Pharmacol.*, 70(1), 132–141, 1992.

160. Wagenmakers, A.J., Beckers, E.J., Brouns, F., Kuipers, H., Soeters, P.B., van der Vusse, G.J., and Saris, W.H., Carbohydrate supplementation, glycogen depletion, and amino acid metabolism during exercise, *Am. J. Physiol.*, 260(6 Pt 1), E883–E890, 1991.

161. MacLean, D.A., Graham, T.E., and Saltin, B., Branched-chain amino acids augment ammonia metabolism while attenuating protein breakdown during exercise, *Am. J. Physiol.*, 267, E1010–E1022, 1994.

162. Colombo, J.P., Cervantes, H., Kokorovic, M., Pfister, U., and Perritaz, R., Effect of different protein diets on the distribution of amino acids in plasma, liver and brain in the rat, *Ann. Nutr. Metab.*, 36, 23–33, 1992.

163. Remesy, C., Morand, C., Demigne, C., and Fafournoux, P., Control of hepatic utilization of glutamine by transport processes or cellular metabolism in rats fed a high-protein diet, *J. Nutr.*, 118, 569–578, 1988.

164. Morens, C., Gaudichon, C., Fromentin, G., Marsset-Baglieri, A., Bensaid, A., Larue-Achagiotis, C., Luengo, C., and Tome, D., Daily delivery of dietary nitrogen to the periphery is stable in rats adapted to increased protein intake, *Am. J. Physiol. Endocrinol. Metab.*, 281, E826–E836, 2001.

165. Morens, C., Gaudichon, C., Meteges, C., Fromentin, G., Baglieri, A., Even, P.C., Huneau, J., and Tome, D., A high-protein meal exceeds anabolic and catabolic capacities in rats adapted to a normal protein diet, *J. Nutr.*, 130, 2312–2321, 2000.

166. Phillips, R.J. and Powley, T.L., Gastric volume rather than nutrients content inhibits food intake, *Am. J. Physiol.*, 271, R766–R769, 1996.

167. Speth, J.D. and Spielmann, K.A., Energy source, protein metabolism, and hunter-gatherer subsistence strategies, *J. Anthropol. Archaeol.*, 2, 1–31, 1983.

168. Rudman, D., DiFulco, T.J., Galambos, J.T., Smith, R.B., Salam, A.A., and Warren, W.D., Maximal rates of excretion and synthesis of urea in normal and cirrhotic subjects, *J. Clin. Invest.*, 52:2241–2249, 1973.

169. Schimke, R.T., The importance of both synthesis and degradation in the control of arginase levels in rat liver, *J. Biol. Chem.*, 239:3808–3817, 1964.

170. Das, T.K. and Waterlow, J.C., The rate of adaptation of urea cycle enzymes, aminotransferases and glutamic dehydrogenase to changes in dietary protein intake, *Br. J. Nutr.*, 32, 353–373, 1974.

171. Jequier, E., Pathways to obesity, *Int. J. Obes. Relat. Metab. Disord.*, 26 Suppl 2, S12–S17, 2002.

172. Volek, J.S., Sharman, M.J., Love, D.M., Avery, N.G., Gomez, A.L., Scheett, T.P., and Kraemer, W.J., Body composition and hormonal responses to a carbohydrate-restricted diet, *Metabolism*, 1(7), 864–870, 2002.

173. Krieger, J.W., Sitren, H.S., Daniels, M.J., and Langkamp-Henken, B., Effects of variation in protein and carbohydrate intake on body mass and composition during energy restriction: A meta-regression, *Am. J. Clin. Nutr.*, 83, 260–274, 2006.

174. Young, C.M., Scanlan, S.S., Im, H.S., and Lutwak, L., Effect on body composition and other parameters in obese young men of carbohydrate level of reduction diet, *Am. J. Clin. Nutr.*, 24, 290–296, 1971.

175. Willi, S.M., Oexmann, M.J., Wright, N.M., Collop, N.A., and Key, L.L. Jr., The effects of a high-protein, low-fat, ketogenic diet on adolescents with morbid obesity: Body composition, blood chemistries, and sleep abnormalities, *Pediatr.*, 101, 61–67, 1998.

176. Manninen, A.H., Metabolic advantage of low-carbohydrate diets: A calorie is still not a calorie, *Am. J. Clin. Nutr.*, 83(6), 1442 – 1443, 2006.

177. Labayen, I., Diez, N., Parra, D., Gonzalez, A., and Martinez, J.A., Basal and postprandial substrate oxidation rates in obese women receiving two test meals with different protein content, *Clin. Nutr.*, 23(4), 571–578, 2004.

178. Volpi, E., Lucidi, P., Cruciani, G., Monacchia, F., Reboldi, G., Brunetti, P., Bolli, G.B., and De Feo, P., Contribution of amino acids and insulin to protein anabolism during meal absorption, *Diabetes*, 45, 1245–1252, 1996.

179. Westman, E.C., Yancy, W.S., Edman, J.S., Tomlin, K.F., and Perkins, C.E., Effect of 6-month adherence to a very low carbohydrate diet program, *Am. J. Med.*, 113(1), 30–36, 2002.

180. Foster, G.D., Wyatt, H.R., Hill, J.O., McGuckin, B.G., Brill, C., Mohammed, B.S., Phillippe, O., Rader, D.J., Edman, J.S., and Klein, S., A randomized trial of a low-carbohydrate diet for obesity, *NEJM*, 348(21), 2082–2090, 2003.

181. Samaha, F.F., Iqbal, N., Seshadri, P., Chicano, K.L., Daily, D.A., McGrory, J., Williams, T., Williams, M., Gracely, E.J., and Stern, L., A low-carbohydrate as compared with a low-fat diet in severe obesity, *N. Engl. J. Med.*, 348 (21), 2074–2081, 2003.

182. Stern, L., Iqbal, N., Seshadri, P., Chicano, K.L., Daily, D.A., McGrory, J., Williams, M., Gracely, E.J., and Samaha, F.F., The effects of low-carbohydrate versus conventional weight loss diets in severely obese adults: One-year follow-up of a randomized trial, *Ann. Intern. Med.*, 140(10), 778–785, 2004.

183. Brehm, B.J., Seeley, R.J., Daniels, S.R., and D'Alessio, D.A., A randomized trial comparing a very low carbohydrate diet and a calorie-restricted low fat diet on body weight and cardiovascular risk factors in healthy women, *J. Clin. Endocrinol. Metab.*, 88, 1617–1623, 2003.

184. Brehm, B.J., Spang, S.E., Lattin, B.L., Seeley, R.J., Daniels, S.R., and D'Alessio, D.A., The role of energy expenditure in the differential weight loss in obese women on low-fat and low-carbohydrate diets, *J. Clin. Endocrinol. Metab.*, 90(3), 1475–1482, 2005.

185. Yancy, W.S. Jr., Olsen, M.K., Guyton, J.R., Bakst, R.P., and Westman, E.C., A low-carbohydrate, ketogenic diet versus a low-fat diet to treat obesity and hyperlipidemia: a randomized, controlled trial, *Ann. Intern. Med.*, 140(10), 769–777, 2004.

186. Halton, T.L., Willett, W.C., Liu, S., Manson, J.E., Albert, C.M., Rexrode, K., and Hu, F.B., Low-carbohydrate-diet score and the risk of coronary heart disease in women, *N. Engl. J.Med.*, 355, 1991–2002, 2006.

187. Lemon, P.W. and Proctor, D.N., Protein intake and athletic performance, *Sports Med.*, 12(5), 313–325, 1991.

188. Wagenmakers, A.J., Amino acid metabolism, muscular fatigue and muscle wasting: Speculations on adaptations at high altitude, *Intern. J. Sports Med.*, 13 Suppl 1, S110–113, 1992.

Section 2

Estimation of Energy Requirements

5 Energy Expenditure of Athletes

Robert G. McMurray and Kristin S. Ondrak

CONTENTS

I. INTRODUCTION

The measurement of metabolic rate can provide important information to athletes concerning their innate abilities and training programs. This is particularly true for high-caliber endurance athletes, but is also true for the everyday fitness enthusiast, since knowledge of metabolism also has health implications. Typically, athletes are interested in four factors. First, they want to know their maximal metabolic rate, an indicator of the body's maximal ability to consume oxygen. Maximal metabolic rate is also referred to as aerobic power or maximal oxygen uptake (VO_{2max}). A higher VO_{2max} means that the athlete can sustain a higher level of work without fatigue. Second, athletes want to know their anaerobic thresholds (AT), or the level of metabolic rate at which there is a rapid rise in lactate concentration. Athletes with high ATs can sustain a higher level of exertion before fatigue ensues. Third, athletes are interested in their economy of motion. Improved economy of motion is related to the mechanics of the activity, be it swim stroke, running stride, or paddling stroke. Highly successful athletes are usually very economical in their use of energy. Fourth, some athletes are interested in their resting metabolic rate, because this knowledge can assist with their weight-loss or -gain programs.

This chapter will explore the issues of the measurement of metabolic rate as they relate to the athlete. The chapter starts with an introduction to the units used to define metabolic rate, followed by a discussion of the varying techniques to measure metabolic rate and their use for athletes. Information on sports-specific means of measuring metabolic rate is presented followed by a more in-depth examination of the four metabolic factors of interest to athletes. Finally, the chapter will conclude with some commentary on estimating of overall energy expenditure for athletes.

The terms metabolic rate and energy expenditure are used synonymously through the literature on metabolism. In the English system of measurement, the basic unit of energy for humans is the *kilocalorie* (kcal). This is the amount of heat required to increase one kilogram of water one degree Celsius. The scientific community, however, has placed considerable emphasis on the use of the *kiloJoule* (kJ) or mega-joule (mJ) over the kcal (S.I. Unit: le Système International d'Unités).[1] Conversion between units is simple: one kcal = 4.184 kJ or 0.00418 mJ. Measuring calories or joules is difficult in humans and requires extremely expensive equipment. Thus, oxygen uptake (VO_2) is more commonly measured and converted to kcal, knowing that there are approximately 4.7–5.1 kcal per liter of oxygen, and then finally to kJ.

II. METHODS FOR THE MEASUREMENT OF METABOLIC RATE

The energy output of humans can be measured using *direct* and *indirect* calorimetry, as well as doubly labeled water.[2-4] The advantages, disadvantages, and uses of the methods are the foci of what follows.

A. Direct Calorimetry

Direct calorimetry assesses heat production, typically requiring a small room with highly insulated walls.[2,4,5] The walls of the unit contain a series of pipes through which water is pumped at a constant rate. The heat generated by the subject is measured by the difference between the incoming and outgoing water temperatures, knowing the volume of water and rate of the water flow. Oxygen is continuously supplied to the subject and carbon dioxide is removed by chemical absorbent. Direct calorimeters range from suit calorimeters, like those used by astronauts, to small chambers and even larger rooms. Using direct calorimetry to measure metabolic rate takes considerable time, as it takes a minimum of 30 minutes to equilibrate heat loss and heat production.[4] The method is highly accurate, but is limited only to resting measures, those activities that have minimal range of movement, or overall energy use for extended periods of time (2–24 hours). The methods will not work for most sports or activities, in varying environments, or in large-scale population studies. Also, most organizations do not have the expensive, complicated facilities and equipment needed to use this method.

B. Indirect Calorimetry

Indirect calorimetry relies on the measurement of VO_2 and is good for measuring metabolic rate over short periods of time for specific activities. The underlying principle for indirect calorimetry is that oxygen is needed for the production of energy and the measurable end-product of metabolism is carbon dioxide production.[2-4] Oxygen uptake and CO_2 production are computed via mathematical computations, knowing the volume of air expired and inspired and expired oxygen and carbon dioxide content of that air (Table 5.1). This method is based on some assumptions.[2] First, the individual is not in a starvation state and proteins make up only a very small portion of the energy and can therefore be ignored. Second, the contribution of anaerobic metabolism to the energy production is quite small. Finally, when using a combination of carbohydrates, fats, and proteins as the source of energy, approximately 4.82 kcal (20 kJ) of energy is liberated per liter of oxygen used.[5]

TABLE 5.1
Computational Model for Oxygen Uptake[4]

V_E (STPD) = (273°C /(273°C + T_V°C)) × ((BP–WVT)/760)

$V_I = V_E \times ((1 - F_E O_2 - F_E CO_2)/0.7904))$

$VO_2 = (V_I \times F_I O_2) - (V_E \times F_E O_2)$

$VCO_2 = (V_E \times F_E CO_2) - (V_I \times F_I CO_2)$

RER = VCO_2/VO_2

RER on chart will give kcal/L oxygen (as well as percent carbohydrates & fats)[12]

kcal/min = (kcal/L O_2) × VO_2 (L/min)

kJ/min = (kcal/min) × 4.184 kJ/kcal

T_V°C: temperature of the expired air volume

BP: barometric pressure

WVT: water vapor tension for the expired (47 mmHg) air at T_V°C

F_I: fraction of inspired gas expressed as a decimal (O_2 = 0.2093 & CO_2 = 0.003)

F_E: fraction of expired gas (O_2 & CO_2) obtained from the gas meters

RER: respiratory exchange ratio

For convenience, the 4.82 kcal/L O_2 has been rounded to 5 kcal or 21 kJ per liter of oxygen. Indirect methods are less expensive, smaller, and more portable than direct calorimetry. Since good agreement (<1% difference) exists between direct and indirect calorimetry and the advantages of indirect calorimetry are considerable, the use of indirect calorimetry is attractive.[4-6] There are actually two general indirect calorimetry methods. One employs a *closed circuit system* while the other uses an *open circuit system.* Both appear to be equally as valid; however, the open circuit system has proven to be more beneficial for activities involving movement.

1. Closed Circuit Spirometry

The closed circuit system of indirect calorimetry uses a spirometer, which is an air-tight cylinder filled with 100% oxygen, and also a separate carbon dioxide absorbent, which is used to remove exhaled CO_2.[7] Since oxygen is assimilated by the body and any CO_2 produced is removed from the spirometer, the volume of gas in the spirometer reduces as the person breathes through the system (Figure 5.1). The difference between the initial and the final volumes of the spirometer is the oxygen uptake. The oxygen uptake is then multiplied by 5 kcal/L to obtain the energy use. There are some problems inherent with this system.[8] The system must be air-tight so volume changes are related only to oxygen uptake. The person must remain on the mouthpiece for the entire test, since any room air entering the system invalidates the test results. The CO_2 absorbent must be adequate or the CO_2 production will simply replace the oxygen uptake and reduce the measured oxygen uptake. The problem with the CO_2 absorbent may be particularly true at high metabolic rates, as it may not be able to keep pace with the respiratory CO_2 output. Inadequate CO_2 absorbent will also increase respiration and reduce any exercise performance. Temperature of the gas affects the volume in the spirometer and since expired air is at a higher temperature than inspired air, metabolic rate could be underestimated. Finally, the spirometer must have the capacity to hold a large volume of oxygen for exercise measures. For example, a person completing a 30-minute exercise session may use 40–90 liters of oxygen. This requires a very large spirometer. Finally, this method does not allow for the determination of the source of the energy, e.g., fats and carbohydrates. These limitations, coupled with the cumbersome size of the equipment and the proximity the subject has to be to the equipment, limits the use of closed-circuit spirometry for exercise studies.

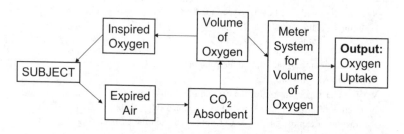

FIGURE 5.1 Schematic of the closed circuit system for measuring energy expenditure.

2. Open Circuit Spirometry

The open-circuit system of indirect calorimetry does not permit subjects to re-breathe their own purified air (Figure 5.2). Instead, subjects inhale room air and exhale their expired gases back into the ambient air. During the exhalation process the gases travel through a system that measures the volume of air and the expired O_2 and CO_2 content of that air.[2-4] The difference between inspired and expired volumes of O_2 is the VO_2.

Variations of open-circuit systems include: (1) a bag system, (2) computerized system, and (3) a portable system.[5] In all three, the subject breathes through a mask or breathing valve that forces the expired air to be directed through into a large balloon, or through a tube and the O_2 and CO_2 is determined using gas analyzers. To measure total air volumes, all three types contain an instrument, either a turbine, pneumotach, or gas meter. The bag system collects the volume of expired air in a large meteorological balloon or a standard rubberized Douglas Bag.[4] The contents of the bag are measured for gas volume and concentrations (%) of O_2 and CO_2.

Values for gas volume and expired air are used to calculate oxygen uptake (Table 5.1). The gas volume is first corrected for temperature and water vapor (V_E and STPD). STPD corrects the volume *from* the ambient conditions *to* 0°C, 760 mmHg (1 atmosphere), and 0% relative humidity (water vapor tension). This correction factor is used so that the measurements obtained on Mt. Everest can be compared with measurements obtained at, or below, sea level. The inspired gas volume is then computed from the expired volume (V_E STPD) and the expired oxygen F_EO_2 and carbon dioxide F_ECO_2 concentration using the Haldane conversion.[5] All these values are inserted into the formulas and VO_2 and carbon dioxide production (VCO_2) are computed. A computerized system uses a similar metering system (F_EO_2, F_ECO_2, and ventilation), but takes an electrical signal from the meters and computes the VO_2.[4] The computerized system has the advantage of using instruments with much faster response times, so that VO_2 can be computed on a breath-by-breath basis. In contrast, the Douglas Bag system usually measures VO_2 in larger increments (30 seconds up to 10 minutes) and cannot measure breath-by-breath.

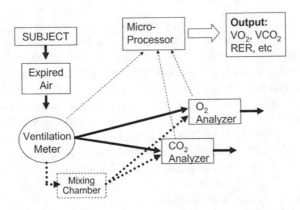

FIGURE 5.2 Schematic for the Open Circuit system for measuring breath-by-breath energy expenditure (bold arrows) and minute-by-minute averaging (dotted line).

Modern technology and microprocessors have resulted in miniaturizing the computerized systems to the point that entire metabolic systems weigh less than 1 kilogram and can be worn on the back or abdomen; thus giving the athlete freedom of movement. These lightweight systems, usually less than 3% of an adult's or adolescent's weight, do not dramatically influence energy expenditure. Thus, they provide a fairly accurate representation of the energy expenditure. Portable metabolic/VO_2 systems have provided a wealth of information on the energy expenditures of physical activities and improved our understanding of athletes in action.[9–17] These breath-by-breath metabolic systems also measure heart rates, making them ideal for endurance athletes attempting to determine their anaerobic thresholds and for estimating the intensities of their workouts. Many of these systems also contain a telemetry system, so that realtime data can be obtained during workouts or competitions. The systems can be set up inside a track and obtain the information with the athlete running unencumbered at his/her own pace, or set up in a car to measure metabolic rates of a cyclist pedaling on the roads. The major drawback of these systems is the high cost (~$30,000 US).

Closed circuit systems use a standard energy equivalent regardless of the source of the energy (carbohydrates or fats). In reality, fats use more O_2 to produce energy than carbohydrates: 213 mLO_2/kcal vs. 198 mLO_2/kcal.[18,19] In addition, fats produce more CO_2 than carbohydrates. Thus, knowing the amount of VCO_2 with respect to VO_2 gives an indication of the specific source of the energy, whether fats or carbohydrates. All open-circuit methods for computing energy expenditure rely on this axiom. The ratio of VCO_2 to VO_2 uptake is called the *respiratory exchange ratio* (RER), respiratory quotient (RQ), or simply the R value.[2–4] Knowing the RER, one can consult standard tables and determine the non-protein energy production per liter of O_2 and insert that value into the equations to determine energy expenditure (Table 5.1).[19]

The RER does not take protein metabolism for energy into consideration; therefore, it is sometimes referred to as the non-protein RER.[2,4] The RER for carbohydrate is 1.0 and the reaction can be summarized by the following equation:

$$C_6H_{12}O_6 + 6O_2 \rightarrow 6CO_2 + 6\ H_2O + \text{energy}.$$

Thus, the oxidation of a single glucose molecule to produce energy requires six O_2 molecules and produces six CO_2 molecules, or a ratio of 6/6 (CO_2/O_2) or 1.0. Conversely, the oxidation of fatty acids results in an RER of ~0.70. For example, 1 molecule of palmitic acid, a typical fatty acid used for energy, requires 23 O_2 molecules and produces 16 CO_2 molecules (16/23 = 0.696). Therefore, as the composition of the energy-producing substrate changes from fat to glucose the RER changes from 0.7 to 1.0. An individual consuming a 50/50 mixture of carbohydrates and fats has an RER of 0.85. The RER relates to kcal production per liter of oxygen.[18,19] Carbohydrates produce 5.047 kcal/liter (21 kJ/L) of oxygen uptake, while fats produce only 4.686 kcal/liter (19.6 kJ/L) of VO_2. So an athlete using 100 liters of oxygen for an activity and a 50/50 mixture of carbohydrates and fats will utilize approximately 486 kcal (2036 kJ) of energy:

$$(50\ LO_2 \times 4.686\ \text{kcal/L}) + (50\ LO_2 \times 5.047\ \text{kcal/L}).$$

Using open-circuit spirometry to measure energy expenditure requires that the person reach a steady state, because the VCO_2 and VO_2 represent only substrate utilization during this time. During steady-state exercise, the VCO_2 is usually less than the VO_2, so the RER is always ≤ 1.0. However, any activity that produces considerable lactic acid (H^+) will increase VCO_2 disproportionate to the oxygen uptake ($H^+ + HCO_3^- \rightarrow H_2O + CO_2$).[2-4] Therefore, open-circuit spirometry cannot be used to measure energy expenditure during high-intensity anaerobic activities or in activities that are of insufficient duration to obtain steady state. Also, some individuals who are uncomfortable with the equipment or perceive the exercise testing as stressful tend to hyperventilate; which increases CO_2 output but does not influence O_2 uptake. In these situations, RER would not be a true representation of substrate utilization. These are the major limitations of indirect calorimetry.

The VO_2 computed from the standard formulas is expressed in units of liters per minute (L/min). This is considered the *absolute* VO_2, which is the measure used to obtain overall energy expenditure. Individuals with large muscle masses have larger absolute VO_2s than individuals with smaller muscle masses. That is because muscle mass is the major metabolically active tissue. Oxygen uptake can also be expressed taking into consideration body mass: milliliters of O_2 per kilogram body weight per minute (mL/kg/min). This is considered the *relative* VO_2. The unit of mL/kg/min is commonly used when trying to compare individuals of differing sizes.

Decades ago D.B. Dill proposed a system of expressing energy expenditure in increments of resting metabolic rate.[20] This proposal has taken root and is the origin of the metabolic equivalent or the *MET*. Research has suggested, but never verified, that an oxygen uptake of 3.5 mL/kg/min or 1 kcal/kg/hr is one MET.[5,21] The MET is commonly used in clinical exercise testing or epidemiological research. Because of the imprecise nature of the MET, its use to represent metabolic rate of athletes is not recommended.

C. Doubly Labeled Water

The calorimetry methods described thus far have limitations. Some methods restrict movements and would not be useful for exercise. Others methods are useful for relatively short periods of time (minutes) or are stationary, thus limiting their utility for athletics. None of the methods can measure energy expenditure during anaerobic exercise (very high intensities), because such activities cannot attain steady-state and CO_2 output can exceed VO_2, producing RER greater than 1.0. To overcome these problems, a technique using doubly labeled water has been developed.[22-25] Doubly labeled water is an isotope that has both the hydrogen and oxygen elements "tagged"; $^2H_2{}^{18}O$. The hydrogen and some of the oxygen ions from the doubly labeled water are eliminated as part of the water molecule in the urine, while additional O_2 is exhaled as part of the CO_2 molecule. Since the same amount of oxygen is eliminated as water and CO_2, simply measuring the hydrogen and oxygen isotope in the body's water can be used to determine the CO_2 production.[25] Energy expenditure is then computed from daily CO_2 output and isotope turnover in the urine (high-precision mass spectrometry), knowing total body water. The overall error of this method for 5–7 days of energy expenditure is about 6%.[25] The subject simply consumes a dose of the labeled water and goes about his/her activities for a period of 5–7 days. The major problem with doubly labeled water is expense; equipment to measure the isotope and total body water and the dosages of $^2H_2^{18}O$ is very costly. Differences in the quality of the isotope exist between producers, which can also lead to errors. Although doubly labeled water is good for estimating overall energy expenditure for multiple days, it is not useful to determine energy expenditure for specific activities, for determining maximal capacity, or economy. The technique has limited use for athletes, except in cases when knowledge of energy balance is needed.

III. ENERGY DURING SPORT AND PHYSICAL ACTIVITY

A. Use of Open Circuit Technology

Energy expenditure during activity is usually measured by open-circuit spirometry. As previously mentioned, a computerized system appears to work best. Some of these systems are stationary and will work only with activities in which the participant strays little from the measurement device. Such systems have been used to measure energy cost of walking and running on treadmills, cycling on cycle ergometers, swimming using a swimming ergometer or swimming flume, rowing using a rowing ergometer, stair stepping using an escalator-type or step ergometer, or arm cranking using an arm ergometer.

The bag technique of open-circuit spirometry has been used to measure VO_2 during ergometry work, as well as during actual cycling, swimming, rope skipping, or household chores. Typically, activities are completed in a confined space. The bag method gives average responses over a period of time, usually 1–10 minutes depending upon the intensity of the activity and the size of the bag. This method is not capable of giving breath-to-breath VO_2. Since the expired air bag is connected to the subject by a breathing tube, this technique requires that the researcher move with the subject, yet not impede any subject movements. In addition, the subject usually has to wear a mouthpiece and support the breathing tube during the collection period. The weight of the breathing tubing, breathing valve, and mouthpiece can be uncomfortable for the subject or cause additional effort to support the apparatus and maintain the mouthpiece in the mouth. Finally, the bags are not totally impermeable to gas exchange. Therefore, if a bag is used for a prolonged period of time, longer than 10–15 minutes, gases may diffuse in or out, dependent upon the concentration gradient, and the results can be unreliable. Therefore, bag measurements are usually taken over periods of time lasting less than 10 minutes and the contents measured as quickly as possible at the end of the collection period. The bag method can be used successfully, but takes preparation, training, and good timing to obtain accurate data.[4,5]

The use of miniaturized portable systems has revolutionized our ability to obtain energy expenditure data during activities. The new systems are sufficiently small to be worn during activity, providing little impairment of motion and little additional weight. The systems have been used to measure energy expenditure of household chores, basketball, tennis, road cycling, and kayaking, to name a few. Some of these systems include good-sized memory or telemetry systems, which allows for obtaining real-time data without being tethered to the subject.

Although these systems have proven to be accurate, there are some minor problems. The additional weight of the apparatus, usually about 1 kg, can increase the energy cost of the activities. The impact of the additional weight on an adult is negligible, since the system's weight may only represent <2% of the body weight; however, for a child, the weight of the system can have a significant impact on the energy cost of the activity. It is also important that the systems be securely attached to the subject. If not, the system can impede motion, which will modify the energy cost. To measured expired gases, most of these systems require that the subject wear a mask, rather than the cumbersome breathing valve and mouthpiece. An improperly fitting mask can result in air leaks that can modify both the measured volume of air and the fractions of expired gases. Experience has also shown that the systems may lose their ability to function via telemetry if they are near an electric field such as a video display. Proper consideration and planning can eliminate these problems and allow the investigator to obtain accurate data.

B. USE OF HEART RATE TO ESTIMATE ENERGY EXPENDITURE

Metabolic equipment is costly, requires considerable training to use properly, and is difficult to use for many sports activities. Thus coaches, athletes, and clinicians have used indirect methods, such as heart rate monitors, to estimate energy expenditure. Heart rates have the potential to provide information on the pattern of activity as well as the energy expenditure,[26] but their use to estimate of energy expenditure requires planning and calibration. The athlete must undergo testing to determine the resting and maximal heart rates, and the heart rate/energy expenditure relationship. Usually this is accomplished by using an ergometer to establish the work, a spirometry system to measure the oxygen uptake, and a heart rate monitor. Once the relationship between the heart rate and metabolic rate are known, the athlete wears a heart rate monitor for his/her workout or competition. The heart rate information is downloaded to a computer and then averaged in 1- to 15-minute time segments. The energy expenditure during each time-segment is estimated by using the previously determined energy expenditure/heart rate relationship.

The major problem with this method is that not all changes in heart rate are related to metabolic activity.[26–28] Emotional stress and body temperature are known to affect heart rate, independent of metabolism. Therefore, some coaches and clinicians believe that heart rates below 120 cannot reliably determine energy expenditure.[28] Also, heart rate is indicative of metabolic rate only during steady-state. Thus, heart rates cannot be used to estimate energy expenditure during anaerobic activities, or activities with an isometric component in which heart rates are elevated above metabolic rate. Finally, the heart rate may not be sufficiently sensitive to respond to short-term activities.[28] Therefore, using heart rates to estimate metabolic rate has limited practicality. However, heart rate can be used to estimate minutes of moderate- to hard-intensity activities.[28]

IV. ERGOMETERS

To facilitate the measurement of metabolic rate for some sports, ergometers or specialized machines have been developed to mimic the actions of the sport. Most ergometers are designed to control the amount of effort, resistance, or speed. Some of the more sophisticated ergometers can control work and power output regardless of speeds. The four most common ergometers are cycle ergometers, rowing ergometers, treadmills, and cross country ski machines. Cycle ergometers have been used in research since the very early 1900s and have been employed for training cyclists for the past 40–50 years. Rowing ergometers, which are relatively new, were actually a development of the fitness industry. Cross-country ski machines were popular in the 1980s and 1990s and can be used as an adjunct to training competitive skiers from countries with limited winter facilities. Treadmills were first used in research settings in the 1940s and quickly were used by competitive runners for training. The problem with treadmills, cycle ergometers, and cross-country ski machines is that they eliminate air resistance. Similarly, swimming and rowing ergometers eliminate water resistance (drag forces, frontal resistance, and skin or surface friction).[29] Water resistance is considerable; therefore, the use of these ergometers may underestimate the true energy expenditure with these activities.

A. Cycle Ergometers

Several types of cycle ergometers are used for physiological testing in athletes. They provide critical information regarding anaerobic and aerobic power. There are two general designs of cycle ergometers: upright and recumbent. Upright models are used more frequently in exercise testing as they mimic the position of real cycling. Furthermore, these ergometers can be fitted with clipless pedals and competitive-style handlebars and seat to further imitate competitive cycling. Recumbent bikes, on the other hand, put the legs in a more horizontal position relative to the trunk, and therefore decrease blood pooling in the legs. Recumbent cycles also reduce the active muscle mass during pedaling, so the cyclist cannot sustain high work rates.[30] The low position of the cyclist in the recumbent cycle improves the comfort, but decreases the cyclist's maximal aerobic power.[30] Recumbent cycles are more frequently used in fitness and rehab situations than for evaluating athletes.

The workload of a cycle ergometer is controlled by the pedal rate, resistance, or type of brake placement on the flywheel. A common brake method is direct friction applied via a strap placed around the flywheel. The workload of the friction-braked design changes with alterations in pedaling rate.[31] Thus, friction cycles require knowledge of the resistance and pedal rate to determine the amount of resistance. The resistance or brakes may also be controlled electronically or electromagnetically. The advent of micro-processors and the use of these types of brakes provide a constant workload regardless of pedaling rate.

Work and power output on cycle ergometers can be expressed in different terms. Most manual-braked, friction-style ergometers apply resistance in terms of kiloponds (kp), or the amount of friction/resistance applied by a kilogram mass. The amount of work is then based on the pedal frequency, the distance theoretically traveled with each rotation of the pedals, and the kps of resistance. Therefore, if pedaling at 60 rpm with 2 kp of resistance, and the distance traveled is 6 m/revolution, the amount of work would be 720 kpm (2 kp × 60 rpm × 6 m/rev). Work on the ergometers has also been expressed in terms of Newton meters or joules, but this is less frequently used. Power, or work per unit of time, is typically expressed in watts. However, in terms of ergometry, no limitation on time is inferred.[32] Watts can be obtained from kpm by simply dividing by 6.12 w/kgm/min. So using the above example, the cyclist would be working at a power output of 118 watts (720 kgm / 6.12 w/kgm).

Oxygen uptake can also be inferred from knowing the work rate in kgm, since there is about 2 mLO$_2$/kgm.[33] For example, an adult cycling at 720 kgm would be using about 1440 mL (1.44 L) O$_2$ per minute for the exercise (2 mL/kgm $\times$ 720 kgm). That would be the VO$_2$ required for the work *only*. To obtain the gross (overall) VO$_2$, a constant for resting VO$_2$ needs to be added. That amounts to approximately 300 mL of VO$_2$ for an adult. Therefore, the total VO$_2$ for the above example would be approximately 1740 mL O$_2$ per minute.

The cycle ergometer is often used to assess anaerobic power, submaximal power and maximal aerobic power. The protocols differ according to the purpose of the test. Tests of anaerobic power are typically very short in duration, 30 seconds or less, and require all-out, supramaximal effort by the rider, using resistance based on body mass.[34] Measures of power are obtained and reported in watts. These measures are commonly classified as peak, mean, maximal, and minimum power in absolute terms, and they may also be expressed relative to one's body mass. A plot of decrements in power is often created, and is a useful measure of the rate of fatigue. On this plot, time is on the x-axis and power is on the y-axis. The slope of the line indicates the rate at which power dropped during the maximal effort.

Submaximal protocols on the cycle ergometer are often utilized to predict VO$_{2max}$. Common submaximal tests include the Astrand-Rhyming, PWC$_{170}$ and YMCA protocols.[35,36] While the stage lengths and loads differ, all submaximal protocols involve gradual increases in workload and terminate prior to the attainment of maximal aerobic power. Submaximal VO$_2$ or HR responses at each workload are entered into prediction equations or nomograms to determine predicted VO$_{2max}$. Moderate to strong correlations have been found between predicted VO$_{2max}$ from submaximal tests and VO$_{2max}$ measured via maximal testing.[35]

Protocols to assess maximal aerobic power on a cycle ergometer typically involve incremental tests with gradual increases in workload at a given pedal rate. The starting workload is selected based on the subject's body mass and fitness level. Normally, these tests last 8 to 15 minutes in duration.[31] To determine the effect of increment length, researchers compared the four exercise protocols.[37] The rate of increase for the workload (watts/stage) was the same for all protocols, however, the length of the increments differed (ramp/continuous increase, 1-, 2-, and 3-minute stages). There were no significant differences between protocols for VO$_{2max}$.[37] This suggests that when the increase in work rate is held constant, the length of the stage does not affect the physiological response to exercise. [37]

Recent developments in computers and electronics have led to the development of small flywheels that can be used with a standard bicycle. The rear wheel of the bicycle is mounted on a stand and the flywheel is attached to the rear wheel. The flywheel is electronically or manually braked, so that the resistance can be adjusted moment-by-moment. Computer programs have been developed that allow a cyclist to simulate specific competitive courses, race distances, flat courses, mountainous courses, or fitness tests, thus providing the cyclist with a "virtual environment" for training. These types of ergometers are much more interesting and fun for the competitive cyclist. Some of these ergometers also have an attachment to monitor heart rate and are capable of using that heart rate to determine the amount of resistance.

B. ROWING ERGOMETERS

Rowing ergometers are designed to mimic the actions of rowing in water while on land. They consist of four parts: a flywheel, a dampening or brake mechanism, a pulley attached to a handle, and an instrument to quantify speed and power. The flywheel spins at a rate proportional to the strength of the pull; it continues to spin and stores potential energy between pulls. The dampening mechanism is attached to the flywheel and provides friction designed to simulate the friction between the water and the boat. In a rowing ergometer, friction is normally applied to the flywheel using air, a weighted belt, or water as resistance. The pulley and handle are attached to the flywheel and are controlled by the operator, similar to oars in the water. Finally, the speed and power monitor measure the rate of flywheel turnover and the force applied to the pulley via a strain gauge.

The two major types of rowing ergometers are static and dynamic. In static ergometers, also referred to as stationary or fixed power heads, the flywheel is fixed and the rower moves his or her body back and forth via a seat sliding on a rail. In contrast, the flywheel on a dynamic ergometer, also called a floating power head, is mounted on the rail and therefore moves in unison with the rower. The latter model is thought to represent more realistic motions of rowing in water. A study comparing fixed to floating designs found that power per stroke and total work did not differ between the models, despite some biomechanical differences[38]

Regardless of the model, rowing ergometers are designed to reproduce the four major components of a rowing stroke: catch, drive, finish and recovery. While the individual performs these actions in a continuous pattern, several variables are calculated for each stroke. Two common variables of interest are power and work. Power (P) is calculated by dividing the energy (E) by time (t) taken to complete the stroke ($P = E/t$) and is expressed in watts. Work (W) is then calculated by dividing power by time ($W = P/t$), and is expressed in joules (1 watt = 1 joule/sec).[8]

Coaches and clinicians use rowing ergometers to test athletic ability and to determine the effectiveness of training.[39] Several protocols have been used to assess aerobic capacity on the rowing ergometer. Three common protocols are a continuous maximal test, a continuous incremental test, and a discontinuous incremental test. Continuous maximal tests or "all-out" tests on a rowing ergometer typically last ~6 minutes, as this time period corresponds closely to a race of 2000 meters.[39] This protocol is favored by some as it simulates true racing conditions. Similarly, the time to complete 2000 m is often measured. High test–retest correlations have been found ($r = 0.96$) for this method,[40] highlighting its reliability for monitoring progress in athletes.

A continuous incremental test, or progressive exercise test, uses gradual increases in exercise intensity until the individual can no longer continue. This allows for the identification of anaerobic threshold, VO_{2max} and examination of the intensity-related rises in cardiovascular, ventilatory, and metabolic parameters.[39]

Finally, discontinuous incremental protocols also involve gradual increases in workload until fatigue, but the individual takes short breaks between each increase. This allows for easy obtainment of blood samples during the rest periods. As a result, clinicians often measure blood lactate levels and are able to identify the lactate threshold during this protocol.

Anaerobic power is another important component of rowing performance. It is quantified on the rowing ergometer using tests of maximal effort sprints of short duration. Using a 30-second test, researchers found strong correlations (r = −0.85 to −0.89) between power (mean, maximal, and minimal) and performance on a 2000-meter rowing competition.[41] In this investigation, peak power accounted for ~76% of the variance in rowing time, demonstrating the importance of this anaerobic phase.

C. TREADMILLS

The treadmill allows the subject to walk or run at specific speeds while maintaining a central location. Thus, the subject is easily attached to the spirometry system. Although the treadmill simulates ambulation, it is not quite the same as normal walking or running. Studies have shown that there are differences in air resistance between treadmill and normal ambulation that may decrease the energy cost of ambulation on treadmill.[42,43]

Motorized treadmills are used frequently for exercise testing and training. The workload is controlled through alterations in speed or grade. Typically, treadmills can reach maximal speeds of 12 miles per hour (19 kpm) and 25% grade. When exercising on a treadmill, the athlete must support and transport his or her own body weight, which subsequently influences the workload. Thus, exercise on a treadmill has been called "weight dependent." Depending upon the model and size of the belt, treadmill can accommodate individuals weighing up to 450 pounds (>200 kg). The dimensions of treadmill belts vary; normal widths range from 16 to 22 inches, with lengths of 45 to 60 inches. These dimensions are important when selecting a treadmill to accommodate a tall person, someone with a long stride length, or an obese person. Athletes who run at high speeds appreciate the larger-sized treadmill. Also, some models have side or front handrails, which are an added safety feature. Some treadmills can measure heart rate using a sensor located on the front rail that does not require placement of a heart rate monitor on the chest. Users place their hands around the sensor for several seconds, a task that may be difficult during a run or high-velocity walk. Treadmills are often used in conjunction with a metabolic system. However, treadmills are space-consuming and difficult to transport. In addition, the sizes of the treadmills needed to accommodate athletes are costly.

D. CROSS-COUNTRY SKI ERGOMETERS

Cross-country ski ergometers are a popular mode for low-impact aerobic exercise. The user stands on two sliding components that simulate the gliding motion of cross-country skis and the alternating arm motion of poling. Arm motion is coordinated to the opposite leg using the corresponding handle and pulley mechanism. This causes the arms to move similarly to cross-country skiing. The intensity of exercise is controlled through variations in elevation and flywheel resistance providing the resistance to leg and arm motions. The resistance for the arm and leg components can be set independently, which allows for workload to be customized. Since there appears to be no standardized testing protocols using these ergometers, they seem to be used more for training than testing.

V. METABOLIC RATE DURING SWIMMING

Obtaining metabolic information during swimming is difficult, since the swimmer moves up and down the pool with flip turns and spends time underwater. Also, the use of electricity around water presents a definite risk to the swimmer. Thus, any metabolic system used in this setting must be portable. Four approaches have been used to obtain metabolic data during swimming: a stationary swimming ergometer, a swimming flume, a circular pool to avoid the problems with turns, and backward extrapolation at the end of the swim. The swimming ergometer (Figure 5.3) has been used for quite some time.[44,45] The swimmer is fitted with a belt, with wires extending back from each side of the swimmer well beyond the length of his or her legs. The wires are kept separate by a floating dowel or bar. A cable extends from that bar through a pulley at water level that redirects the cable upward and around another fixed pulley stationed above the swimmer. A weight is suspended from the free end of the cable. The concept is that the swimmer swims sufficiently hard to keep the weight suspended. More or less weight can be added or subtracted to make the swimmer work harder or easier. Since the swimmer is now fairly stationary, a breathing tube can be extended to capture expired gases, and VO_2 can be computed using a standard metabolic system stationed on the pool deck. The system works well, but it does change the body position and dynamics of the swimmer, making the person kick harder than normal to maintain alignment.

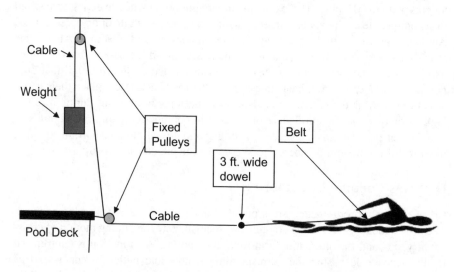

FIGURE 5.3 Schematic of the side and top view of a swimming ergometer.

The swimming flume has also been available since the early 1970s.[46] The flume recycles a current of water past the swimmer at a specific velocity and the swimmer once again tries to maintain a stationary position in the small tank. Since the swimmer is fairly stationary, metabolic measures are obtained similar to the swimming ergometer. The swim flume allows swimmers to use their natural swimming stroke in a more natural position than the swim ergometer would. However, swimming flumes are very expensive, beyond the budgets of many athletic facilities.

Circular pools have been used in which the swimmer simply swims continuously around the pool. The metabolic system is housed on a central platform inside the circular pool. An arm with a breathing tube extends to the swimmer, similar to the swim ergometer. Pace can be set by an auditory signal or by lights situated on the bottom of the pool. Like the swim ergometer, the connection of the breathing tube to the mouth changes the body position of the swimmer, except when swimming breaststroke. Also, since the swimmer is always circling, there is greater use of one side of the body than the other, so the swim stroke is not normal. These circular pools are very expensive, but have been used successfully to obtain metabolic data.[47]

Swimming usually requires the participant to traverse the length of the pool, using underwater, or flip turns at each end to change direction. Metabolic systems capable of measuring these actions are presently not available. Also, the use of any breathing apparatus during swimming changes the body position in the water and head rotation, increasing resistance and drag forces and increasing energy expenditure at a given speed. To overcome these problems, practitioners and researchers have used a backward extrapolation method.[48,49] This method uses standard open-circuit spirometry. In this method, the swimmer usually swims 200–400 meters. At the completion of the swim a stopwatch is started and as quickly as possible the breathing mask or mouthpiece from the spirometry system is placed on the face (or in the mouth). VO_2 is then measured for three 20-second periods. VO_2 can then be computed using the first 20-second measure (VO_2m) and the formula:

$$VO_2(L/min) = (0.916 \times VO_2m) + 0.426.$$

The result can be converted to kcal using the following formula:

$$kcal/min = VO_2 (L/min) \times 4.86 Kcal/L.$$

Alternatively a curve can be constructed from the three 20-second VO_2 measures and extrapolated backward to what the VO_2 would have been during the last minute of swimming.

Specificity of testing mode is important when testing in athletes. The same individual may have significantly different responses to an exercise test, depending on the apparatus on which it was conducted. The maximal aerobic power measured on a treadmill is often greater than that measured on a cycle ergometer.[50-53] During treadmill exercise, athletes transport their body mass and have a greater amount of active muscle mass compared with cycling, during which body mass is supported by the bike seat. In a comparison of treadmill and bike protocols, Faulkner et al.[51] attributed the higher treadmill VO_{2max} to a larger stroke volume and greater muscle mass in use. A comparison of cardiovascular responses during graded exercise test on a treadmill with rowing demonstrated that the HR during the treadmill test was greater than during rowing for a given lactate level, while the VO_{2max} during rowing was greater than on the treadmill.[54] The authors attributed these differences to posture and increased venous return during rowing. Finally, greater maximal aerobic power has been seen during treadmill tests than in swimming.[50] Interestingly, when trained swimmers completed a maximal test during cycling and swimming, higher values were attained during swimming.[55] Triathletes, on the other hand, had higher maximal aerobic power during the cycling test than in swimming.[55] This demonstrates the importance of considering the athlete's training when selecting the testing mode.

VI. MAXIMAL METABOLIC RATE

Maximal metabolic rate is also referred to as maximal aerobic capacity, maximal aerobic power, or VO_{2max}. VO_{2max} is dependent upon the physiologic systems, the respiratory, cardiovascular, and muscle metabolic systems, acting in consort to produce work. A problem in any of the three systems can limit VO_{2max}. For example, a person with emphysema cannot get oxygen into the blood, thus limiting oxygen availably for energy production in the muscle. A person who has had a heart attack can usually get the oxygen into the blood (respiratory system), but has the reduced capacity to pump the blood to the muscles; thus, also limiting oxygen availably for energy production in the muscle. Sedentary, untrained individuals usually have limited capacities in all three physiologic systems, which compromises VO_{2max} compared with highly trained endurance athletes.

Because VO_{2max} is commonly expressed per kilogram body weight (ml/kg/min), it can be used to compare a variety of different-sized individuals. VO_{2max} is also expressed in absolute terms (Liters/minute), but it is harder to compare individual of differing sizes, because higher absolute VO_{2max} levels can simply reflect a larger muscle mass. Generally, large individuals have higher VO_{2max} expressed in *L/min* than smaller individuals because of the muscle mass, but have lower values for VO_{2max} when expressed per kilogram body mass. For example, a football player may weigh 300 pounds (136 kg) and have 20% body fat. His VO_{2max} expressed per LO_2/min may be 5 L/min, which is extremely high. Yet when expressed per unit body mass, his VO_{2max} would only be 36.8 mL/kg/min, similar to a sedentary adult. The reason a larger individual has lower VO_{2max} when expressed per kilogram body mass, is that larger individuals have more supporting tissues (bone, tendon, adipose) that are not related to energy output. The reverse is also true; smaller individuals have lower absolute VO_{2max}, but higher relative VO_{2max} than large individuals.

To eliminate the influence of fat mass, some researchers have suggested expressing VO_{2max} per unit of fat free mass (ml/kg$_{FFM}$/min). This method has been used, for example, to evaluate the validity of true gender differences in VO_{2max}, because women are genetically endowed to have more fat mass than men.[56] In general, the higher the VO_{2max}, expressed as either mL/kg/min or ml/kg$_{FFM}$/min, the more work that can be performed aerobically. For example, a person with a VO_{2max} of 40 ml/kg/min has the capacity to run at about 7 mph, whereas an individual with the capacity of 60 ml/kg/min can run at 10.5 mph.[57] The advantage of a high VO_{2max} to an endurance athlete is obvious.

Maximal aerobic capacity is influenced by a number of factors. VO_{2max} generally declines with age. Hence, children have higher VO_{2max} per kilogram of body mass than adults, due in some part to the ration of their size to muscle mass, or the inactive lifestyle of adults having reduced physiologic mechanisms.[58] Adult men usually have greater capacities than women. The normal range for weight-adjusted VO_{2max} is about 40–45 ml/kg/min for men and 35–40 ml/kg/min for women.[59] These gender differences may be related to body composition or hemoglobin concentrations. Women have greater fat mass than men, which contributes to overall energy demands during exercise, but not to energy production. If body fat content is removed from the equation, differences between men and women are significantly reduced.[56] Circulating hemoglobin concentration of men is about 10–20% higher than women's, increasing men's ability to get oxygen to the muscle. Figure 5.4 presents estimated ranges of VO_{2max} for highly trained male athletes based on a compilation of values seen in the literature and what we have measured here at the University of North Carolina. Highly conditioned endurance athletes have aerobic powers above 55 ml/kg/min, upwards to over 80 ml/kg/min.[60] The higher aerobic capacities of these individuals may be related to genetics, which has endowed these individuals with highly developed respiratory, cardiovascular, and metabolic systems, and the plasticity of these systems to improve even more through rigorous training. Conversely, the VO_{2max} of athletes who compete in anaerobic-type sports or resistance training are usually less than endurance athletes but higher than sedentary individuals.[60]

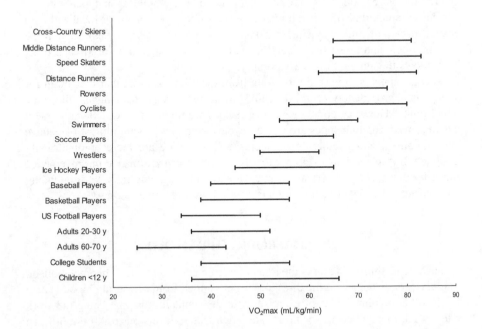

FIGURE 5.4 Maximal aerobic power (VO_{2max}) of various populations of elite athletes and normal adults. These data are for men; women usually have lower values by approximately 10 mL/kg/min.[34,52,60,100]

Interestingly, the VO_{2max} of top athletes has not increased over what was reported in 1960 but endurance performances have improved. Some changes in techniques have caused improvements in performances, but even so the lack of improvement in VO_{2max} combined with improvements in sports performance implies that training is improving other characteristics of endurance athletes such as their anaerobic threshold or economy of movement, discussed in sections 5.7 and 5.8.

Maximal oxygen uptake is usually obtained by having the person complete some form of incremental exercise protocol with progressively increasing work intensities and simultaneously measuring VO_2 by open-circuit spirometry. A variety of testing protocols are available, some of which have been described elsewhere.[34] In addition, a variety of ergometers have been utilized to obtain the work (see section 5.4). In some instances, practitioners have simply used progressive speed while running on a track or swimming in a pool to obtain the work intensities. The mode of exercise used for the test should be related to the sport of the athlete; the concept of specificity. For example, a highly trained runner who completes the maximal test on a cycle ergometer will have a lower maximal capacity than if the runner used a treadmill for the test. Likewise, a highly trained swimmer will have a lower VO_{2max} running than during a swimming protocol. Therefore, there is no optimal test protocol that should be used for all athletes. The beginning workloads/speeds should be low intensity (25–30% VO_{2max}), to serve as a warm-up. Each successive stage should be small enough to avoid lactate build-up, which will cause premature fatigue unrelated to VO_{2max}. The test should be designed to reach maximal capacity in approximately 10–15 minutes. Shorter tests may be invalid due to lactate build-up and local fatigue. Longer tests could also be invalid because the subject gets bored or localized pain ensues (back pain during cycling or from running up very steep grades). Also, if the plan is to test and retest the athlete, the same protocol should be used each time. This allows the athlete to directly compare performances.

VO_{2max} appears to have limits. Data from the 1960s suggest that the zenith for VO_{2max} is approximately 85 mL/kg/min.[60] More recent data also suggest the same upper limit.[61] However, endurance performances are improving. Athletic equipment has improved; running shoes are lighter, cycles weigh less, swimming strokes have been modified, and paddles for canoeing and kayaking are more ergometrically designed. But these changes do not totally account for performance improvements. Since levels of VO_{2max} have not increased, endurance training must be influencing other factors. Two such factors are anaerobic threshold and economy.[62–64]

VII. ANAEROBIC THRESHOLD

The anaerobic threshold marks the transition from aerobic to anaerobic metabolism. In precise terms the anaerobic threshold is determined from measuring blood lactate levels at various intensities of exercise, with the standard outcome being the work rate, speed, metabolic rate, or heart rate when lactate levels reach 4.0 mmol/L. In practical terms, the anaerobic threshold is known as the ventilatory threshold. The reason for the different terminology is that the lactate threshold is highly correlated with the ventilatory threshold, and the ventilatory threshold is easier to measure and does not require blood samples. Other than directly obtaining blood lactate levels at each progressive stage, the anaerobic threshold is identified indirectly during the progressive exercise test using one of the following methods:

1. Indirectly by a disproportionate rise in V_E relative to VO_2 or VCO_2
2. A decrease in $P_{ET}O_2$ with no change in $P_{ET}CO_2$
3. A non-linear increase in V_E/VO_2 relative to V_E/VCO_2.[65,66]

Above this threshold, the increase in anaerobic metabolism leads to the accumulation of blood lactate and fatigue. Lactate is buffered by HCO_3^-, which leads to an increase in CO_2 production and a state of metabolic acidosis due to the excess H^+ remaining. These changes are illustrated by the following two equations:

$$Lactic\ Acid + Na^+ \rightarrow NaLactate + H^+$$

$$H^+ + HCO_3^- \rightarrow H_2CO_3 \rightarrow H_2O + CO_2.$$

Both the excess H^+ and CO_2 stimulate the chemoreceptors to increase ventilation above what is needed for metabolism, with the outcome being that the CO_2 is removed by ventilation. Hence, this is the reason that VCO_2 is used as an indirect marker for lactate production.

Identification of the AT is particularly important to endurance athletes. In some instances, research has shown that the AT can increase without an increase in maximal capacity.[67,68] Thus, the endurance athlete can improve performance (speed) by exercising at a higher percentage of VO_{2max} without the deleterious effects of lactic acid. In fact, most of the literature shows that endurance athletes have anaerobic thresholds well above 75% of VO_{2max} and possibly as high as 95% of VO_{2max}.[5] In contrast, the AT of sprinters is lower 60–70% of VO_{2max} and college-aged individuals have AT about 65% of VO_{2max}.[5] The mechanisms responsible for this difference include improved lactate removal and increased mitochondria function and enzyme activity in trained individuals. These training adaptations lead to improved production of energy from aerobic sources, permitting the athlete to exercise at a higher intensity before turning to anaerobic energy sources and the concomitant increase in blood lactate levels.[66] As a result, endurance exercise performance may improve drastically. In contrast, periods of detraining result in a loss of this adaptation, as anaerobic threshold returns to baseline pre-training levels.[65] Knowing one's anaerobic threshold also has important implications for training. Training at a workload just below the anaerobic threshold allows athletes to exercise at the highest possible intensity before lactate accumulation ensues. Since fatigue during this type of training is not related to the build up of lactate, the athlete can exercise longer and receive the maximal aerobic training effect.

Several methods are used to determine anaerobic threshold. The most common is through a graded exercise test on a treadmill or cycle ergometer. During the graded exercise test, the intensity of exercise increases in predetermined intervals by gradually increasing the speed and grade on a treadmill or resistance on a cycle ergometer.

Ventilatory measurements are collected throughout the test and blood lactate measurements may be taken during each stage. The most common method is to find the point at which V_E increases disproportionately to VO_2. The simplest way to identify this point is to plot V_E and VO_2 on a graph, with workload on the x-axis and V_E/VO_2 on the y-axis. The workload that corresponds to the anaerobic threshold is the point at which the line increases in a nonlinear fashion. When blood lactate levels are obtained, a similar plot with lactate and VO_2 or heart rate can be created. The point at which blood lactate levels begin to rise in a curvilinear fashion is termed the lactate threshold or onset of blood lactate accumulation (OBLA). A threshold value of 4.0 mM/L is often identified, although this value differs from person to person. The AT has been expressed in terms of the absolute VO_2 (L/min), as the percentage of VO_{2max} at which the AT occurs (relative AT), and practically speaking, in terms of heart rate at the AT.[65,69] For athletes, the AT as related to heart rate has the most application to their training, since VO_2 is not commonly measured during a training session, but heart rates are easily attainable in all training situations.

To confirm that the correct workload was identified, a second graded exercise test is often performed. In this confirmatory test, athletes exercise for equal periods of time at intensities slightly lower than, equal to, and slightly greater than their anaerobic threshold. If the anaerobic threshold was correctly identified, the athlete's V_E/VO_2 and blood lactate will remain steady at the lower intensity, begin to rise at the intensity corresponding to the AT and rise drastically during the highest intensity. If the V_E/VO_2 and blood lactate fail to rise markedly in any of the three stages, the AT has not been met.

Another method used to identify AT involves measuring speed during running and the corresponding heart rate.[70] This method is fast, simple, and easy to administer outside of a laboratory. Using this method, the point at which the speed–heart rate relationship becomes nonlinear is thought to be the AT. A study comparing the AT obtained by this method found strong correlations ($r = 0.99$) between this deflection in HR and AT measured through blood lactate.[70] However, this method has been questioned by other researchers who note that this heart rate deflection is not always associated with the lactate threshold.[66]

VIII. ECONOMY OF HUMAN MOVEMENT

Economy is related to the energy expenditure to complete a given distance or energy expenditure to maintain a given speed. An athlete with good economy uses less oxygen at a given submaximal speed, or for a given distance. Economy relates more to prolonged exercise performance, when the maintenance of the lowest VO_2 prolongs glycogen stores, delaying fatigue. A study using highly trained runners has shown that the oxygen uptake is lower at a given pace for endurance-trained runners compared with sprinters.[71] Although the authors reported the differences were small (5–11%), this difference in energy cost can have a cumulative effect for prolonged exercise. McArdle et al. suggest that variation in running economy in a homogeneous group can explain the majority of performance difference in a 10K run.[5] Therefore, knowing economy can be beneficial for endurance athletes, such as runners, cyclists, swimmers, rowers, and paddlers.

Economy is related to a number of factors. Gender influences economy, with women being less economical during high-speed running.[72] Although the reason for the gender differences is not clear, it may be related to differences in body composition, anatomical biomechanics, or training. An effective muscle recruitment pattern improves economy. The more an athlete reproduces an action, the better the motor pattern is learned and extraneous muscle activity (which costs energy) is eliminated.[73] This is particularly true for activities that involve a skill, such as swimming or paddling strokes for canoeing and kayaking. Muscle fiber type also influences economy. Type I fibers are more mechanically efficient than type II fibers and are more efficient for aerobic energy production.[74] Physical structure, e.g., leg length and upper body size, influences the number of strides or strokes and activity needed to complete a distance. Typically, more strides, or strokes, cause more energy expenditure. Equipment can also influence economy. For example, during cycling, the use of toe clips improves efficiency, while standing decreases economy.[75]

The major concern with economy is that there are no sport-specific standards for comparisons and there is no one "perfect pace,"[76] so coaches and athletes typically use repeated measures of economy to show that training is producing the desired improvements. Athletes usually complete a set of exercises at different submaximal velocities and the oxygen uptake is measured when steady-state is obtained; the outcome being VO_2 per unit speed.

IX. RESTING ENERGY EXPENDITURE

Knowledge of resting energy expenditure (REE) is most useful for athletes who are trying to lose or gain weight, since the REE accounts for a major portion of the daily energy expenditure. Resting energy expenditure is not basal metabolic rate, or BMR. The BMR is the minimal amount of energy necessary to sustain conscious life — keep the heart beating, maintain respiration, cell metabolism, nerve transmission, body temperature, etc. The BMR requires that the person have no additional physiologic or psychologic stimulation, such as digestion, excess temperature regulation, psychological tension, or any form of movement.[77] BMR is measured in the supine resting position, after a normal night's sleep, and 12 hours postprandial.[77] REE is the energy expenditure required to maintain normal body functions at rest.[3,5] The REE is typically measured in the morning, after a normal night's sleep, with the individual lying down or sitting, in a thermo-neutral environment, after a minimum of 3 hours' fast, and no exercise for the previous 12 hours. Since the two states are relatively close in definition, and since the difference between the BMR and the REE is less than 10%, both terms appear to be used interchangeably.[78] And, if the REE is measured in a 12-hour post absorptive condition, it is the same as BMR.[3] The BMR is difficult to precisely measure and requires more controls than the REE. Thus, the REE is usually obtained. BMR and REE are generally expressed as kilocalories per hour (kcal/h) or kiloJoules per hour (kJ/h). The rate varies as much as ±20% from individual to individual.[5,7]

A. MEASUREMENT OF RESTING ENERGY EXPENDITURE

All calorimetry methods can be used to measure REE. The procedure for REE involves obtaining two 5–7-minute continuous measures of VO_2 and VCO_2, or one single 15-minute collection period with the first 5 minutes of measurement discarded.[77] The person reclines in a supine position for 30–45 minutes in a quiet, thermo-neutral environment. To reduce anxiety caused by the equipment, the mask or mouthpiece from the spirometry system is inserted so that the subject becomes comfortable breathing through the apparatus. At the end of the rest period the measurements are obtained. The measurement of BMR is more restrictive to reduce anxiety and the gas measurements are obtained with the subject inside a transparent hood or a room calorimeter.[3,77] Also, the BMR is typically measured over a 20–30-minute period rather than the two 5–7-minute measurements.[77]

Since REE takes considerable equipment, time, and knowledge, methods have been derived to estimate REE based on weight (body mass), height, and age. Adult males will use 1.0 kcal/kg/h or 4.186 kJ/kg/h, while females will use 0.9 kcal/kg/h or 3.77 kJ/kg/h.[79,80] Energy expenditure per hour is simply obtained by multiplying the constant by body mass. The World Health Organization (WHO) has developed age- and gender-specific prediction equations[80] and other formulas have also been developed. The problem is that there is over a 15% difference between methods of estimation and there is no simple way to determine which formula is most accurate for which person. Although the majority of formulas take into consideration gender and age,[80,81] many of the standardized formulas ignore other factors that influence resting energy expenditure.

B. Factors Influencing REE

Athletes typically have a greater lean body mass or a greater proportion of lean mass to fat mass than non-athletes.[3] Lean body mass, or muscle mass, is a major contributor to REE.[80] If two individuals have the same gender, height, and weight, the one with the greater muscle mass and less fat mass will have the higher REE. Standard REE formulas fail to account for lean body mass, which can lead to erroneous results. For example, studies have reported that highly active subjects have REEs greater than sedentary controls.[82,83] Yet, when the energy expenditure was reported based on lean body mass, the groups were found to be similar. Furthermore, the size of the individual will modify that relationship. Size is concerned with height for a given weight.[80] Thus, if two individuals have the same body mass (weight), the taller person will have a higher REE than the shorter person. The taller leaner person has more surface area through which heat is lost and needs to produce more heat to maintain thermo-balance.

Prolonged exposure to either temperature extremes can increase the REE. During acute cold exposure, REE can more than double.[84] In our society, climatic effects on REE are relatively minor because most of the exposures to these extremes by athletes are limited. Also, during acute exposures, high-technology clothing reduces the direct effects of the cold or improves heat dissipation in the heat. Air conditioning of training facilities and competition arenas reduces prolonged exposure to high temperatures. Thus, climatic influences may be minimal in westernized cultures, but are of importance for many less developed societies.

The pattern of food intake can directly affect metabolic rate. Skipping meals results in a lower REE,[3] while overfeeding increases REE.[85] The pattern of food intake can also influence dietary-induced thermogenesis.[3] After feeding, the process of digestion and absorption, as well as assimilation of substrates in the liver (proteins, glycogen) requires energy. This process is about 65–95% efficient, dependent upon the type of food ingested.[5] These calories are referred to as dietary-induced thermogenesis (DIT). The DIT varies by substrate. Carbohydrate metabolism increases REE about 4–5%, proteins increase REE by 20–30%, ethanol about 22%.[3,7] Conversely, fats increase DIT by about 2%. A typical mixed meal increases REE by ~10%. DIT peaks about an hour after eating, but if the meal is high in protein, DIT can last 3–5 hours. The thermogenesis seems to be more dependent upon the feeding pattern than the total caloric intake, as feeding four meals produces a larger increase in thermogenesis than feeding one meal of the same caloric content.[86] Gorging significantly elevates the thermogenesis;[87,88] however, the effect may not be as significant for obese individuals.[89] This is thought to be in some way related to their body fat.[90] Other factors that may influence dietary-induced thermogenesis include genetics, caffeine, nicotine, and diseases such as obesity or diabetes mellitus that affect insulin.[3]

The hormones thyroxin, epinephrine (adrenalin), and insulin increase REE.[3,5,7] Thyroxin increases cell mitochondrial metabolic rate, while epinephrine has a direct effects on glycolysis, as well as increasing muscle, respiratory, and circulatory metabolic demands. Insulin, although increasing the cellular storage of glucose, also increases the cellular metabolism of glucose, especially after consuming a meal.

Prolonged exercise training appears to influence REE, but the findings of studies have been inconsistent. Some reports indicated a greater REE per unit lean body mass in athletes compared with sedentary controls,[81,82,91–93] while others disagree.[82,86,94–96] The disparity of findings may be related to differing methodologies that (1) have not controlled for an effect of the previous exercise, which can persist up to 12–13 hours after prolonged strenuous exercise; (2) the thermic effect of subsequent food intake; or (3) have used cross sectional samples of varying size and body compositions.[3,82,84,91,93,94] Evidence is accumulating from longitudinal data that aerobic training does increase REE. For example, a 10-week exercise program in lean, initially sedentary females resulted in an elevation in REE.[97] Also, the trained individuals usually have more lean body mass at a given weight, thus increasing absolute REE.[3] Although REE may increase, endurance training may also lower the dietary-induced thermogenesis compared with untrained subjects.[91,94,98] The reduced thermogenesis could help conserve energy during periods of intense physical training.

X. DAILY ENERGY EXPENDITURE OF ATHLETES

The energy expenditure of daily life is greater than the REE and is dependent upon lifestyle, occupation, and exercise. Lifestyle can account for 30–90% more energy above REE depending upon the occupation of the person. For example, someone with a sedentary occupation and little extraneous activity may only need 10–20% more calories than the REE where as a roofer or bricklayer may need an additional 80–90% more calories. A typical college student uses about 40–50% more calories a day then his/her REE. This does not account for their exercise program. In general, an adult exercising about 30–45 minutes a day requires only an additional caloric intake of about 10–14% above the caloric intake that is needed for rest, lifestyle and

TABLE 5.2
Energy Requirements of Various Sports Determined from Over 100 Sources

Sport	Men Kilocalories	Men Megajoules	Women Kilocalories	Women Megajoules
Baseball/softball	2200–3500	5.25–8.36	1800–2800	4.30–6.70
Basketball	3000–5500	7.17–13.1	1800–3800	4.30–9.08
Crew	2400–7000	5.73–16.73	1300–3600	3.11–8.60
Cross-Country Runners	2600–3900	6.21–9.32	2500–3400	5.98–8.12
Cross-country Skiers	6000–15000	14.34–36.0	6569–8400	15.7–20.0
Cyclists	2800–3900	6.70–9.32	2500–3300	5.98–7.89
Fencing	2400–4000	5.73–9.56	2100–3200	5.02–7.64
Figure Skating	2300–3100	5.50–7.41	1500–2100	3.59–5.02
Gymnastics	1600–4000	3.82–9.56	1200–2200	2.87–5.26
Lacrosse	2400–5000	5.73–11.95	1500–3000	3.59–7.17
Long Distance Runners	2600–4000	6.21–9.56	2200–3500	5.26–8.36
Power Athletes*	2500–4000	5.98–9.56	-----------	-----------
Soccer	2100–3700	5.01–8.84	1700–2600	4.06–6.21
Swimming	2500–4500	5.98–10.75	2000–4000	4.78–9.56
Tennis	-----------	-----------	1300–2500	3.10–5.98
Track	2800–6500	6.69–15.54	1800–2900	4.30–6.93
Ultra-endurance	2500–6000	5.98–14.34	1800–3100	4.30–7.41
US Football	3300–7000	7.89–16.73	-------------	-----------
Volleyball	2700–3500	6.45–8.36	1800–2400	4.30–5.74
Weight lifting	3000–5000	7.17–11.95	-------------	-----------
Wrestling	2600–3800	6.21–9.08	-------------	-----------

* power athletes = shotput, javelin, high jump, pole vault, divers

occupation. However, for athletes who exercise 3–5 hours a day the energy demand of the exercise would be considerably greater than the total allowance for REE plus lifestyle needs. Tables of energy expenditure during numerous activities have been developed.[99] In general Table 5.2 can be used as an estimate of additional energy needs of individuals training for specific sports. This table was developed from over 140 references and represents ranges of energy needs. These estimates of energy needs should not be taken as absolutes, because they will vary considerably based on duration of the exercise, the intensity of training and size, age and gender of the athlete. Some sports, like recreational basketball, may require only slightly more than normal amounts of energy, while others, like competitive endurance cycling, or ultra-marathon running, can require an enormous amount of additional energy. Measured REE can be used to improve these estimates.

Knowledge of the REE can then be combined with the estimated expenditure for lifestyle and the exercise program to obtain an estimate of the total daily energy expenditure. Armed with this information and combined with knowledge of caloric intake, athletes, coaches, or clinicians can determine the energy consumption needed to obtain the desired nutritional balance. For example, a 20-year-old female runner who weighs 112 pounds (~51 kg) works as a receptionist and trains 5 days a week for about 2 hours per day and her weight is stable. Stable weight would indicate that she is in energy balance: intake = output. Her REE was measured to be 1100 kcal/24 h. Her daily activity was estimated to be an additional 330 kcal (REE × 30% for her relatively sedentary job). Measured during her workout using a portable spirometry system, her metabolic rate was was about 7 kcal/min. Thus, her aerobic program would expend about 840 kcals (7 kcal/min × 120 min), and on the days she exercises her total energy expenditure was about 2270 kcal (1100 + 330 + 840), while on her non-exercising days she expended 1430 kcal (1100 + 330). If she wants to gain 5 pounds (2.267 kg) of muscle over the next 3 months, theoretically she will need to increase her caloric intake by about 100 kcal of carbohydrate or protein per day using the following computations:

$$\text{Weight gain} = 2.267 \text{ kg} = 2267 \text{ gm}$$

There are approximately 4 kcal/g of protein or carbohydrate

$$4 \text{ cal/g} \times 2267 \text{ g} = 9067 \text{ kcal}$$

$$9067 / 90 \text{ days} = 101 \text{ kcal/d}$$

On workout days her intake should be about 2370, where as on her non-workout days her intake should be about 1530 kcal. Conversely, if she wanted to lose 5 pounds over the same time period she would need to decrease energy intake by 101 kcal/d. This is a theoretical example and in reality, many factors will influence the total caloric needs. But by knowing the REE and exercise EE, a coach or clinician can more precisely determine the needs of the athlete.

XI. SUMMARY

Four energy expenditure measures may be useful for endurance athletes: maximal aerobic power (VO_{2max}), economy of movement, REE, and estimates of AT. Athletes with high aerobic power are generally more successful at endurance sports than athletes with lower power. However, success in endurance sports is not totally dependent on aerobic power. If two endurance athletes have the same aerobic power, but one has a higher anaerobic threshold or is more economical in movement than the other, than there is a strong likelihood that the athlete with these latter traits will prevail.

The measurement of energy expenditure, although a complex process, is important to high-level endurance athletes. Direct calorimetry, in which the person is placed in a closed chamber and heat production is directly measured, is too confining to be applicable to athletes, except for the measurement of resting metabolic rate. Indirect calorimetry appears to be more applicable to athletes. Indirect calorimetry measures VO_2 and CO_2 production to compute the energy use for short periods of time (e.g., minutes, hours). Indirect calorimetry has evolved to the point where systems are miniaturized so that metabolic rate can be measured during unhindered exercise and outside of the laboratory. These characteristics make this method most applicable for measuring VO_{2max} and economy of motion, and for estimating anaerobic threshold. Also, to obtain accurate energy expenditures, the activity must be completed in an aerobic state, or low-to-moderate intensities. At present, we have a limited capability to estimate energy cost of very high-intensity exercise, which results in the production of considerable lactic acid.

Because indirect calorimetry is not appropriate to obtain a measure of energy expenditure over a period of days, doubly labeled water techniques have evolved. This method uses a double-isotope of water ($^2H_2^{18}O$) and is most applicable when measuring overall (total) energy expenditure over days. Doubly labeled water will not work to measure the specific energy cost of a given activity, or for maximal aerobic power testing, estimating anaerobic threshold, or economy of motion. Thus, indirect calorimetry is presently our best method for measuring energy expenditure during specific activities, while the doubly labeled water is best to estimate overall daily energy use. In addition, doubly labeled water is expensive and probably out of the range to be used routinely by athletes.

Knowledge of REE is probably important for athletes who are trying to lose or gain weight, or if they are having difficulty maintaining weight. REE makes up about 50–65% of daily energy expenditure for athletes. In general, the REE is dependent upon the amount of metabolically active tissue and lean body mass, and athletes typically have greater lean body mass and less fat mass than non-athletes. However, other factors such as age, gender, size, climate, caloric intake, hormones, and exercise training will modify the REE. REE can be measured by a variety of means ranging from room calorimeters to simply measuring oxygen uptake. Presently, the easiest and least costly methods for measuring REE are the portable, indirect calorimetry systems. Ultimately, to estimate the individual daily energy expenditure three factors must be summed: (1) the REE for the 24-hr period, (2) the energy expenditure based on lifestyle (work/school), and (3) the energy expenditure from any exercise program.

Endurance athletes can gain much knowledge from measurements of metabolic rate, which can aid in their training program, track their training status, and assess their potential in their specific sport. As the availability of the miniaturized metabolic system increases, costs will hopefully decline and athletes with have greater access to these measurements of metabolic rate.

REFERENCES

1. Young, D.S., Implementation of SI units for clinical laboratory data, *Ann. Intern. Med.* 106, 14–129, 1987.
2. Schutz, Y., The basis of direct and indirect calorimetry and their potentials, *Diabetes/Metabol. Rev.* 11, 383–408, 1995.
3. Schutz, Y. and Jéquier, E., Resting energy expenditure, thermic effect of food, and total energy expenditure. In *Handbook of Obesity*, Bray, O.J., Bouchard, C., and James, W.P.T. Eds., Marcel Dekker, Inc., New York, 1998, 433–455.
4. Consolazio, C.F., Johnson, R.E., and Pecora, L.J., *Physiological Measurements of Metabolic Functions in Man*, McGraw-Hill Book Company, New York, 1963, 1–98.

5. McArdle, W.D., Katch, F.I., and Katch, V.L., *Exercise Physiology: Energy, Nutrition and Human Performance,* Williams & Wilkins, Baltimore, 1996, 139–213.

6. Krogh, A. and Lindhard, J., The relative value of fat and carbohydrate as sources of muscular energy, *Biochem. J.* 14, 290–363, 1920.

7. Bell, G.H., Emslie-Smith, D., and Paterson, C.R., *Textbook of Physiology and Biochemistry,* Churchill Livingstone, New York, 1976, 57–64.

8. Mellerowicz, H. and Smodlaka, V.N., *Ergometry: Basics of Medical Exercise Testing,* Urban & Schwarzenberg: Munich, 1981, 1–23.

9. McLaughlin, J.E., King, G.A., Howley, E.T., Bassett, D.R., and Ainsworth, B.E., Validation of the Cosmed K4b2 portable metabolic system, *Int. J. Sports Med.* 22, 280–284, 2001.

10. Harrell, J.S., McMurray, R.G., Baggett, C.D., Pennell, M.L., Pearce, P.F., and Bangdiwala, S.I., Energy costs of physical activities in children and adolescents. *Med. Sci. Sports Exerc.* 37, 329–336, 2005.

11. Barbosa, T.M., Fernandes, R., Keskinen, K.L., Colaco, P., Cardoso, C., Silva, J., and Vilas-Boas, J.P., Evaluation of the Energy Expenditure in Competitive Swimming Strokes, *Int. J. Sports Med.* Apr 11, Epub ahead of print, 2006.

12. Duffield, R., Dawson, B., Pinnington, H.C., and Wong, P., Accuracy and reliability of a Cosmed K4b2 portable gas analysis system, *J. Sci. Med. Sport.* 7, 11–22, 2004.

13. Maiolo, C., Melchiorri, G., Iacopino, L., Masala, S., and De Lorenzo, A., Physical activity energy expenditure measured using a portable telemetric device in comparison with a mass spectrometer, *Br. J. Sports Med.* 37, 445–447, 2003.

14. Strath, S.J., Bassett, D.R., Swartz, A.M., Thompson, D.L., Simultaneous heart rate-motion sensor technique to estimate energy expenditure, *Med. Sci. Sports Exerc.* 33, 2118–2123, 2001.

15. Bigard, A.X. and Guezennec, C.Y., Evaluation of the Cosmed K2 telemetry system during exercise at moderate altitude, *Med. Sci. Sports Exerc.* 27, 1333–1338, 1995.

16. Gray, G.L., Matheson, G.O., and McKenzie, D.C., The metabolic cost of two kayaking techniques, *Int. J. Sports Med.* 16, 250–254, 1995.

17. Smekal, G., Baron, R., Pokan, R., Dirninger, K., and Bachl, N., Metabolic and cardiorespiratory reactions in tennis players in laboratory testing and under sport-specific conditions, *Wien. Med. Wochenschr.* 145, 611–615, 1995.

18. Zuntz, N. and Schumburg, N.A.E.F., *Studien zu Einer Pphysiologie des Macsches.* A. Hirschwald, Berlin, 1901.

19. Carpenter, T.M., Tables, Factors and Formulas for Computing Respiratory Exchange and Biological Transformations of Energy. Carnegie Institution of Washington, Washington, DC, 1964, 104.

20. Dill, D.B., The economy of muscular exercise. *Physiol. Rev.,* 16, 263–291, 1936.

21. Bassett, D.R., Ainsworth, B.E., Swartz, A.M., Strath, S.J., O'Brien, W.L., and King, G.A., Validity of four motion sensors in measuring moderate intensity physical activity, *Med. Sci. Sports Exerc.* 32, S471–480, 2000.

22. Klein, P.D., James, W.P.T., Wong, W.W., Irving, C.S., Murgatroyd, P.R., Cabrera, M., Dallosso, H.M., Klein, E.R., and Nichols, B.L., Calorimetric validation of the doubly labeled water method for determination of energy expenditure in man, *Human Nutr. Clin. Nutr.* 38C, 95–106, 1984.

23. Schoeller, D.A., Energy expenditure from doubly labeled water: Some fundamental considerations in humans, *Am. J. Clin. Nutr.* 38, 999–1005, 1983.

24. Schoeller, D.A. and Webb, P., Five-day comparison of doubly labeled water method with respiratory gas exchange, *Am. J. Clin. Nutr.* 40, 153–158, 1984.

25. Schoeller, D.A., Measurement of energy expenditure in free-living humans by using doubly labeled water, *J. Nutr.* 118, 1278–1289, 1988.
26. Wareham, N.J., Hennings, S.J., Prentice, A.M., and Day, N.E., Feasibility of heart-rate monitoring to estimate total level and pattern of energy expenditure in a population-based epidemiological study: The Ely young cohort feasibility study 1994–5. *Br. J. Nutr.* 78, 889–900, 1997.
27. Major P., Subtle physical activity poses a challenge to the study of heart rate. *Physiol. Behav.* 63, 381–384, 1997.
28. Ott, A.E., Pate, R.R., Trost, S.G., Ward, D.S., and Saunders, R., The use of uniaxial and triaxial accelerometers to measure children's free play physical activity, *Pediatr. Exerc. Sci.* 12, 360–370, 2000.
29. Councilman, J.E., *The Science of Swimming*, Prentice Hall, Englewood Cliffs, 1968, 1–5.
30. Saitoh, M., Matsunaga, A., Kamiya, K., Ogura, M.N., Sakamoto, J., Yonezawa, R., Kasahara Y., Watanabe, H., and Masuda, T., Comparison of cardiovascular responses between upright and recumbent cycle ergometers in healthy young volunteers performing low-intensity exercise: Assessment of reliability of the oxygen uptake calculated by using the ACSM metabolic equation, *Arch. Phys. Med. Rehabil.* 86,1024–1029, 2005.
31. Paton, C.D. and Hopkins, W.G., Tests of cycling performance, *Sports Med.* 31, 489–496, 2001.
32. Knuttgen, H.G., Force, work, power and exercise, *Med. Sci. Sports Exerc.* 10, 227–228, 1978.
33. American College of Sports Medicine. *ACSM's Resource Manual for Guidelines for Exercise Testing and Prescription.* Baltimore:Williams & Wilkins, 1998.
34. MacDougall, J.D., Wenger, H.A., and Green, H.J., *Physiological Testing of the High-Performance Athlete.* Champaign: Human Kinetics, 1991.
35. Howley, E.T. and Franks, B.D., *Health Fitness Instructor's Handbook.* Champaign: Human Kinetics, 1997.
36. American College of Sports Medicine. *Guidelines for Exercise Testing and Prescription. Physical Fitness Testing and Interpretation*, 6th Edition, Baltimore: Lippincott Williams & Wilkins, 2000, pp. 57–90.
37. Zhang, Y.Y., Johnson, M.C., Chow, N., and Wasserman, K., Effect of exercise testing protocol on parameters of aerobic function, *Med. Sci. Sports Exerc.* 23, 625–630, 1991.
38. Bernstein, I.A., Webber, O., and Woledge, R., An ergonomic comparison of rowing machine designs: Possible implications for safety, *Br. J. Sports Med.* 36, 108–112, 2002.
39. Mahler, D.A., Andrea, B.E., and Andresen, D.C., Comparison of 6-min "all-out" and incremental exercise tests in elite oarsmen, *Med. Sci. Sports Exerc.* 16, 567–571, 1984.
40. Schabort, E.J., Hawley, J.A., Hopkins, W.G., and Blum, H., High reliability of performance of well-trained rowers on a rowing ergometer, *J. Sports Sci.* 17, 627–632, 1999.
41. Riechman, S.E., Zoeller, R.F., Balasekaran, G., Goss, F.L., and Robertson, R.J., Prediction of 2000 m indoor rowing performance using a 30 s sprint and maximal oxygen uptake, *J. Sports Sci.* 20, 681–687, 2002.
42. Herk, H., Mader, A., Hess, G., Mucke, S., Muller, R., and Hollmann, W., Justification of the 4-mmol/l lactate threshold, *Int. J. Sports Med.* 6, 117–130, 1985.

43. McMurray, R.G., Berry, M.J., Vann, R.T., Hardy, C.J., and Sheps, D.S., The effect of running in an outdoor environment on plasma beta endorphin, *Ann. Sports. Med.* 3, 230–233, 1988.

44. Costill, D.L., Use of a swimming ergometer in physiological research, *Res. Quart.* 37, 564–567, 1966.

45. McMurray, R.G., Effects of body position and immersion on recovery after swimming exercise, *Res. Quart.* 40, 738–742, 1969.

46. Holmer, I., Physiology of swimming man. *Acta Physiol. Scand.* Suppl 407, 1–55, 1974.

47. Pendergast, D.R., diPrampero, P.E., Craig, A.B., Wilson, D.R., and Rennie, D.W., Quantitative analysis of the front crawl in men and women, *J. Appl. Physiol.* 43, 475–479, 1977.

48. Leger, L.A., Seliger, V. and Brassard, L., Backward extrapolation of VO_{2max} values from the O_2 recovery curve, *Med. Sci. Sports Exerc.* 12, 24–27, 1979.

49. Costill, D.L., Kovaleski, J., Porter, D., Kirwan, J., Fielding, R., and King, D., Energy expenditure during front crawl swimming: predicting success in middle distance events, *Int. J. Sports Med.* 6, 266–270, 1985.

50. Astrand, P.O. and Saltin, B., Maximal oxygen uptake and heart rate in various types of muscular activity, *J. Appl. Physiol.* 16, 977–981, 1961.

51. Faulkner, J.A., Roberts, D.E., Elk, R.L., and Conway, J., Cardiovascular responses to submaximum and maximum effort cycling and running, *J. Appl. Physiol.* 30, 457–461, 1971.

52. McArdle, W.D., Katch, F.I., and Pechar, G.S., Comparison of continuous and discontinuous treadmill and bicycle tests for max VO_2, *Med. Sci. Sports* 5, 156–160, 1973.

53. Wicks, J.R., Sutton, J.R., Oldridge, N.B., and Jones, N.L., Comparison of the electrocardiographic changes induced by maximum exercise testing with treadmill and cycle ergometer, *Circulation.* 57, 1066–1070, 1978.

54. Yoshiga, C.C. and Higuchi, M., Heart rate is lower during ergometer rowing than during treadmill running, *Eur. J. Appl. Physiol.* 87, 97–100, 2002.

55. Roels, B., Schmitt, L., Libicz, S., Bentley, D., Richalet, J.P., and Millet, G., Specificity of VO_{2max} and the ventilatory threshold in free swimming and cycle ergometry: Comparison between triathletes and swimmers. *Br. J. Sports Med.* 39, 965–968, 2005.

56. Keller, B. and Katch, F.I., It is not valid to adjust gender differences in aerobic capacity and strength for body mass or lean body mass, *Med. Sci. Sports Exerc.* 23, S167, 1991.

57. Swain, D.P. and Leutholtz, B.C., *Metabolic Calculations Simplified.* Baltimore: Williams & Wilkins, 1997.

58. Rowland T.W., *Developmental Exercise Physiology.* Champaign: Human Kinetics, 1996.

59. Shvartz, E. and Reibold, R.C., Aerobic fitness norms for males and females aged 6 to 75 years: A review, *Aviat. Space Environ. Med.* 61, 3–11, 1990.

60. Saltin B. and Astrand P.O., Maximal oxygen uptake of athletes, *J. Appl. Physiol.* 23, 353–358, 1967.

61. Rusko, H.K., Development of aerobic power in relation to age and training in cross-country skiers, *Med. Sci. Sports Exerc.* 24, 1040–1047, 1992.

62. Beneke, R. and Hutler, M., The effect of training on running economy and performance in recreational athletes, *Med. Sci. Sports Exerc.* 37, 1794–1799, 2005.

63. Jones, A.M. and Carter, H. The effect of endurance training on parameters of aerobic fitness, *Sports Med.* 29, 373–386, 2000.

64. Powers, S.K., Dodd, S., Deason, R., Byrd, R., and McKnight, T., Ventilatory threshold, running economy and distance running performance of trained athletes, *Res. Quart.* 54, 179–182, 1983.

65. Ready, A.E. and Quinney, H.A., Alterations in anaerobic threshold as the result of endurance training and detraining, *Med. Sci. Sports Exerc.* 14, 292–296, 1982.

66. Wasserman, K., Whipp, B.J., Koyl, S.N., and Beaver, W.L., Anaerobic threshold and respiratory gas exchange during exercise, *J. Appl. Physiol.* 35, 236–243, 1973.

67. Denis, C., Fouquet, R., Poty, P., Geyssant, A., and Lacour, J.R., Effects of 40 weeks of endurance training on anaerobic threshold, *Int. J. Sports Med.* 3, 208–214, 1982.

68. Kohrt, W.M., O'Conner, J.S., and Skinner, J.S., Longitudinal assessment of responses by triathletes to swimming, cycling and running, *Med. Sci. Sports Exerc.* 21, 569–575, 1989.

69. McLellan, T.M. and Jacobs, I., Active recovery, endurance training, and the calculation of the individual anaerobic threshold, *Med. Sci. Sports Exerc.* 21, 586–592, 1989.

70. Conconi, F., Ferrari, M., Ziglio, P.G., Droghetti, P., and Codeca, L., Determination of the anaerobic threshold by a noninvasive field test in runners, *J. Appl. Physiol.* 52, 869–873, 1982.

71. Svedenhag, J. and Sjodin, B., Maximal and submaximal oxygen uptakes and blood lactate levels in elite male middle- and long-distance runners, *Int. J. Sports Med.* 5, 255–261, 1984.

72. Daniels, J. and Daniels, N., Running economy of elite male and elite female runners, *Med. Sci. Sports Exerc.* 24, 483–489, 1992.

73. Alexander, R.M., Walking and running, *Am. Scientist.* 72, 348–354, 1984.

74. Coyle, E.F., Sidossis, L.S., Horowitz, J.F. and Beltz, J.D., Cycling efficiency is related to the percentage of type 1 muscle fiber, *Med. Sci. Sports Exerc.* 24, 782–788, 1992.

75. Tanaka, K., Nakadomo, F., and Moritani, T., Effects of standing cycling and the use of toe stirrups on maximal oxygen uptake, *Eur. J. Appl. Physiol.* 56, 699–703, 1987.

76. Burfoot, A. and Billing, B., The perfect pace. *Runner's World*, Nov, 1985, pp. 39+

77. Bursztein, S., Elwyn, D.H., Askanazi, J., and Kinney, J.M., *Energy Metabolism, Indirect Calorimetry, and Nutrition.* Williams & Wilkins, Baltimore, 1989.

78. Matthews, C.E. and Freedson, P.S., Field trial of a three-dimensional activity monitor: comparison with self report, *Med. Sci. Sports Exerc.* 27, 1071–1078, 1995.

79. Arciero, P.J., Goran, M.I., and Poehlman E.T. Resting metabolic rate in lower in women than men, *J. Appl. Physiol.* 75, 2514–2520, 1993.

80. National Research Council. *Recommended Dietary Allowances.* 10th edition, National Academy Press, Washington DC, 1989.

81. Altman, P.L. and Dittmer, D.S., Metabolism. *Fed. Am. Soc. Exper. Biol.*, Bethesda, 1968.

82. Horton, T.J., and Geissler, C.A., Effects of habitual exercise on daily energy expenditure and metabolic rate during standardized activity, *Am. J. Clin. Nutr.* 59, 13–19, 1994.

83. Toth, M.J., and Poehlman, E.T., Effect of exercise on daily energy expenditure, *Nutr. Rev.* 54, S140–148, 1996.

84. Jacobs, I., Martineau, L., and Vallerand, A.L., Thermoregulatory thermogenesis in humans during cold exposure, *Exerc. Sport Sci. Rev.* 22, 221–250, 1994.

85. Lammert, O. and Hansen, E.S., Effects of excessive caloric intake and caloric restriction on body weight and energy expenditure at rest and light exercise, *Acta Physiol. Scand,* 114, 135–141, 1982.

86. LeBlanc, J. and Mercier, I., Components of postprandial thermogenesis in relation to meal frequency in humans, *Canad. J. Physiol. Pharm.,* 71, 879–883, 1993.

87. Miller, D.S., Gluttony 2: Thermogenesis in overeating man, *Am. J. Clin. Nutr.* 20, 1233–1239, 1967.

88. Verboeket-Van de Venne, W.P.H.G., Westerterp, K.R., and Kester, A.D.M., Effect of the pattern of food intake on human energy metabolism, *Br. J. Nutr.* 70, 103–115, 1993.

89. Zahorska-Markiewicz, B., Thermic effects of food and exercise in obesity, *Eur. J. Appl. Physiol.* 44, 231–235, 1980.

90. Shetty, P.S., Jung, R.T., James, W.P., Barrand, M.A., and Callingham, B.A., Post-prandial thermogenesis in obesity, *Clin. Sci.* 60, 519–525, 1981.

91. Poehlman, E.T., Melby, C.L. and Badylek, S.F., Resting metabolic rate and post prandial thermogenesis in highly trained and untrained males, *Am. J. Clin. Nutr.* 47, 793–798, 1988.

92. Horton, E.S., Metabolic aspects of exercise and weight reduction, *Med. Sci. Sports Exerc.* 18, 10–18, 1986.

93. Tremblay, A.E., Fontaine, E., Poehlman, E.T., Mitchell, D., Perron, L., and Bouchard, C., The effect of exercise-training on resting metabolic rate in lean and moderately obese individuals, *Int. J. Obes.* 10, 511–517, 1986.

94. Davis, J.R., Tagiaferro, A.R., Kertzer R., Gerardo, T., Nichols, J., and Wheeler, J., Variation in dietary-induced thermogenesis and body fatness with aerobic capacity, *Eur. J. Appl. Physiol.* 50, 319–329, 1983.

95. Wilmore, J.H., Stanforth, P.R., Hudspeth, L.A., Gagnon, J., Warwick Daw, E., Leon, A.C., Rao, D.C., Skinner, J.S., and Bouchard, C., Alterations in resting metabolic rate as a consequence of 20 wk of endurance training: the Heritage Family Study, *Am. J. Clin. Nutr.* 68, 66–71, 1998.

96. Dolezal, B.A. and Potteiger, J.A., Concurrent resistance and endurance training influence basal metabolic rate in nondieting individuals, *J. Appl. Physiol.* 85, 695–700, 1998.

97. Lawson, S., Webster, J.D., Pacy, P.J., and Garrow, J.S., Effect of a 10-week aerobic exercise programme on metabolic rate, body composition and fitness in lean sedentary females, *Brit. J. Clin Pract.* 41, 684–688, 1987.

98. Thorbek, G., Chwalibog, A., Jakobsen, K., and Henckel, S., Heat production and quantitative oxidation of nutrients by physically active humans, *Ann. Nutr. Metabol.* 38, 8–12, 1994.

99. Ainsworth, B.E., Haskell, W.L., Whitt, M.C., Irwin, M.L., Swartz, A.M., Strath, S.J., O'Brien, W.L., Bassett, D.R., Schmitz, K.H., Emplaincourt, P.O., Jacob, D.R., and Leon, A.S., Compendium of physical activities: an update of activity codes and MET intensities, *Med. Sci. Sports Exerc.* 32, S498–S504, 2000.

100. Short, S.H. and Short, W.R., Four-year study of university athletes' dietary intake, *J. Am. Diet. Assoc.* 82, 632–645, 1983.

6 The Measurement of Energy Expenditure and Physical Activity

Kelley K. Pettee, Catrine Tudor-Locke, and Barbara E. Ainsworth

CONTENTS

I. INTRODUCTION

Regular, moderate- to high-intensity physical activity confers substantial health-related[1] and performance-related[2] benefits. The specific activity-related physiologic adaptations and the degree to which these adaptations occur is dependent on the interaction of the frequency, duration, and intensity of the activity being performed.[3] This interaction is often quantified as "energy expenditure" (EE). It should be noted that total daily EE is the sum of energy expended at rest (resting metabolic rate) (~50–70% of total EE), while eating and digesting a meal (thermic effect of food) (~7–10% of total EE), and during and after bouts of physical activity (activity-related EE).[4] However, although resting metabolic rate may account for the largest percentage of daily EE, differences in physical activity-related EE represent the largest source of variability in the energy requirements of a given individual as well as among groups of individuals.[4] A 2000 position statement on nutrition and athletic performance emphasized the relation between energy intake and activity-related EE to enhance athletic performance, maintain total and lean body mass, govern metabolic and endocrine factors associated with the regulation of energy stores, and to enhance recovery between exercise bouts.[5]

To appropriately match athletes' energy intake with their EE, valid measures are needed to precisely quantify and track physical activity and exercise patterns and their associated energy costs. Because physical activity is a complex multidimensional behavior, precise measurement remains a challenge for researchers and practitioners, especially among free-living individuals.[6,7] Feasibility considerations both in terms of expense and administrative burden result in the need for low-cost, reliable indirect methods of assessing activity-related EE as a part of a holistic approach to meeting the energy requirements of athletes. The objective of this chapter is to review current methods used to quantify free-living physical activity-related EE. First, important terminology will be introduced as an entrée to the presentation of a conceptual framework that will guide the discussion on measuring physical activity and EE. Following will be a discussion of measurement techniques with an emphasis on field methods that can be used to assess activity-related EE among athletic populations.

II. DEFINITIONS

Before a specified construct (e.g., cardiorespiratory fitness) can be operationalized into a measurable variable (e.g., maximal oxygen consumption, VO_{2max}, measured in units of $mL \cdot O_2 \cdot kg^{-1} \cdot min^{-1}$) for research or exercise training purposes, precise conceptual definitions must be established for the construct of interest.[8] Conceptually different terms pertaining to the measurement of physical activity and EE have often been used interchangeably by researchers and practitioners. This has resulted in confusion, inconsistent study designs, limitations to inter-study comparisons, and a lack of standardized measurement practices.[3,9,10] Attempts to standardize terminology have been made.[10,11] These efforts were aimed at developing a universal framework from which definitions can be drawn to aid in operationalizing constructs into measurable study variables and within which more precise data interpretations and comparisons can be made among studies that relate physical activity to health or performance variables. Table 6.1 presents several definitions of terms related to the measurement of physical activity and EE.

It is important to recognize that physical activity and EE are not synonymous terms. Physical activity is a behavioral process characterizing body movement that results from skeletal muscle contraction, of which a product is EE.[7] Several types or categories of physical activity exist (Figure 6.1) and likely overlap to some extent, depending on an individual's purpose for performing the activity. For example, a brisk walk to and from the store may be a form of transportation for one individual, whereas the same brisk walk may be part of a planned exercise program aimed at managing blood pressure for another. Exercise training and competitive sport compose a subcategory of physical activity that is systematically structured for the primary objective of enhancing one or more dimension of physical fitness or sport

TABLE 6.1
Definitions of Terms Related to the Measurement of Energy Expenditure and Physical Activity

Energy	The capacity to do work.
Energy Expenditure	The exchange of energy required to perform biological work.
Physical Activity	Bodily movement that is produced by the contraction of skeletal muscle and that substantially increases energy expenditure.
Physical Fitness	A set of attributes (e.g., muscle strength and endurance, cardiorespiratory, flexibility, etc.) that people have to achieve that relate to the ability to perform physical activity.
Exercise	Planned, structured, and repetitive bodily movement done to improve or maintain one or more components of physical fitness. Exercise is a specific sub-category of physical activity.
Calorimetry	Methods used to calculate the rate and quantity of energy expenditure when the body is at rest and during physical activity.
Calorie	A unit of energy that reflects the amount of heat required to raise the temperature of 1 gram of water by 1°C.
Kilocalories (kcal)	1,000 calories, 4.184 kilojoules.
Kilojoules (kj)	The unit of energy in the International System of Units. 1,000 Joules, 0.238 kcal.
Metabolic Equivalent (MET)	A unit used to estimate the metabolic cost (oxygen consumption) of physical activity. One MET equals the resting metabolic rate of approximately 3.5 ml $O_2 \cdot kg^{-1} \cdot min^{-1}$, or 1 $kcal \cdot kg^{-1} \cdot hr^{-1}$.
Duration	The dimension of physical activity referring to the amount of time an activity is performed.
Frequency	The dimension of physical activity referring to how often an activity is performed.
Intensity	The dimension of physical activity referring to the rate of energy expenditure while the activity is performed.
Hours/Minutes	Typical units of time used in quantifying the rate of energy expenditure or the period of physical activity measurement (e.g., kcal per minute or $kcal \cdot min^{-1}$).
MET-minutes	The rate of energy expenditure expressed as METS per minute, which is calculated by multiplying the minutes a specific activity is performed by the corresponding energy cost of the activity.
MET-hours	The rate of energy expenditure expressed as METS per hours, which is calculated by multiplying the hours a specific activity is performed by the corresponding energy cost of the activity.
Unitless Indices	A unitless number that is computed as an ordinal measure of physical activity or energy expenditure.
Dose-Response	A relationship where increasing levels or "doses" of physical activity result in corresponding changes in the expected levels of the defined health parameter.

Sources: Brooks, Fahey, and White, 1996[12], pp. 15–25; Caspersen, Powell, and Christenson, 1985[10]. pp.126–131; Corbin, Pangrazi, and Franks, 2000[11], pp.1–9; Montoye, Kemper, Saris, and Washburn, 1996[13]; pp. 3–14.

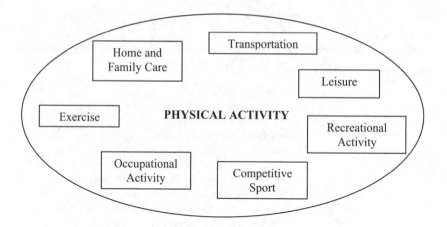

FIGURE 6.1 Physical activity and its related components.

specific skills to optimize an individual's sport-related performance. Because the subcategories of physical activity overlap, they are very difficult to measure as independent categories.[9] Additional categorization of physical activities can be based on the intensity or rate of EE attributed to a specific activity.[14–17] Activities can be self-rated as *light, moderate,* or *vigorous* intensity,[18] or can be described according to objective published intensity categories.[14–17] Hence, physical activity may be classified by purpose, such as sports, occupation, and home care, or by intensity, as in light, moderate, and vigorous. Seasonal and day-to-day intra-individual variation in physical activity patterns[19–21] and discordance between self-rated and actual activity intensity[18,22] have been shown to affect the precision of measuring activity and EE. Further, because the subcategories of physical activity have different meanings according to sex, race-ethnicity, and cultural perspectives,[23,24] self-report activity instruments must reflect the specific demographics and lifestyle of the targeted population. Accordingly, these issues should be considered when choosing a method of assessing physical activity and its related EE. It is critical to consider all sources of daily habitual physical activity to precisely quantify activity-related EE to accurately meet an individual's energy requirements.

Physical activity is typically quantified in terms of its frequency (number of bouts) and its duration (e.g., minutes per bout). The resulting EE is a direct function of all metabolic processes involved with the exchange of energy required to support the skeletal muscle contraction associated with a given physical activity. Energy expenditure reflects the intensity or metabolic cost of a given physical activity and is a product of the frequency, duration, and energy cost of the specific activity. For example, if a 55-kg female runner completes a 45-minute tempo run at a 6-min/mile pace (4 min/km), her EE would be about 660 kcal based on the following computation:

frequency (1) × duration (45 min) × the energy cost of running a 6-min/mile pace ($\sim$0.267 kcal·kg^{-1}·min^{-1}).[25]

This calculation determined the *gross* EE for running 45 minutes at a 6-min/mile pace (4 min/km). This value, however, reflects both the activity-related and resting EE.[26] To account for only the energy expended during the running activity, one must compute the *net* EE. To do so, the amount of energy assumed to be expended to sustain resting metabolic functions within the specified activity duration must be subtracted from the gross EE. A 55-kg individual has a resting EE of about 55 kcal · hr^{-1} or 0.92 kcal · min^{-1}. Therefore, the amount of energy expended within the 45-min running bout attributed to resting metabolism would be about 41.2 kcal (0.92×45). After subtracting this value from the previously computed gross EE of 660 kcal, a net EE of about 619 would be attributed to the 45 minutes of running activity. Net EE should be used when comparing the energy cost of one activity with another and when comparing activity-related EEs between individuals.[26]

Another important consideration pertaining to quantifying activity-related EE is the use of absolute vs. relative scales to index the energy cost of specific activities. Although several factors may influence EE on a relative scale (e.g., age, body size, fitness level), if one assumes a fairly constant human mechanical efficiency to perform physical work (~23%),[27] then absolute EE is generally constant for a given activity. Therefore, it is possible to standardize methods of assigning energy costs to specific activities for the purpose of assessing activity-related EE among large populations of free-living individuals. Factors such as age, sex, and fitness level will undoubtedly influence the precision by which a standardized activity-specific absolute energy cost reflects a given individual's relative intensity level (e.g., percentage of actual maximal capacity).[28] For example, a 3.5 mph (5.6 km/hr) walk carries an absolute energy cost of 3.8 kcal·kg^{-1}·hr^{-1}. For a healthy individual with a maximal capacity of about 12 kcal·kg^{-1}·hr^{-1} the relative intensity is about 32% of maximal capacity; whereas for an older individual with a maximal capacity of 7 kcal·kg^{-1}·hr^{-1} the relative intensity is about 55%. The issue of absolute vs. relative intensity is probably more important when prescribing exercise or when categorizing individuals into intensity-specific levels of activity (e.g., moderately vs. vigorously active). Feasibility considerations related to individualized measures of relative EE limit assessment methods among large free-living populations limit the use of absolute energy cost scales. However, because EE is closely related to body size, it is essential to account for this factor when quantifying activity-related EE. It is therefore preferable to express EE per unit of body mass, for example, as kcal per kilogram of body mass per minute (kcal·kg^{-1}·min^{-1}). Returning to the 55-kg female runner who completes a 45-minute run at a 6-min/mile pace (4 min/km), the absolute net EE was 619 kcal, whereas the net EE relative to the individual's body mass would be about 11.25 kcal·kg^{-1} during the 45-minute bout of running activity. A 75-kg runner who completes the same running task would have an absolute net EE of 844.75 kcal, but when expressed per kg of body weight, the EE is the same (11.26 kcal·kg^{-1}) as that computed for the lighter runner.

An alternative unit of quantifying activity-related EE is the metabolic equivalent, or MET.[14] The MET represents the ratio of work to resting metabolic rate.[13] It is accepted that resting EE is approximately 1 MET, which is equivalent to 3.5 mL·O$_2$·kg^{-1}·min^{-1}, or about 1 kcal·kg^{-1}·hr^{-1}.[13] To compute the MET level of a given physical activity, multiply the associated MET level for a given activity by the duration (e.g., minutes) for which the activity was performed. This results in the MET-minute.

This index quantifies the rate at which energy is expended for the duration an activity is performed, while accounting simultaneously for body size and resting metabolism.[14,29,30] To standardize the quantification of EE and reduce potential sources of extraneous variation in physical activity research, a systematic approach for assigning MET levels of EE to specific physical activities has been published.[14,15] The *Compendium of Physical Activities*[14,15] provides researchers and practitioners with a standardized linkage between specific activities, their purpose and their estimated energy cost expressed in METS. A sample entry from the Compendium is listed below:

Code	MET	Activity	Examples
12120	16	running	running, 10 mph

Column 1 shows a five-digit code that indexes the general class or purpose of the activity. In this example, 12 refers to running and 120 refers specifically to running a 6 min/mile (4 min/km) pace. Column 2 shows the energy cost of the activity in METs. Columns 3 and 4 show the type of activity (running) and a specific example related with the activity code. Much of the original work to standardize the energy cost of physical activity was calibrated for a 60-kg person.[14] Therefore, the conversion between MET minutes and kcal of EE is approximated by multiplying MET minutes by the quotient of an individual's body mass divided by 60.[14] For a 60-kg person, the caloric equivalent will be slightly higher and, for those weighing less than 60 kg, the caloric equivalent will be slightly lower than the MET-minute value. The caloric equivalent of 150 MET-minutes of walking for a 70-kg person is about 75 kcal, for a 60-kg person the caloric equivalent is about 150 kcal, and for a 50-kg person, about 125 kcal. Returning to the 55-kg runner, completing the 45-minute bout of running at 6-min/mile (4 min/km) pace would result in 720 MET-minutes (16 MET activity × 45 minutes) or 660 kcal (720 MET-min × [55/60]). Kcal energy expenditure also can be estimated using MET-hr as follows: MET × hrs × kg body weight.

Defining and standardizing terms associated with physical activity measurement is a critical step in reducing unwanted sources of variation and producing unbiased estimates of activity-related EE.[13–15,29] It should be apparent from the previous discussion that, although the use of a standardized compendium to index activity-specific energy costs results in potentially large differences between individuals in terms of absolute net EE, after accounting for body size, EE estimates for a given activity are quite small. The *Compendium of Physical Activities* may not resolve every issue related to individual vs. population-based assessment of activity-related EE. It does, however, provide a standardized measurement method for use in research and practical settings, which should enhance the consistency of EE assessment in terms of precision and reproducibility.

III. CONCEPTUAL FRAMEWORK FOR QUANTIFYING ENERGY EXPENDITURE

To incorporate the terminology described above into a framework that can guide the measurement of EE under laboratory and field conditions, it could be argued that the construct of interest within the activity-EE measurement paradigm might best be defined as "movement". Movement can be operationalized into two measurable variables:

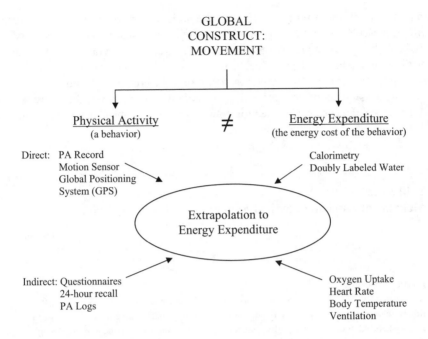

FIGURE 6.2 Conceptual Framework for defining and assessing physical activity and energy expenditure. Adapted with permission from M.J. LaMonte and B.E. Ainsworth, Quantification of energy expenditure and physical activity in the context of dose response, *Med. Sci. Sports Exerc.* 2001; 33 (6 suppl): S370–S378.

physical activity (a behavior) and EE (the energy cost of the behavior) (Figure 6.2). Direct and indirect measures exist for both physical activity and EE. However, because researchers and practitioners are ultimately interested in matching energy intake with EE, researchers typically extrapolate activity measures to units of EE prior to evaluating potential effects on energy balance. Energy expenditure is often estimated from physical activity questionnaires or other indirect measures that reflect patterns of activities in various settings. Indirect measures of activity or EE may provide acceptable estimates, depending on the degree of concordance with more direct measures of EE. Following is a review of methods to assess physical activity and EE, with emphasis placed on direct and indirect techniques that can be used to quantify EE among free-living populations. Laboratory-based methods for assessing physical activity and EE are covered elsewhere in this volume. Comprehensive reviews of free-living and laboratory methods used to assess activity-related EE can be found elsewhere.[6,7,13,31–40]

IV. METHODS OF ASSESSING PHYSICAL ACTIVITY AND ENERGY EXPENDITURE

The primary objective of measuring activity-related EE is to obtain a reliable and accurate estimate of the energy cost for a given activity or series of activities. The EE score can then be applied within the context of designing and tracking exercise training and nutrition programs to optimize athletic performance (e.g., endurance, power, muscular strength). The practical application of linking physical activity and EE is predicated upon precise measures of both variables. Several direct and indirect methods exist to assess physical activity and EE in laboratory and field settings.[6,7,13,31-40] Table 6.2 lists the most common measurement techniques.

Direct measures of physical activity include the use of physical activity records and diaries and mechanical or electronic motion sensors to obtain detailed information

---

TABLE 6.2
Methods of Assessing Physical Activity and Energy Expenditure

	Dimension Measured	Units	Technical/ Administrative Burden
Direct Measures			
Observation	Physical Activity	Frequency, Duration, Type	Moderate
Room Calorimetry	Energy Expenditure	kcal of heat production	High
Doubly Labeled Water	Energy Expenditure	kcal from CO_2 production	High
Biochemical Forces	Energy Expenditure	kcal from VO_2 – force curves	High
Acceleration Vectors (e.g., Accelerometery)	Physical Activity	Frequency, Duration	Moderate
	Energy Expenditure	kcal, METs from VO_2 regressions	Moderate
Motion Sensors (e.g., Pedometry)	Physical Activity		Low
	Energy Expenditure		Low
PA Records or Diaries	Physical Activity	Frequency, Duration, Type	High
	Energy Expenditure	kcal, METs from Compendium of Physical Activities	High
Indirect Measures			
Indirect Calorimetry	Energy Expenditure	kcal, METs from CO_2 production	High
Physiologic Measures (e.g., Heart Rate)	Energy Expenditure	kcal, METs from relation with VO_2	Moderate
PA Surveys or Questionnaires, Recall Interviews, Logs	Physical Activity	Frequency, Duration, Type	Low
	Energy Expenditure	kcal, METs from Compendium of Physical Activities	Low
Surrogate Reports (e.g., Energy Intake)	Energy Expenditure	kcal, assumes weight stable	Low

pertaining to the frequency, duration, or pattern of physical activities performed over a defined observation period. Indirect physical activity measures involve the use of questionnaires, logs, and 24-hour recall instruments that require respondents to recall their usual activity habits during a period in the far or recent past. Indirect methods typically produce less detail than direct physical activity measures, but offer substantially less administrative burden and cost.

Precise measures of EE are difficult without the use of expensive laboratory procedures involving metabolic chambers or radioactive isotope tracers.[6,13] Activity-related EE can be estimated indirectly from field measures of physiologic variables or physical activity;[7,9] however, the error associated with estimated EE may limit the precision needed for application on an individual level.[41]

A. Measuring Energy Expenditure

The complex biochemical processes that drive the transfer of metabolic energy required for skeletal muscle contraction during physical activity result in a large amount of heat energy.[12] The rate of heat production is directly proportional to the net activity-related EE; therefore, EE can be precisely quantified by measuring body heat at rest or during exercise.[42] The oxidation of food substrate is a primary source of energy production at rest, during and following physical activity. Therefore, activity-related EE can be estimated by measuring the fractional considerations of expired CO_2 and O_2 during physical activity and calculating EE based on some assumptions about the energy cost of substrate oxidation.[42] Laboratory methods for direct measures of heat production (e.g., room calorimetry) and ventilatory gas exchange (e.g., indirect calorimetry) have been described elsewhere in this volume. Following is an overview of the field methods used to assess activity-related EE in a variety of settings.

1. Direct Measures of Energy Expenditure

a. Doubly Labeled Water (DLW)

Energy Expenditure estimated from DLW is based on the rate of metabolic carbon dioxide production (VCO_2).[43,44] The DLW solution consists of the stable water isotopes ^2H_2O and $H_2^{18}O$ and is administered according to body size. Urinary isotope excretion is tracked using an isotope-ratio mass spectrometer prior to dosing, shortly after dosing, and over several days thereafter. Labeled hydrogen (^2H_2O) is excreted as water alone, while labeled oxygen ($H_2^{18}O$) is lost as water and CO_2 ($C^{18}O_2$) through the carbonic anhydrase system. The difference in the isotope turnover rate provides a measure of metabolic VCO_2.[44] Oxygen uptake (VO_2) and total body EE are extrapolated from measured VCO_2 and an estimate of the respiratory quotient (RQ) based on established equations.[45] Under steady-state conditions, RQ reflects the relative percentage of carbohydrate and fat oxidation and is calculated as VCO_2/VO_2. Inherent error will exist in DLW EE estimates when RQ is estimated and when measurements are made under non-steady-state conditions such as exercise.[13]

Differences in EE estimates between DLW and indirect calorimetry measures have been as high as 20%.[41,46-48] Discrepancies between DLW and indirect calorimetry may reflect a greater amount of activity-related EE under free-living conditions that can be simulated and measured under controlled laboratory conditions. Although DLW provides precise estimates of free-living EE over prolonged periods (e.g., weeks), this technique is limited to studies of total EE and does not differentiate the duration, frequency, or intensity of specific physical activity.

A "physical activity level" index (PAL) has been computed as the DLW total daily EE divided by measured or estimated resting metabolic rate.[49] The PAL reflects the energy requirements of adult population groups and is classified by the 1985 FAO/WHO/UNU expert consultation[50] as sedentary or light activity (1.53), active or moderately active (1.76) or vigorous or vigorously active (2.25), depending on one's occupational and leisure time activity. The 24-hour PAL is based on the physical effort demanded by occupational work and the effort expended in leisure time activity. The PAL can be used to calculate energy requirements by multiplying the PAL by an individual's BMR using the examples below:

- *Sedentary or light activity:* If this PAL was from a female population, 30 to 50 years old, with mean weight of 55 kg and mean BMR of 5.40 $MJ \cdot d^{-1}$ (1,290 $kcal \cdot d^{-1}$), TEE = 1.53 × 5.40 = 8.26 MJ (1,975 kcal), or 150 kJ (36 $kcal \cdot kg^{-1} \cdot d^{-1}$).

- *Active or moderately active:* If this PAL was from a female population, 20 to 25 years old, with mean weight of 57 kg and mean BMR of 5.60 $MJ \cdot d^{-1}$ (1,338 $kcal \cdot d^{-}$), TEE = 1.76 × 5.60 = 9.86 MJ (2,355 kcal), or 173 kJ (41 $kcal \cdot kg^{-1} \cdot d^{-1}$).

- *Vigorous or vigorously active:* If this PAL was from a male population, 20 to 25 years old, with mean weight of 70 kg and mean BMR of 7.30 $MJ \cdot d^{-1}$ (1,745 $kcal \cdot d^{-1}$), TEE = 2.25 × 7.30 = 16.42 MJ (3,925 kcal), or 235 kJ (56 $kcal \cdot kg^{-1} \cdot d^{-1}$).

The lack of information as to the type, duration, and frequency of activities resulting in the expended energy, as well potential errors with estimating resting metabolic rate, challenge the utility of the PAL. The expense of the isotopes and mass spectrometry analysis may limit this method of assessing EE exclusively to research settings.

b. Labeled Bicarbonate

The labeled bicarbonate ($NaH^{14}CO_3$) method, which is very similar to DLW, has been used to measure free-living total daily EE over shorter observation periods (e.g., days) than in studies of DLW.[51] A known amount of isotope is infused at a constant rate that will eventually be diluted by the body's CO_2 pool. Labeled carbons are recovered from expired air, blood, urine, or saliva. Metabolic VCO_2 is determined from the degree to which the isotope was diluted. Total EE can be calculated from VCO_2 based on assumptions made about RQ. Controlled experimental studies of this method have demonstrated EE estimates within <6% of that measured in a respiratory chamber.[51,52] Labeled bicarbonate measures of EE are limited by similar concerns as described for the DLW method.

2.   Indirect Measures of Energy Expenditure

a.   Oxygen Uptake

Activity-related EE measured with indirect calorimetry procedures is based on assumed relations between oxygen uptake and the caloric cost of substrate oxidation.[12,13,42] Based on the gas concentrations and volume of expired air, rates of VCO_2 and VO_2 can be determined. RQ is typically estimated by the respiratory exchange ratio (RER) as VCO_2 / VO_2. Then VO_2 and RQ can be used to estimate EE in kcal according to Weir's equation.[53]

$$EE \ (kcal) = VO_2 \ (3.9 + 1.1 \ RQ) \qquad (6.1)$$

Differences between actual and estimated RQ can result because of unreliable assumptions regarding the caloric cost of specific substrate oxidation, bicarbonate buffering of metabolic CO_2 during exercise and post-exercise oxygen consumption kinetics. Therefore, measured RQ, which involves urinary nitrogen collection,[42] is required for precise estimates of activity-related EE using indirect calorimetry methods.

It is likely that free-living activity patterns are altered during laboratory simulations, methods for performing indirect calorimetry outside the laboratory setting. These techniques are based on the same principles described above and utilize small, portable, indirect calorimeters that integrate O_2 and CO_2 analyzers, a ventilation flow-volume meter and a microcomputer to process expired air collected through a fitted hood, face mask, or mouthpiece.[54] Devices such as the Cosmed K4b have allowed for field assessment of VO_2 and, thus, measures of gross activity-related EE during a variety of free-living activities.[55,56] Cost issues, the necessity of wearing cumbersome and obtrusive instrumentation, the potential for altered patterns of physical activity and lack of testing under a variety of field settings limit the usefulness of this approach to measuring free-living activity related EE outside of the research setting.

b.   Heart Rate

Activity-related EE has been estimated from HR based on the assumption of a strong linear relation between HR and VO_2.[57,58] However, variation in the HR–VO_2 relationship during low- and very high-intensity PA and considerable between-person HR–VO_2 variability[59,60] have led some researchers to recommend using individual HR–VO_2 calibration curves to estimate activity related EE.[60,61] One such method requires establishing a heart rate "threshold" prior to estimating activity-related EE from the HR–VO_2 calibration curve.[62] This threshold is referred to as the "FLEX HR" and is determined from laboratory-based indirect calorimetry studies at various work intensities. Activities eliciting an HR below the FLEX HR are assigned an activity-related energy cost based on resting EE. Activities eliciting an HR above the FLEX HR are assigned an activity-related energy cost using the individual HR–VO_2 calibration curve. Other techniques have been used to estimate activity-related EE from the HR response during physical activity.[60,63,64]

Correlations of 0.53 and 0.73 have been reported between total EE estimated from DLW and HR values based on individual HR–VO_2 calibrations.[65] Although activity-related EE estimates based on individual HR–VO$_2$ curves correlate reasonably well with an objective EE measure such as DLW, measurement variability is high. Livingstone et al.[62] reported differences scores of –22% to +52% between total EE estimated from DLW and FLEX HR. However, Strath et al.[64] showed a strong correlation between activity-related EE estimated from HR reserve and indirect calorimetry ($r = 0.87$; SEE 0.76 METs) among adults performing moderate-intensity lifestyle activities. Energy expenditure estimates based on relative vs. absolute HR measures may reduce between-person sources of variation related with age, sex, and fitness level, which may improve the precision of estimating activity-related EE from HR responses during physical activity.

The HR–VO$_2$ relationship is not linear during low- and very high-intensity activity.[32,59] Because many daily activities are low to moderate intensity,[15] HR monitoring may not provide precise estimates of habitual daily activity-related EE under free-living conditions. Imprecise estimates of activity-related EE may also be attributed to several factors that influence HR without having substantial effects on oxygen uptake, such as day-to-day HR variability, body temperature, size of the activity muscle mass (e.g., upper vs. lower body), type of exercise (static vs. dynamic), stress and medication.[7,13,32] The need to develop individual HR–VO$_2$ calibration curves and instrumentation costs ($150 per unit) make HR monitoring a less suitable surrogate activity-related EE outside the research setting. HR measurements may best be utilized as part of an integrated physical activity and heart rate monitoring system (e.g., Actiheart) rather than as a single measure of activity-related EE among free-living individuals.[66]

c. Body Temperature and Ventilation

Because a close relationship between EE and core body temperature and ventilation has been reported under laboratory conditions,[13] continuous monitoring of these variables could provide a means of extrapolating activity-related EE under certain conditions. However, body temperature and ventilation measures of EE may be limited by time requirements, several confounding factors, and inconvenient measurement techniques.[7] Similar to HR, these measurements may best be utilized as part of an integrated monitoring system rather than as single measures of activity-related EE among free-living individuals.[66]

B. MEASURING PHYSICAL ACTIVITY

1. Direct Measures of Physical Activity

a. Physical Activity Records

Physical activity records are detailed accounts of activity types and patterns recorded in diary format during a defined period of time.[6] Their level of detail ranges from recording each activity and its associated duration[67] to recording activities performed at specified time intervals (e.g., every 15 minutes).[68] Respondents record information about the type (e.g., sleep, running, weightlifting), purpose (e.g., exercise, transportation), duration (e.g., minutes), self-rated intensity (light, moderate, vigorous), and body position (reclining, sitting, standing, walking) for every activity completed within a defined observation period (typically 24 hours). Seasonal records (e.g., winter, summer) can be kept to obtain information about habitual physical activity levels and patterns and related seasonal variations in these behaviors.[20,21] Because entries are recorded in the activity record at the time the behavior is executed, there is little concern over the effects of recall bias on the precision of quantifying activity-related EE. A completed physical activity record including codes from the *Compendium of Physical Activities* would be used to assign an energy cost to each activity for scoring purposes. Once scored, the physical activity record provides a detailed account of the minutes spent and estimated energy expended in various types, intensities, and patterns of physical activity. The physical activity record is a highly objective and reproducible method[69] of tracking the specific types (e.g., walking, running, occupation) and patterns (e.g., single continuous bouts, sporadic intermittent bouts) of activity that account for individual or population (e.g., entire sport teams) activity-related EE. For example, an athlete thought to be in a chronic negative energy balance could complete a series of physical activity records over a defined time frame, from which estimates of total EE as well as activity-specific EE can be obtained. It may be discovered that the athlete in question is expending a large amount of energy in non-sport activities (e.g., occupational or recreational activity) that are not being met with a compensatory increase in energy intake. Using data from the activity record, nutritional counseling, and training modifications can be implemented to reestablish energy balance in this athlete.

Physical activity records have been used in field settings to obtain comprehensive detailed accounts of free-living physical activities and related EE.[18,41,67,69–73] Various forms of physical activity records are accessible on the World Wide Web to monitor one's exercise patterns (i.e., American Heart Association's *Just Move Program*).[74] The precision of physical activity record's measurement of free-living EE has been studied. Conway et al.[41] reported a difference of only 7.9 ± 32% between a 7-day physical activity record and doubly labeled water estimates of free-living activity-related EE in men. Richardson et al.[75] observed moderate to strong age-adjusted correlations (r = 0.35 – 0.68) between total MET-min per day of EE from the physical activity record and an electronic accelerometer among free-living men and women. Physical activity records have also been used to study activity patterns among free-living individuals. Ainsworth et al.[67] characterized the types and patterns of physical activity and related EE among Caucasian, African-American, and Native American women living in the southeastern and southwestern regions of the U.S. as a part of the NIH-funded Women's Health Initiative.[76] Data from the physical activity record were then used to develop population-specific physical activity surveys that would precisely measure habitual daily activity-related EE among these population sub-groups of women. Focus groups[24] or individual debriefing pertaining to recorded information have been used to enhance the richness and interpretation of data gleaned from physical activity records. Together, these methods can be used to obtain information required to identify athletes at risk for overtraining,[2,77] chronic energy imbalance,[5] and related declines in athletic performance and overall health status.[2,4,5,78]

Similar to their dietary counterpart aimed at assessing energy intake,[79] physical activity records provide a very detailed and comprehensive method of assessing an important determinant of energy balance. As with dietary records, feasibility is limited by cost, the potential for altered behavior, and administrative burden on the practitioner and participant. For these reasons, physical activity records may best be suited for use with individuals considered to be at high risk for energy imbalance or as a criterion measure for validating simpler field surveys of physical activity and related EE.

b. Movement Monitors

The use of mechanical and electronic body-worn motion sensors as a direct measure of free-living physical activity has become increasingly popular.[7,80,81] Energy expenditure is often extrapolated from the activity data under the assumption that movement (or acceleration) of the limbs and torso is closely related to whole-body activity-related EE.[32] There are several types of motion sensors that differ in cost, technology, and data output (Figure 3).

i. Pedometers

Pedometers have gained widespread popularity in research and practice settings to quantify ambulation in terms of accumulated steps in free-living settings. Pedometers are small, inexpensive devices (~$20) used to directly quantify ambulatory activity in terms of accumulated steps per unit of time (e.g., per day).[6,8] Battery-operated digital pedometers (e.g., Yamax Digiwalker) are smaller and may be more reliable than earlier models.[82,83] Pedometers are worn at the waist and are triggered by the vertical accelerations of the hip that cause a horizontal spring-suspended level arm to move up and down. Movement of the lever arm opens and closes an electrical circuit. Each time the circuit closes, a "step" is counted. Step registration, in theory, should reflect only the vertical forces of the hip; however, any vertical force through the hip are (e.g., sitting down hard onto a chair) can trigger the device. An estimate of distance walked is obtained by calibrating the pedometer to an individual's stride length during a short walking trial over a known distance; however, distance estimates are less valid than the direct measurement of steps.[82,83]

Pedometers have demonstrated reasonable precision for use in research and clinical settings where walking is the primary type of physical activity.[54,81,82,84–87] Correlations of $r = 0.84$–0.93[84] and $r = 0.48 - 0.80$[55] have been reported between pedometer steps per day and EE estimates from electronic accelerometers. Investigators have also shown pedometer steps per day to be moderately correlated with measured oxygen uptake ($r = 0.49$[55]) and self-reported total daily activity-related EE ($r = 0.21$ to 0.49[81,88]). Moreover, their ease of administration makes pedometers a practical assessment tool for individuals encompassing nearly all age groups.[31,89,90] Finally, pedometers have the ability to promote behavior change and have been increasingly used in intervention settings as an intervention tool.[91–93]

A major limitation to using pedometers as an objective field measure of activity-related EE is that pedometers lack temporal information on the type, duration, and intensity of activities performed while steps were being recorded.[7,32] Although some pedometers include an estimate of net EE based on an assumed relation of about 100 kcal per mile walked, empirical data is lacking as to the precision of these estimates compared with measured EE.[83] Similar to other motion sensors, pedometers do not have the capability to quantify upper body movements[94] and have difficulty accurately assessing activity levels in individuals moving at slower speeds.[82]

Because researchers recommend using the "raw steps" data as opposed to distance traveled or estimated EE to represent ambulatory activity,[94] pedometry may not be a suitable method of assessing activity-related EE among athletes. Pedometers may, however, serve as an inexpensive method of monitoring ambulatory activity among athletes who are rehabilitating sport-related injuries wherein walking is a major part of the rehabilitation, or is being restricted due to the specific nature of the injury. Used in conjunction with a detailed self-report of physical activity (e.g., activity log), pedometers may provide a simple, cost-effective way to monitor both the quantity and quality of certain types of physical activity.

ii. Accelerometers

Accelerometers are small, battery-operated electronic motion sensors that, in theory, measure the rate and magnitude of that which the body's center of mass displaces during movement. Accelerometers are typically worn at the waist and measure movement in single (uniaxial — Actigraph) or multiple planes (triaxial — Tritrac) by way of piezoelectric signaling. Activity or EE data are stored in solid-state memory for computer downloading and processing at a later time. Solid-state technology integrates and sums the absolute value and frequency of acceleration forces over a defined observation period. Data is output as an activity "count," an approximation of both the number of independent forces detected and their acceleration Regression equations have been developed from controlled laboratory experiments to allow for the estimation of activity-related EE from the integral of accelerometer count.[95–99]

The Actigraph, formerly known as Computer Science and Applications (CSA) and Manufacturing Technology Inc. (MTI) (Actigraph, LLC Fort Walton Beach, FL) has become increasingly popular for field studies of physical activity and EE because of its small size and ability for time-interval sampling (e.g., minute by minute) and data storage. Data are presented as counts per unit sampling time, and regression equations have been developed to estimate EE from raw count data.[95,96,99] These equations were generated from controlled studies of treadmill exercise or limited simulations of lifestyle physical activities. The most common equations are those developed by Freedson et al.,[95,100] which are preprogrammed into the unit:

$$\text{METs} = 1.439008 + (0.000795 \times \text{counts·min}^{-1}) \qquad (6.2)$$

$$\text{kcal·min}^{-1} = (0.00094 \times \text{counts·min}^{-1}) + (0.1346 \times \text{mass in kg}) \qquad (6.3)$$

The precision of each equation was $R^2 = 0.82$ (SEE = 1.12 METs) for METs and $R^2 = 0.82$ (SEE = 1.4 kcal·min^{-1}) for kilocalories during treadmill exercise at 80, 106, and 162 m·min^{-1}.[95]

Several studies have assessed the ability of the Actigraph to determine activity-related EE.[55,80,96,99–103] Actigraph counts have varied significantly with monitor placement at three different ipsilateral hip locations.[80] Melanson and Freedson[100] showed Actigraph counts·min^{-1} were correlated with VO$_2$ during treadmill walking (r = 0.82), but unrelated to treadmill grade (r = 0.03). Actigraph counts·min^{-1} were sensitive to changes in ambulatory velocity across three walking speeds (p < 0.0001) but inter-instrument reliability was substantially lower during slower (53 m·min^{-1}, R = 0.55) vs. faster (107 m·min^{-1}, R = 0.91).[102] Correlations between VO_2 and Actigraph counts·min^{-1} have been stronger during controlled laboratory activity (e.g., r = 0.80 to 0.95)[80,100] than during simulated or actual field conditions or lifestyle activities (e.g., r = 0.40 to 0.60).[80,101] Hendelman et al.[96] showed large differences (e.g., 30–57%) between measured and predicted METs for a variety of daily lifestyle activities. Regression equations used to estimate EE from lifestyle activities have shown lower precision (R^2 = 0.32 – 0.35, SEE = 0.96 to 1.2 METs)[96,99] compared with equations from controlled laboratory activity (R^2 = 0.82–0.89, SEE = 1.1 METs).[95,102] Discrepancies in the time spent (e.g., min·day^{-1}) in defined EE categories were large between detailed physical activity logs and Actigraph data based on cutpoints derived from three different regression equations.[101] These issues and other topics related to the use of accelerometers was the topic of a consensus conference held in 2004 with the proceedings published in a supplement issue of *Medicine and Science in Sports and Exercise*.[103]

The Tritrac (Hemokinetics Inc., Madison, WI) is a triaxial accelerometer that provides count data for the anterior-posterior, medial-lateral, and vertical planes, as well as an integrated vector magnitude (Vmag) of counts for all three planes combined. Energy expenditure can be estimated through regression equations that account for body mass and resting EE. Resting EE is calculated as follows:[98]

$$\text{Men: } (0.00473 \times \text{wt kg}) + (0.00971 \times \text{ht cm}) - (0.00513 \times \text{age yr}) + 0.04687 \tag{6.4}$$

$$\text{Women: } (0.00331 \times \text{wt kg}) + (0.00352 \times \text{ht cm}) - (0.00513 \times \text{age yr}) + 0.49854 \tag{6.5}$$

A regression equation (R^2 = 0.90, SEE = 0.014 kcal·kg^{-1}·min^{-1} has been developed during treadmill walking and running to estimate activity-related EE from the Tritrac Vmag:[98]

$$\text{kcal·kg}^{-1}\text{·min}^{-1} = 0.018673 + (0.000029051 \times \text{Vmag·min}^{-1}) \tag{6.6}$$

Oddly, the preceding regression equation predicts EE using a triaxial monitor based on experimental activity that results in acceleration from essentially one plane (e.g., vertical). Measurement in three planes should theoretically account for more sources of bodily movement and therefore provide more precise estimates of activity-related EE, particularly under lifestyle conditions. Studies have shown that triaxial devices have only slightly better correlations with both laboratory ($r_{triaxial}$ = 0.84 – 0.93 vs. $r_{uniaxial}$ = 0.76 – 0.85) and lifestyle activity ($r_{triaxial}$ = 0.59 – 0.62 vs. $r_{uniaxial}$ = 0.48 – 0.59) related EE.[80,96]

Numerous types of accelerometers are available for use to assess physical activity (e.g., Sensewear [Bodymedia; Pittsburgh], AMP [Dynastream Innovations; Cochrane, Alberta,], Actiwatch and Actical [Minimitter Physiological and Behavioral Monitoring; Bend, Oregon], Stepwatch [Cyma Corporation; Mountlake Terrace, CA]). While all brands provide data about human movement or energy expenditure, the sensitivity and utility of the information obtained may vary by instrument. In general, accelerometers can be used to assess frequency, duration, and intensity of physical activity, however, the specific type of physical activity is unknown. Accelerometers tend to overestimate walking-related EE and underestimate lifestyle activity-related EE. Furthermore, activity-related EE owed to upper extremities or increased resistance to body movement (e.g., uphill walking) is not accounted for. Subject compliance issues, potentially altered physical activity patterns and the cost of more sophisticated instruments (uniaxial ~$300, triaxial ~$550 per unit) limit the practicality of using accelerometers to measure activity-related EE among free-living athletes. If used together with a detailed activity log, accelerometers may be useful to quantify physical activity patterns and their related EE for an athlete at high risk for energy imbalance.

2. Indirect Measures of Physical Activity

a. Physical Activity Recalls

Physical activity recalls are typically conduced as interviews (telephone or in person) and are aimed at detailing an individual's activity level during the past 24 hours or longer.[6] Activity recalls are similar to physical activity records in that they can identify the type, duration, purpose, and related EE of activities performed during the recall frame. The physical activity recall was developed after methods used in the 24-hr recalls and takes from 20–45 minutes to complete.[79,104] Multiple random 24-hr activity recalls have been used to profile activity patterns and estimate EE among adults in a 1-year cohort study of blood lipid variability[104] and to validate a global physical activity questionnaire.[105] In the blood lipid study by Matthews et al.[104] the range of test–retest reliability coefficients for the 24-hr recall was very large and the magnitude of the coefficients was moderate at best ($r = 0.22$ to 0.58). Criterion validity correlations between total MET-hr·d^{-1} from the 24-hr recalls and activity data from an electronic accelerometer were $r = 0.74$ and $r = 0.32$ for men and women, respectively. Based on the feasibility, reasonable reliability and validity, minimal participant effort, and potential reductions in response bias and altered activity patterns during assessment, the researchers advocated using the 24-hr recalls to assess activity-related EE among free-living populations. However, this method may not be suitable in populations with limited telephone access, may be hampered by individuals who are unwilling or unable to complete the phone interview and may utilize a time frame (e.g., past 24 hr) that does not capture an individual's true habitual physical activity pattern or level. On the other hand, this method may be useful during tapering periods of the yearly training plan, where small acute changes in an athlete's total exercise volume and its associated energy requirements might be highly influential on performance in an upcoming competition.

b. Physical Activity Logs

A modified version of the physical activity record is the physical activity log. These instruments aim to provide detailed accounts of habitual daily activities, their associated duration, and EE.[6] The activity log is structured as a checklist of activities specific to the target population's usual activity patterns.[6,24,101] The Bouchard Physical

Activity Log[68] is designed to allow respondents to check the type and intensity of activity they are performing every 15 minutes during a specific period. The Ainsworth Physical Activity Log[79] is a modifiable form that includes a list of 20 to 50 activities that reflect population-specific PA interests (Figure 6.3). At the end of the day, respondents complete the single-page checklist by identifying the type and duration of activities performed that day. Activity-related EE is computed by assigning intensity values from the *Compendium of Physical Activities* to each activity selected by the respondent. The log takes only a few minutes to complete and can be quickly scored to provide information about the type, time, and estimated energy cost of physical activities performed during specified periods (e.g., 7 days). Summary scores for daily activity-related EE (e.g., MET min·day^{-1}) or for specific categories of activity (e.g., exercise or sport, sleep, occupation) can be tracked for individual or groups of athletes. Because the log is completed at the end of the day, the degree of recall bias associated with this method of quantifying activity-related EE is likely higher than with the physical activity record, but considerably less than more traditional approaches (e.g., questionnaires).[106]

Physical activity logs may be more convenient to complete and process than physical activity records as they are less time consuming for the respondent and contain less information for data processing. Alternatively, activity logs may underestimate actual activity-related EE if participants engage in activities other than those listed on the log.

c. Physical Activity Questionnaires

Self-report questionnaires are the most frequently used method of assessing physical activity levels among free-living individuals. Based on their level of detail and subject burden, activity questionnaires are generally classified as global, recall, and quantitative history instruments.[6,13] Table 6.3 provides a list of questionnaires that have been used to estimate physical activity and EE in various studies. To date, there has been no self-reported physical activity questionnaires designed specifically for athletic populations.

i. Global Questionnaires

Global activity questionnaires are typically one to four items long and provide an estimate of an individual's general physical activity level (Figure 6.3). They are short and easy to complete, but global questionnaires provide little detail on specific types and patterns of physical activity. Therefore, global questionnaires allow for only simple classifications of activity status (e.g., active vs. inactive)[107,126] and do not generally allow for precise assessment of activity-related EE. Global questionnaires are preferred in physical activity surveillance systems[112] where samples sizes are very large, administrative time is limited, and the goal for assessment may be to merely classify respondents as inactive or active at levels recommended for health benefits. The accuracy and reproducibility of global activity instruments have been reported.[29,101,108] Age-adjusted test–retest correlations of 0.90 and 0.81 for men and women, respectively, and an age-sex-adjusted coefficient of determination of 0.29 between the activity score and maximal aerobic capacity have been reported for the two-point (e.g., active vs. inactive) Lipid Research Clinic's global activity question.[108] Lack of detail on the type, frequency, duration, and intensity of physical activity render global questionnaires inadequate for estimating activity-related EE.

TABLE 6.3
Self-Report Questionnaires Used to Quantify Levels of Physical Activity and Energy Expenditure in Free-Living Populations

Method/Questionnaire	Physical Activity Domains	Recall Time Frame	Expression of Physical Activity Score	Reference
Global				
Lipid Research Clinics	JOB, EX	Usual day	2- and 4-point scale	Siscovick et al. 1988[107] Ainsworth et al. 1993[108]
Minnesota Heart Health	EX, JOB	General	$MET \cdot min^{-1} \cdot d^{-1}$	Sidney et al. 1991[109]
Stanford Usual	MOD & VIG Lifestyle PA	Usual Day	MOD – 6 point scale VIG – 5 point scale	Sallis et al. 1985[30]
Behavioral Risk Factor Surveillance System (BRFSS) Occupational	JOB	Usual Day	1-item selection	Yore et al. 2006[110]
Short Telephone Activity Recall (STAR)	MOD & VIG Lifestyle PA	Usual Week	$min \cdot wk^{-1}$	Matthews et al. 2005[105]
Recall Questionnaires				
Baecke Habitual Physical Activity	JOB, EX, LEIS	General	Indices for Work, Sport, Leisure, Total	Baecke et al. 1982[111]
Behavioral Risk Factor Surveillance System (BRFSS)	MOD & VIG Lifestyle PA	Usual Week	3-point scale	Macera et al. 2000[112]
International Physical Activity Questionnaire (IPAQ) – Short Form	MOD & VIG Lifestyle PA, WALK, INAC	Past 7 Days	3-point scale	Craig et al. 2003[113]
IPAQ – Long Form	JOB, HH, EX/REC/LEIS TRANS, INAC	Past 7 Days	3-point scale	Craig et al. 2003[113]
Behavioral Risk Factor Surveillance System (BRFSS) Walking	Lifestyle WALK	Usual Week	3-point scale	Addy et al. 2004[114]
Occupational Physical Activity Questionnaire (OPAQ)	JOB	Usual week	$hr \cdot wk^{-1}$	Reis et al. 2005[115]
Stanford 7-Day Recall	JOB, EX, LEIS	Past 7 Days	$kcal \cdot kg^{-1} \cdot d^{-1}$	Blair et al. 1985[116]
College Alumnus	EX, LEIS, STAIR	Past 7 Days	$kcal \cdot wk^{-1}$	Paffenbarger, 1978[117]
Kuopio 7-Day Recall	EX	Past 7 Days	$kcal \cdot wk^{-1}$	Lakka et al. 1992[118]

(Continued)

TABLE 6.3 (CONTINUED)
Self-Report Questionnaires Used to Quantify Levels of Physical Activity
and Energy Expenditure in Free-Living Populations

Method/Questionnaire	Physical Activity Domains	Recall Time Frame	Expression of Physical Activity Score	Reference
Kuopio Occupational	JOB	Typical Day	$kcal \cdot d^{-1}$	Lakka et al. 1992[118]
Typical Week Survey	JOB, EX, LEIS, TRAN, HH	Typical week in past month	$MET \cdot min^{-1} \cdot d^{-1}$	Ainsworth et al. 2000[70]
Quantitative History:				
Minnesota Leisure Time	EX, SP, LEIS, HH	Past Year	$AMI \cdot d^{-1}$	Taylor et al. 1978[119]
Tecumseh Occupation	JOB, TRANS	Past Year	$MET \cdot hr \cdot wk^{-1}$	Montoye et al. 1971[120]
Modifiable Activity Questionnaire	EX, LEIS, JOB, TRAN	Past Year	$MET \cdot hr \cdot wk^{-1}$	Kriska et al. 1990[121]
Modifiable Activity Questionnaire for Adolescents	EX	Past Year	$MET \cdot hr \cdot wk^{-1}$	Aaron et al. 1995[122]
Kuopio Leisure Time	EX, LEIS	Past Year	$kcal \cdot mon^{-1}$	Lakka et al. 1993[123]
CHAMPS	EX, LEIS, INAC, HH	Past 4 weeks	$Kcal \cdot wk^{-1}$ Frequency/week	Stewart et al. 2001[124]
Historical PA	SP, LEIS	Lifetime	Ordinal Scale in $hr \cdot wk^{-1}$ and $kcal \cdot wk^{-1}$	Kriska et al. 1988[125]

EX = Exercise; LEIS = Leisure; JOB = Occupational; INAC = Inactivity; TRAN = Transportation; HH = Household and Yard; STAIR = Stair Climbing; MOD = Moderate Intensity; VIG = Vigorous; PA = Physical Activity, SP = Sport, AMI = Activity Metabolic Index.

ii. Recall Questionnaires

Recall instruments are more burdensome (7–20 items) to complete than their global counterparts, but these questionnaires ask for details on the frequency, duration, and types of physical activity performed during the past day, week, or month (Figure 6.3). Scoring systems vary among recall questionnaires, ranging from simple ordinal scales (e.g., 1–5 representing low to high levels of physical activity),[111] to comprehensive summary scores of continuous data (e.g, kcal, kJ, or $MET \cdot min \cdot d^{-1}$).[88,116,127] The advantage of the latter measure is the ability to quantify time spent (e.g., $min \cdot d^{-1}$) performing specific physical activities, as well as their related EE.

Recall surveys have demonstrated acceptable levels of accuracy and repeatability.[29,70,73,88,116,128] The International Physical Activity Questionnaire (IPAQ) is an example of a recall questionnaire that has both short and long versions.[113] The IPAQ questionnaires are printed in various languages and are available for download at www.ipaq.ki.se.[129] The short version of the IPAQ has seven items that assess the duration (hr·d^{-1}) and frequency (d·wk^{-1}) spent in occupational-, moderate- and vigorous-intensity lifestyle physical activities, walking activities, and inactivity. Spearman correlations are on the order of 0.66 to 0.88 for 1-week test-retest reliability and 0.02 to 0.47 for validity as compared with the Actigraph accelerometer.[113] The long version of the IPAQ separates the various domains of physical activity (i.e. occupational, household, transportation, walking, moderate- and vigorous-intensity exercise activity, and inactivity). Spearman rank order correlations for the long form were 0.70 to 0.91 for 1-week test–retest reliability and 0.05 to 0.52 for validity as compared with the Actigraph accelerometer.[113]

With regard to other recall questionnaires, the 1-month test–retest correlations for activity-related EE computed from self-reported walking, stair climbing, and sport activity were 0.61 and 0.75 for men and women, respectively, who completed the College Alumnus questionnaire.[128] Criterion validity correlations between activity-related EE and an accelerometer METs·d^{-1} and kcal·d^{-1} were 0.29 and 0.17, respectively for all participants. Richardson et al.[73] observed age-adjusted test–retest correlations of 0.60 and 0.36 for total MET·min·d^{-1} of EE among men and women, respectively, who completed the Stanford 7-Day Activity Recall twice over 26 days apart. Age-adjusted criterion validity correlations for total daily EE between the 7-day recall and the accelerometer were 0.54 and 0.20 for men and women, respectively and, between the 7-day recall and 48-hr physical activity records, were 0.58 and 0.32 for men and women, respectively.

Recall surveys typically do a poor job of assessing non-occupational, non-leisure activity-related EE (e.g., household or transportation),[7,29,88] which may be particularly relevant sources of health-related EE among women and minorities[24,130] and may partially explain the lower correlations between self-reported and objectively measured activity levels among women. Ainsworth et al.[70] have reported data from a comprehensive Typical Week Survey administered to middle-aged minority women. This survey is very detailed and requires respondents to recall frequency and duration of several types of activities including items for house and family care, exercise and sport, and occupation. Age-adjusted test–retest correlations were 0.43 and 0.68 summary scores for total, light, moderate, and vigorous MET-min·d^{-1} of activity-related EE, and age-adjusted criterion validity correlations were 0.45 and 0.54 between detailed physical activity records and logs and the activity summary scores. Despite being one of the most detailed and comprehensive recall questionnaires, the validity and reliability characteristics of the Typical Week Activity Survey[70] were similar or better than other more frequently used recall questionnaires.[73,111,116,127]

There are two primary limitations to physical activity recall instruments. First, the physical activity estimate is subject to errors in recall that may result in biased measures of activity-related EE.[131–133] This bias seems to be intensity-related in that recall error is typically highest for light- and moderate-intensity physical activities that are habitual in nature (e.g., walking, housework).[29,73,104,132] This may be particularly relevant when trying to quantify activity-related EE among athletic populations who have little trouble remembering planned bouts of vigorous sports activity, but pay little attention to other sources of habitual daily EE (e.g., walking on campus or at work) that may contribute substantially to an individual's total energy requirements. Second, the structure of the instrument may not include relevant population-specific sources of activity-related EE, which would likely lead to an under-representation of an individual's actual physical activity level and related EE.[7,9]

iii. Quantitative History Questionnaires

Quantitative histories (Figure 6.3) are detailed (e.g., >20 items) records of the frequency and duration of leisure-time or occupational physical activities over the past year[119,120] or lifetime.[125] Activity scores are usually expressed as a continuous variable (e.g., kcal·kg^{-1}·min^{-1}), allowing for the evaluation of activity-related EE. The most frequently used quantitative history is the Minnesota Leisure Time Physical Activity Questionnaire (MNLTPA),[119] which uses a 1-year recall frame to identify the frequency (events per year) and average duration (hr or min per event) of 74 activity items in categories of walking, conditioning, hunting and fishing, water, winter, sports, home repair, and household maintenance activities. Richardson et al.[75] reported age-adjusted 1-year test–retest correlations for total, light, moderate, and heavy MET-min·d^{-1} of activity-related EE of 0.69, 0.60, 0.32, and 0.71, respectively, among adults responding to the MNLTPA. These investigators also showed age-adjusted criterion validity correlations of 0.75. 0.72. 0.70 and 0.75 between MNLTPA and 4-week activity history summary scores of total, light, moderate, and heavy MET-min·d^{-1}.

Similar to the "remote diet recall" used to assess past dietary habits,[79] quantitative activity histories are useful in settings where investigators and practitioners are interested in detailing activity-related EE patterns over long periods of time (e.g., 12 months). The intensive administrative burden (e.g., 60 min) and recall effort required by the respondent limits the feasibility of these instruments.

V. MEASURES OF PHYSICAL INACTIVITY

Physical inactivity is defined as a state in which body movement is minimal.[134] Inactivity can be categorized into behaviors that are modifiable, such as television viewing and recreational computer use vs. necessary sedentary behaviors such as sleeping, sitting while engaging in homework (children), or occupational activities. Although the U.S. Surgeon General has determined that physical inactivity is a major health risk factor for various chronic diseases, the quantification of physical inactivity has received far less attention than physical activity participation. Furthermore, there is limited published evidence in current literature regarding the reliability and validity of measures that can be used to accurately assess sedentary behavior.[135]

Researchers often focus on modifiable sedentary activities when quantifying physical inactivity. In both children and adults, researchers often examine the average amount of time spent viewing television or videos and playing computer/video games, and sometimes even include reading or napping.[135–145]

There has also been considerable interest in assessing physical inactivity through the use of objective monitoring, such as accelerometers.[105] As mentioned previously, accelerometers have the capability of providing information relating to patterns of physical activity. Data is output as counts per minute, which is an expression of change in acceleration during a 1-minute time period. Therefore, a count of zero may indicate time spent in sedentary activity, especially if zero counts are accumulated over longer periods of time. For example, zero counts accumulated over a 30-minute span may indicate that the individual was inactive during that time period. However, since a zero count may also be reflective of removal of the monitor, this information should be used with caution. The use of a supplemental activity diary indicating wear time may allow the investigator to better differentiate between monitor removal or inactivity.

VI. SUMMARY

Many direct and indirect methods are available to measure physical activity and its related EE under free-living conditions. These measurements exist along a continuum of precision, cost, and administrative burdens. Sophisticated laboratory measures of EE are not feasible for studying large numbers of individuals under free-living conditions, but may not be appropriate to evaluate individual athletes thought to be at high risk for energy imbalance and the related consequences on performance and health parameters. The utility of direct laboratory procedures for measuring EE as a means of validating field techniques for assessing activity-related EE, however, should not be understated.

Field measures are often used to assess activity-related EE with an acknowledged trade-off between precision and practicality. Each method is limited by between- and within-person variation in the measured variable, as well as ancillary factors that may confound each method's true association with activity-related EE. Portable indirect calorimeters may be the most accurate indirect method for assessing activity-related EE in the field, but costs, restricted movement, and the potential for altered usual behavior limit using this technique as the gold-standard field measure. Development of small, non-obtrusive integrated systems that employ multiple indirect measures of activity-related EE (e.g., HR, body temperature, ventilation, acceleration, steps) may improve the accuracy and feasibility of estimating EE under field conditions. Physical activity records and questionnaires are the least expensive and least burdensome methods that allow for detailed assessment of activity-related EE under free-living conditions, although how well an instrument represents population-specific activity behaviors and recall biases are concerns. Use of standardized methods for assigning energy costs to self-reported (e.g., activity log, recall questionnaire) or objectively measured (e.g., accelerometer), free-living physical activities will improve the accuracy and reproducibility of these field measures.

ACKNOWLEDGMENT

The authors would like to acknowledge Kristi L. Storti, PhD, for her contribution to this chapter.

REFERENCES

1. *Physical Activity and Health: A Report of the Surgeon General.* Atlanta, U.S. Department of Health and Human Services, Centers for Disease Control and Prevention National Center for Chronic Disease Prevention and Health Promotion, 1996.

2. Pate, R. R. and Branch, J. D., Training for endurance sport, *Med Sci Sports Exerc* 24 (9 Suppl), S340–3, 1992.

3. Haskell, W. L., *Dose–Response Issues from a Biological Perspective*, Human Kinetics, Champaign, IL, 1994.

4. Hill, J. O., Melby, C., Johnson, S. L., and Peters, J. C., Physical activity and energy requirements, *Am J Clin Nutr* 62 (5 Suppl), 1059S–1066S, 1995.

5. Joint Position Statement: Nutrition and athletic performance. American College of Sports Medicine, American Dietetic Association, and Dietitians of Canada, *Med Sci Sports Exerc* 32 (12), 2130–45, 2000.

6. Ainsworth, B. E., Montoye, H. J., and Leon, A. S., *Methods of Assessing Physical Activity During Leisure and Work*, Human Kinetics, Champaign, IL, 1994.

7. Lamonte, M. J. and Ainsworth, B. E., Quantifying energy expenditure and physical activity in the context of dose response, *Med Sci Sports Exerc* 33 (6 Suppl), S370–8; discussion S419–20, 2001.

8. Thomas, J. R. and Nelson, J. K., *Research Methods in Physical Activity*, 3rd ed. Human Kinetics, Champaign, IL, 1996.

9. Ainsworth, B. E., *Barrow and McGee's Practical Measurement and Assessment*, 5th ed. Lippincott, Williams and Wilkens, Baltimore, MD, 2000.

10. Caspersen, C. J., Powell, K. E., and Christenson, G. M., Physical activity, exercise, and physical fitness: definitions and distinctions for health-related research, *Public Health Rep* 100 (2), 126–31, 1985.

11. Corbin, C. B., Pangrazi, R. P., and Franks, B. D., Definitions: Health, fitness and physical activity, *Res. Dig.* 3, 1, 2000.

12. Brooks, G. A., Fahey, T. D., and White, T. P., *Exercise Physiology: Human Bioenergetics and its Application*, 2nd edition ed. Mayfield Publishing, Mountain View, CA, 1996.

13. Montoye, H. J., Kemper, H. C. G., Saris, W. H. M., and Washburn, R. A., *Measuring Physical Activity and Energy Expenditure,* Human Kinetics, Champaign, IL, 1996.

14. Ainsworth, B. E., Haskell, W. L., Leon, A. S., Jacobs, D. R., Jr., Montoye, H. J., Sallis, J. F., and Paffenbarger, R. S., Jr., Compendium of physical activities: Classification of energy costs of human physical activities, *Med Sci Sports Exerc* 25 (1), 71–80, 1993.

15. Ainsworth, B. E., Haskell, W. L., Whitt, M. C., Irwin, M. L., Swartz, A. M., Strath, S. J., O'Brien, W. L., Bassett, D. R., Jr., Schmitz, K. H., Emplaincourt, P. O., Jacobs, D. R., Jr., and Leon, A. S., Compendium of physical activities: an update of activity codes and MET intensities, *Med Sci Sports Exerc* 32 (9 Suppl), S498–504, 2000.

16. American College of Sports Medicine Position Stand. The recommended quantity and quality of exercise for developing and maintaining cardiorespiratory and muscular fitness, and flexibility in healthy adults, *Med Sci Sports Exerc* 30 (6), 975–91, 1998.

17. Pate, R. R., Pratt, M., Blair, S. N., Haskell, W. L., Macera, C. A., Bouchard, C., Buchner, D., Ettinger, W., Heath, G. W., King, A. C., and et al., Physical activity and public health. A recommendation from the Centers for Disease Control and Prevention and the American College of Sports Medicine, *JAMA* 273 (5), 402–7, 1995.

18. Stolarczyk, L. M., Addy, C. L., Ainsworth, B. E., Chang, C., and Heyward, V., Accuracy of self–reported physical activity intensity in minority women., *Med Sci Sports Exerc* 30 (5 (supplement)), S10, 1998.

19. Gretebeck, R. J. and Montoye, H. J., Variability of some objective measures of physical activity, *Med Sci Sports Exerc* 24 (10), 1167–72, 1992.

20. Levin, S., Jacobs, D. R., Jr., Ainsworth, B. E., Richardson, M. T., and Leon, A. S., Intra-individual variation and estimates of usual physical activity, *Ann Epidemiol* 9 (8), 481–8, 1999.

21. Uitenbroek, D. G., Seasonal variation in leisure time physical activity, *Med Sci Sports Exerc* 25 (6), 755–60, 1993.

22. Robertson, R. J., Caspersen, C. J., Allison, T. G., Skrinar, G. S., Abbott, R. A., and Metz, K. F., Differentiated perceptions of exertion and energy cost of young women while carrying loads, *Eur J Appl Physiol Occup Physiol* 49 (1), 69–78, 1982.

23. Ainsworth, B. E., Richardson, M. T., Jacobs, D. R., and Leon, A. S., Gender differences in physical activity, *Women Sports Phys. Activ. J.* 1, 1, 1993.

24. Henderson, K. A. and Ainsworth, B. E., Sociocultural perspectives on physical activity in the lives of older African American and American Indian women: A cross cultural activity participation study, *Women Health* 31 (1), 1–20, 2000.

25. McArdle, W. D., Katch, F. I., and Katch, V. L., *Exercise physiology: Energy, nutrition and human performance*, 3rd ed. Lea & Febiger, Philadelphia, PA, 1991.

26. Howley, E. T., You asked for it. Question authority, *ACSM's Hlth Fitness J* 3, 12, 1999.

27. Sparrow, W. A., *Energetics of Human Activity,* Human Kinetics, Champaign, IL, 2001.

28. Arroll, B. and Beaglehole, R., Potential misclassification in studies of physical activity, *Med Sci Sports Exerc* 23 (10), 1176–8, 1991.

29. Jacobs, D. R., Jr., Ainsworth, B. E., Hartman, T. J., and Leon, A. S., A simultaneous evaluation of 10 commonly used physical activity questionnaires, *Med Sci Sports Exerc* 25 (1), 81–91, 1993.

30. Sallis, J. F., Haskell, W. L., Wood, P. D., Fortmann, S. P., Rogers, T., Blair, S. N., and Paffenbarger, R. S., Jr., Physical activity assessment methodology in the Five-City Project, *Am J Epidemiol* 121 (1), 91–106, 1985.

31. Bassett, D. R., Validity and reliability in objective monitoring of physical activity, *Res. Q. Exerc. Sport.* 71, 30, 2000.

32. Freedson, P. S. and Miller, K., Objective monitoring of physical activity using motion sensors and heart rate., *Res. Q. Exerc. Sport.* 71, 21, 2000.

33. Washburn, R. A. and Montoye, H. J., The assessment of physical activity by questionnaire, *Am J Epidemiol* 123 (4), 563–76, 1986.

34. Ainsworth, B. E. and Coleman, K. J., *Physical Activity Measurement,* Taylor & Francis, Boca Raton, FL, 2006.

35. Lamonte, M. J., Ainsworth, B. E., and Tudor-Locke, C. E., *Assessment of Physical Activity and Energy Expenditure,* Human Kinetics, Champaign, IL, 2003.

36. Berlin, J. E., Storti, K. L., and Brach, J. S., Using activity monitors to measure physical activity in free-living conditions, *Phys Ther* 86 (8), 1137–45, 2006.

37. Steele, B. G., Belza, B., Cain, K., Warms, C., Coppersmith, J., and Howard, J., Bodies in motion: Monitoring daily activity and exercise with motion sensors in people with chronic pulmonary disease, *J Rehabil Res Dev* 40 (5 Suppl 2), 45–58, 2003.

38. Vanhees, L., Lefevre, J., Philippaerts, R., Martens, M., Huygens, W., Troosters, T., and Beunen, G., How to assess physical activity? How to assess physical fitness?, *Eur J Cardiovasc Prev Rehabil* 12 (2), 102–14, 2005.

39. Bjornson, K. F., Physical activity monitoring in children and youths, *Pediatr Phys Ther* 17 (1), 37–45, 2005.

40. Chen, K. Y. and Bassett, D. R., Jr., The technology of accelerometry-based activity monitors: current and future, *Med Sci Sports Exerc* 37 (11 Suppl), S490–500, 2005.

41. Conway, J. M., Seale, J. L., Irwin, M. L., Jacobs, D. R., and Ainsworth, B. E., Ability of 7-day physical activity diaries and recalls to estimate free-living EE, *Obesity Research* 7 (Supplement 1), 107S, 1999.

42. Ferrannini, E., The theoretical bases of indirect calorimetry: A review, *Metabolism* 37 (3), 287–301, 1988.

43. Lifson, N., Gordon, G. B., and Mc, C. R., Measurement of total carbon dioxide production by means of D2O18, *J Appl Physiol* 7 (6), 704–10, 1955.

44. Speakman, J. R., The history and theory of the doubly labeled water technique, *Am J Clin Nutr* 68 (4), 932S–938S, 1998.

45. Black, A. E., Prentice, A. M., and Coward, W. A., Use of food quotients to predict respiratory quotients for the doubly-labelled water method of measuring energy expenditure, *Hum Nutr Clin Nutr* 40 (5), 381–91, 1986.

46. Schultz, S., Westerterp, K., and Bruck, K., Comparison of EE by the doubly labeled water technique with energy intake, heart rate and activity recording in man., *Am J Clin Nutr* 49, 1146, 1989.

47. Seale, J. L., Rumpler, W. V., Conway, J. M., and Miles, C. W., Comparison of doubly labeled water, intake-balance, and direct- and indirect-calorimetry methods for measuring energy expenditure in adult men, *Am J Clin Nutr* 52 (1), 66–71, 1990.

48. Westerterp, K. R., Brouns, F., Saris, W. H., and ten Hoor, F., Comparison of doubly labeled water with respirometry at low- and high-activity levels, *J Appl Physiol* 65 (1), 53–6, 1988.

49. Black, A. E., Coward, W. A., Cole, T. J., and Prentice, A. M., Human energy expenditure in affluent societies: An analysis of 574 doubly-labelled water measurements, *Eur J Clin Nutr* 50 (2), 72–92, 1996.

50. 2004.

51. Elia, M., Fuller, N. J., and Murgatroyd, P. R., Measurement of bicarbonate turnover in humans: applicability to estimation of energy expenditure, *Am J Physiol* 263 (4 Pt 1), E676–87, 1992.

52. Elia, M., Jones, M. G., Jennings, G., Poppitt, S. D., Fuller, N. J., Murgatroyd, P. R., and Jebb, S. A., Estimating energy expenditure from specific activity of urine urea during lengthy subcutaneous NaH14CO3 infusion, *Am J Physiol* 269 (1 Pt 1), E172–82, 1995.

53. Weir, J. B., New methods for calculating metabolic rate with special reference to protein metabolism, *J Physiol* 109 (1–2), 1–9, 1949.

54. Davis, J. A., *Direct Determination of Aerobic Power,* Human Kinetics, Champaign, IL, 1996.

55. Bassett, D. R., Jr., Ainsworth, B. E., Swartz, A. M., Strath, S. J., O'Brien, W. L., and King, G. A., Validity of four motion sensors in measuring moderate intensity physical activity, *Med Sci Sports Exerc* 32 (9 Suppl), S471–80, 2000.

56. King, G. A., McLaughlin, J. E., Howley, E. T., Bassett, D. R., Jr., and Ainsworth, B. E., Validation of Aerosport KB1-C portable metabolic system, *Int J Sports Med* 20 (5), 304–8, 1999.

57. Berggren, G. and Hohwu Christensen, E., Heart rate and body temperature as indices of metabolic rate during work, *Arbeitsphysiologie* 14 (3), 255–60, 1950.

58. Wilmore, J. H. and Haskell, W. L., Use of the heart rate-energy expenditure relationship in the individualized prescription of exercise, *Am J Clin Nutr* 24 (9), 1186–92, 1971.

59. Christensen, C. C., Frey, H. M., Foenstelien, E., Aadland, E., and Refsum, H. E., A critical evaluation of energy expenditure estimates based on individual O_2

consumption/heart rate curves and average daily heart rate, *Am J Clin Nutr* 37 (3), 468–72, 1983.

60. Washburn, R. and Montoye, H. J., Validity of heart rate as a measure of daily EE, *Exercise Physiology* 2, 161, 1986.

61. Haskell, W. L., Yee, M. C., Evans, A., and Irby, P. J., Simultaneous measurement of heart rate and body motion to quantitate physical activity, *Med Sci Sports Exerc* 25 (1), 109–15, 1993.

62. Livingstone, M. B., Prentice, A. M., Coward, W. A., Ceesay, S. M., Strain, J. J., McKenna, P. G., Nevin, G. B., Barker, M. E., and Hickey, R. J., Simultaneous measurement of free-living energy expenditure by the doubly labeled water method and heart-rate monitoring, *Am J Clin Nutr* 52 (1), 59–65, 1990.

63. Andrews, R. B., Net heart rate as a substitute for respiratory calorimetry, *Am J Clin Nutr* 24 (9), 1139–47, 1971.

64. Strath, S. J., Swartz, A. M., Bassett, D. R., Jr., O'Brien, W. L., King, G. A., and Ainsworth, B. E., Evaluation of heart rate as a method for assessing moderate intensity physical activity, *Med Sci Sports Exerc* 32 (9 Suppl), S465–70, 2000.

65. *Human Body Composition,* Human Kinetics, Champaign, IL, 1996.

66. Healey, J., Future possibilities in electric monitoring of physical activity, *Res Q Exerc Sport* 71, 137, 2000.

67. Ainsworth, B. E., Irwin, M. L., Addy, C. L., Whitt, M. C., and Stolarczyk, L. M., Moderate physical activity patterns of minority women: The Cross-Cultural Activity Participation Study, *J Wom Hlth Gend Based Med* 8 (6), 805–13, 1999.

68. Bouchard, C., Tremblay, A., Leblanc, C., Lortie, G., Savard, R., and Theriault, G., A method to assess energy expenditure in children and adults, *Am J Clin Nutr* 37 (3), 461–7, 1983.

69. Lamonte, M. J., Durstine, J. L., Addy, C. L., Irwin, M. L., and Ainsworth, B. E., Physical activity, physical fitness and Framingham 10-year risk score: The Cross-Cultural Activity Participation Study, *J. Cardiopulm. Rehab.* 21, 1, 2001.

70. Ainsworth, B. E., Lamonte, M. J., Drowatzky, K. L., Cooper, R. S., Thompson, R. W., Irwin, M. L., Whitt, M. C., and Gilman, M., Evaluation of the CAPS Typical Week Physical Activity Survey among minority women, in *Proc. Community Prevention Res. in Women's Health Conference*, Bethesda, MD, 2000.

71. Fogelholm, M., Hiilloskorpi, H., Laukkanen, R., Oja, P., Van Marken Lichtenbelt, W., and Westerterp, K., Assessment of energy expenditure in overweight women, *Med Sci Sports Exerc* 30 (8), 1191–7, 1998.

72. Richardson, M. T., Leon, A. S., Jacobs, D. R., Jr., Ainsworth, B. E., and Serfass, R., Ability of the Caltrac accelerometer to assess daily physical activity levels, *J Cardio Rehab* 15 (2), 107–13, 1995.

73. Richardson, M. T., Ainsworth, B. E., Jacobs, D. R., and Leon, A. S., Validation of the Stanford 7-day recall to assess habitual physical activity, *Ann Epidemiol* 11 (2), 145–53, 2001.

74. American Heart Association. Start! http://www.americanheart.orgpresenter.jhtml?identifier=304077 Retrieved May 22, 2007.

75. Richardson, M. T., Leon, A. S., Jacobs, D. R., Jr., Ainsworth, B. E., and Serfass, R., Comprehensive evaluation of the Minnesota Leisure Time Physical Activity Questionnaire, *J Clin Epidemiol* 47 (3), 271–81, 1994.

76. Finnegan, L. P., The NIH Women's Health Initiative: Its evolution and expected contributions to women's health, *Am J Prev Med* 12 (5), 292–3, 1996.

77. Lehmann, M., Foster, C., and Keul, J., Overtraining in endurance athletes: A brief review, *Med Sci Sports Exerc* 25 (7), 854–62, 1993.

78. Brownell, K. D., Steen, S. N., and Wilmore, J. H., Weight regulation practices in athletes: Analysis of metabolic and health effects, *Med Sci Sports Exerc* 19 (6), 546–56, 1987.
79. Willett, W. C., *Nutritional Epidemiology*, 2nd ed. Oxford Press, New York, NY, 1998.
80. Welk, G. J., Blair, S. N., Wood, K., Jones, S., and Thompson, R. W., A comparative evaluation of three accelerometry-based physical activity monitors, *Med Sci Sports Exerc* 32 (9 Suppl), S489-97, 2000.
81. Welk, G. J., Differding, J. A., Thompson, R. W., Blair, S. N., Dziura, J., and Hart, P., The utility of the Digi-walker step counter to assess daily physical activity patterns, *Med Sci Sports Exerc* 32 (9 Suppl), S481–8, 2000.
82. Bassett, D. R., Jr., Ainsworth, B. E., Leggett, S. R., Mathien, C. A., Main, J. A., Hunter, D. C., and Duncan, G. E., Accuracy of five electronic pedometers for measuring distance walked, *Med Sci Sports Exerc* 28 (8), 1071–7, 1996.
83. Crouter, S. E., Schneider, P. L., Karabulut, M., and Bassett, D. R., Jr., Validity of 10 electronic pedometers for measuring steps, distance, and energy cost, *Med Sci Sports Exerc* 35 (8), 1455–60, 2003.
84. Leenders, N., Sherman, W. M., and Nagaraja, H. N., Comparisons of four methods of estimating physical activity in adult women, *Med Sci Sports Exerc* 32 (7), 1320–6, 2000.
85. Nelson, T. E., Leenders, N., and Sherman, W. M., Comparison of activity monitors worn during treadmill walking, *Med Sci Sports Exerc* 30 (5 Supplement), S11, 1998.
86. Tudor-Locke, C. E., Williams, J. E., Reis, J. P., and Pluto, D., Utility of pedometers for assessing physical activity: Convergent validity, *Sports Medicine* 32 (12), 795–808, 2002.
87. Tudor-Locke, C. E., Williams, J. E., Reis, J. P., and Pluto, D., Utility of pedometers for assessing physical activity: Construct validity, *Sports Medicine* 34 (5), 281–291, 2004.
88. Ainsworth, B. E., LaMonte, M. J., Whitt, M. C., Irwin, M. L., and Drowatzky, K. L., Development and Validation of a Physical Activity Questionnaire to Assess Moderate Intensity Activity in Minority Women, Ages 40 and Older, in *Proc. NIH Women's Health Community Research Conference*, 2000.
89. Scruggs, P. W., Beveridge, S. K., Eisenman, P. A., Watson, D. L., Shultz, B. B., and Ransdell, L. B., Quantifying physical activity via pedometry in elementary physical education, *Med Sci Sports Exerc* 35 (6), 1065–71, 2003.
90. Macko, R. F., Haeuber, E., Shaughnessy, M., Coleman, K. L., Boone, D. A., Smith, G. V., and Silver, K. H., Microprocessor-based ambulatory activity monitoring in stroke patients, *Med Sci Sports Exerc* 34 (3), 394–9, 2002.
91. Dunn, A. L., Garcia, M. E., Marcus, B. H., Kampert, J. B., Kohl, H. W., and Blair, S. N., Six-month physical activity and fitness changes in Project Active, a randomized trial, *Med Sci Sports Exerc* 30 (7), 1076–83, 1998.
92. Dunn, A. L., Marcus, B. H., Kampert, J. B., Garcia, M. E., Kohl, H. W., 3rd, and Blair, S. N., Reduction in cardiovascular disease risk factors: 6-month results from Project Active, *Prev Med* 26 (6), 883–92, 1997.
93. Kohl, H. W., 3rd, Dunn, A. L., Marcus, B. H., and Blair, S. N., A randomized trial of physical activity interventions: Design and baseline data from project active, *Med Sci Sports Exerc* 30 (2), 275–83, 1998.
94. Tudor-Locke, C. E. and Myers, A. M., Methodological considerations for researchers and practitioners using pedometers to measure physical (ambulatory) activity, *Res Q Exerc Sport* 72 (1), 1–12, 2001.
95. Freedson, P. S., Melanson, E., and Sirard, J., Calibration of the Computer Science and Applications, Inc. accelerometer, *Med Sci Sports Exerc* 30 (5), 777–81, 1998.

96. Hendelman, D., Miller, K., Baggett, C., Debold, E., and Freedson, P., Validity of accelerometry for the assessment of moderate intensity physical activity in the field, *Med Sci Sports Exerc* 32 (9 Suppl), S442–9, 2000.

97. Montoye, H. J., Washburn, R., Servais, S., Ertl, A., Webster, J. G., and Nagle, F. J., Estimation of energy expenditure by a portable accelerometer, *Med Sci Sports Exerc* 15 (5), 403–7, 1983.

98. Nichols, J. F., Morgan, C. G., Sarkin, J. A., Sallis, J. F., and Calfas, K. J., Validity, reliability, and calibration of the Tritrac accelerometer as a measure of physical activity, *Med Sci Sports Exerc* 31 (6), 908–12, 1999.

99. Swartz, A. M., Strath, S. J., Bassett, D. R., Jr., O'Brien, W. L., King, G. A., and Ainsworth, B. E., Estimation of energy expenditure using CSA accelerometers at hip and wrist sites, *Med Sci Sports Exerc* 32 (9 Suppl), S450–6, 2000.

100. Melanson, E. L., Jr. and Freedson, P. S., Validity of the Computer Science and Applications, Inc. (CSA) activity monitor, *Med Sci Sports Exerc* 27 (6), 934–40, 1995.

101. Ainsworth, B. E., Bassett, D. R., Jr., Strath, S. J., Swartz, A. M., O'Brien, W. L., Thompson, R. W., Jones, D. A., Macera, C. A., and Kimsey, C. D., Comparison of three methods for measuring the time spent in physical activity, *Med Sci Sports Exerc* 32 (9 Suppl), S457–64, 2000.

102. Nichols, J. F., Morgan, C. G., Chabot, L. E., Sallis, J. F., and Calfas, K. J., Assessment of physical activity with the Computer Science and Applications, Inc., accelerometer: Laboratory versus field validation, *Res Q Exerc Sport* 71 (1), 36–43, 2000.

103. Rost, S. G., McIver, K., Pate, R. R., Objective monitoring of physical activity: Closing the gaps in the science of accelerometry, *Med Sci Sports Exerc* 37 (Suppl. 11), S487–S588, 2005.

104. Matthews, C. E., Freedson, P. S., Hebert, J. R., Stanek, E. J., 3rd, Merriam, P. A., and Ockene, I. S., Comparing physical activity assessment methods in the Seasonal Variation of Blood Cholesterol Study, *Med Sci Sports Exerc* 32 (5), 976–84, 2000.

105. Matthews, C. E., Ainsworth, B. E., Hanby, C., Pate, R. R., Addy, C., Freedson, P. S., Jones, D. A., and Macera, C. A., Development and testing of a short physical activity recall questionnaire, *Med Sci Sports Exerc* 37 (6), 986–94, 2005.

106. Kriska, A. M. and Caspersen, C. J., Introduction to a Collection of Physical Activity Questionnaire, *Med Sci Sports Exerc* 29 (Supplement 6), S5–S9, 1997.

107. Siscovick, D. S., Ekelund, L. G., Hyde, J. S., Johnson, J. L., Gordon, D. J., and LaRosa, J. C., Physical activity and coronary heart disease among asymptomatic hypercholesterolemic men (the Lipid Research Clinics Coronary Primary Prevention Trial), *Am J Public Health* 78 (11), 1428–31, 1988.

108. Ainsworth, B. E., Jacobs, D. R., Jr., and Leon, A. S., Validity and reliability of self-reported physical activity status: The Lipid Research Clinics questionnaire, *Med Sci Sports Exerc* 25 (1), 92–8, 1993.

109. Sidney, S., Jacobs, D. R., Jr., Haskell, W. L., Armstrong, M. A., Dimicco, A., Oberman, A., Savage, P. J., Slattery, M. L., Sternfeld, B., and Van Horn, L., Comparison of two methods of assessing physical activity in the Coronary Artery Risk Development in Young Adults (CARDIA) Study, *Am J Epidemiol* 133 (12), 1231–45, 1991.

110. Yore, M. M., Bowles, H. R., Ainsworth, B. E., Macera, C. A., and Kohl, H. W., Single- Versus Multiple-Item Questions on Occupational Physical Activity, *J Phys Act Health* 1, 102–111, 2006.

111. Baecke, J. A., Burema, J., and Frijters, J. E., A short questionnaire for the measurement of habitual physical activity in epidemiological studies, *Am J Clin Nutr* 36 (5), 936–42, 1982.

112. Macera, C. A. and Pratt, M., Public health surveillance of physical activity., *Res. Q. Exerc. Sport.* 71, 97, 2000.

113. Craig, C. L., Marshall, A. L., Sjostrom, M., Bauman, A. E., Booth, M. L., Ainsworth, B. E., Pratt, M., Ekelund, U., Yngve, A., Sallis, J. F., and Oja, P., International physical activity questionnaire: 12-country reliability and validity, *Med Sci Sports Exerc* 35 (8), 1381–95, 2003.

114. Addy, C. L., Wilson, D. K., Kirtland, K. A., Ainsworth, B. E., Sharpe, P., and Kimsey, D., Associations of perceived social and physical environmental supports with physical activity and walking behavior, *Am J Public Health* 94 (3), 440–3, 2004.

115. Reis, J. P., Dubose, K. D., Ainsworth, B. E., Macera, C. A., and Yore, M. M., Reliability and validity of the occupational physical activity questionnaire, *Med Sci Sports Exerc* 37 (12), 2075–83, 2005.

116. Blair, S. N., Haskell, W. L., Ho, P., Paffenbarger, R. S., Jr., Vranizan, K. M., Farquhar, J. W., and Wood, P. D., Assessment of habitual physical activity by a seven–day recall in a community survey and controlled experiments, *Am J Epidemiol* 122 (5), 794–804, 1985.

117. Paffenbarger, R. S., Jr., Wing, A. L., and Hyde, R. T., Physical activity as an index of heart attack risk in college alumni, *Am J Epidemiol* 108 (3), 161–75, 1978.

118. Lakka, T. A. and Salonen, J. T., Intra-person variability of various physical activity assessments in the Kuopio Ischaemic Heart Disease Risk Factor Study, *Int J Epidemiol* 21 (3), 467–72, 1992.

119. Taylor, H. L., Jacobs, D. R., Jr., Schucker, B., Knudsen, J., Leon, A. S., and Debacker, G., A questionnaire for the assessment of leisure time physical activities, *J Chronic Dis* 31 (12), 741–55, 1978.

120. Montoye, H. J., Estimation of habitual physical activity by questionnaire and interview, *Am J Clin Nutr* 24 (9), 1113–8, 1971.

121. Kriska, A. M., Knowler, W. C., LaPorte, R. E., Drash, A. L., Wing, R. R., Blair, S. N., Bennett, P. H., and Kuller, L. H., Development of questionnaire to examine relationship of physical activity and diabetes in Pima Indians, *Diabetes Care* 13 (4), 401–11, 1990.

122. Aaron, D. J., Kriska, A. M., Dearwater, S. R., Cauley, J. A., Metz, K. F., and LaPorte, R. E., Reproducibility and validity of an epidemiologic questionnaire to assess past year physical activity in adolescents, *Am J Epidemiol* 142 (2), 191–201, 1995.

123. Lakka, T. A. and Salonen, J. T., Moderate to high intensity conditioning leisure time physical activity and high cardiorespiratory fitness are associated with reduced plasma fibrinogen in eastern Finnish men, *J Clin Epidemiol* 46 (10), 1119–27, 1993.

124. Stewart, A. L., Mills, K. M., King, A. C., Haskell, W. L., Gillis, D., and Ritter, P. L., CHAMPS physical activity questionnaire for older adults: Outcomes for interventions, *Med Sci Sports Exerc* 33 (7), 1126–41, 2001.

125. Kriska, A. M., Sandler, R. B., Cauley, J. A., LaPorte, R. E., Hom, D. L., and Pambianco, G., The assessment of historical physical activity and its relation to adult bone parameters, *Am J Epidemiol* 127 (5), 1053–63, 1988.

126. Belloc, N. B. and Breslow, L., Relationship of physical health status and health practices, *Prev Med* 1 (3), 409–21, 1972.

127. Paffenbarger, R. S., Jr., Hyde, R. T., Wing, A. L., and Hsieh, C. C., Physical activity, all-cause mortality, and longevity of college alumni, *N Engl J Med* 314 (10), 605–13, 1986.

128. Ainsworth, B. E., Leon, A. S., Richardson, M. T., Jacobs, D. R., and Paffenbarger, R. S., Jr., Accuracy of the College Alumnus Physical Activity Questionnaire, *J Clin Epidemiol* 46 (12), 1403–11, 1993.

129. International Physical Activity Questionnaire. http://www.ipaq.ki.se. Retrieved May 22, 2007.

130. Weller, I. and Corey, P., The impact of excluding non-leisure energy expenditure on the relation between physical activity and mortality in women, *Epidemiology* 9 (6), 632–5, 1998.

131. Baranowski, T., Validity and reliability of self-report measures of physical activity: An information-processing perspective., *Res. Q. Exerc. Sport.* 59, 314, 1988.

132. Durante, R. and Ainsworth, B. E., The recall of physical activity: Using a cognitive model of the question-answering process, *Med Sci Sports Exerc* 28 (10), 1282–91, 1996.

133. Lichtman, S. W., Pisarska, K., Berman, E. R., Pestone, M., Dowling, H., Offenbacher, E., Weisel, H., Heshka, S., Matthews, D. E., and Heymsfield, S. B., Discrepancy between self-reported and actual caloric intake and exercise in obese subjects, *N Engl J Med* 327 (27), 1893–8, 1992.

134. Dietz, W. H., The role of lifestyle in health: The epidemiology and consequences of inactivity, *Proc Nutr Soc* 55 (3), 829–40, 1996.

135. Gordon-Larsen, P., McMurray, R. G., and Popkin, B. M., Determinants of adolescent physical activity and inactivity patterns, *Pediatrics* 105 (6), E83, 2000.

136. Fitzgerald, S. J., Kriska, A. M., Pereira, M. A., and de Courten, M. P., Associations among physical activity, television watching, and obesity in adult Pima Indians, *Med Sci Sports Exerc* 29 (7), 910–5, 1997.

137. Gordon-Larsen, P., Adair, L. S., and Popkin, B. M., Ethnic differences in physical activity and inactivity patterns and overweight status, *Obes Res* 10 (3), 141–9, 2002.

138. Fung, T. T., Hu, F. B., Yu, J., Chu, N. F., Spiegelman, D., Tofler, G. H., Willett, W. C., and Rimm, E. B., Leisure-time physical activity, television watching, and plasma biomarkers of obesity and cardiovascular disease risk, *Am J Epidemiol* 152 (12), 1171–8, 2000.

139. Andersen, R. E., Crespo, C. J., Bartlett, S. J., Cheskin, L. J., and Pratt, M., Relationship of physical activity and television watching with body weight and level of fatness among children: Results from the Third National Health and Nutrition Examination Survey, *Jama* 279 (12), 938–42, 1998.

140. Hu, F. B., Li, T. Y., Colditz, G. A., Willett, W. C., and Manson, J. E., Television watching and other sedentary behaviors in relation to risk of obesity and type 2 diabetes mellitus in women, *JAMA* 289 (14), 1785–91, 2003.

141. Manson, J. E., Greenland, P., LaCroix, A. Z., Stefanick, M. L., Mouton, C. P., Oberman, A., Perri, M. G., Sheps, D. S., Pettinger, M. B., and Siscovick, D. S., Walking compared with vigorous exercise for the prevention of cardiovascular events in women, *N Engl J Med* 347 (10), 716–25, 2002.

142. Feldman, D. E., Barnett, T., Shrier, I., Rossignol, M., and Abenhaim, L., Is physical activity differentially associated with different types of sedentary pursuits? *Arch Pediatr Adolesc Med* 157 (8), 797–802, 2003.

143. Jakes, R. W., Day, N. E., Khaw, K. T., Luben, R., Oakes, S., Welch, A., Bingham, S., and Wareham, N. J., Television viewing and low participation in vigorous recreation are independently associated with obesity and markers of cardiovascular disease risk: EPIC-Norfolk population-based study, *Eur J Clin Nutr* 57 (9), 1089–96, 2003.

144. Utter, J., Neumark-Sztainer, D., Jeffery, R., and Story, M., Couch potatoes or french fries: Are sedentary behaviors associated with body mass index, physical activity, and dietary behaviors among adolescents?, *J Am Diet Assoc* 103 (10), 1298–305, 2003.

145. Evenson, K. R. and McGinn, A. P., Test-retest reliability of adult surveillance measures for physical activity and inactivity, *Am J Prev Med* 28 (5), 470–8, 2005.

Section 3

Physiological Aspects of Energy Metabolism

7 Influence of Dietary Fiber on Body Weight Regulation

Daniel D. Gallaher

CONTENTS

I. INTRODUCTION

The prevalence of obesity in the United States has reached alarming levels. As of 2004, the Centers for Disease Control estimated that 33 states had an obesity prevalence (BMI $\geq$ 30) of between 20–24% and that nine states had a prevalence $\geq$ 25%.[1] Further, the rate of increase in obesity shows little evidence of slowing. Even more alarming is the high incidence of obesity among youth, as obesity in childhood is highly predictive of adult obesity. The causes of being overweight or obese are complex, but certainly involve factors such as reduced physical activity, overconsumption of energy-dense highly palatable foods, and low socioeconomic status. The primary concern regarding obesity is, of course, the greater risk for a number of chronic diseases experienced by overweight and obese individuals. These include hypertension, type 2 diabetes, and coronary heart disease. Indeed, the rapidly increasing occurrence of type 2 diabetes is undoubtedly due to the increase in the pervasiveness of obesity.

Although no single dietary component, either by its lack or excess, is solely responsible for the dramatic increase in obesity, a number of dietary components, or their relative lack, are receiving scrutiny as playing a role in the imbalance in energy that leads to obesity. One such component is dietary fiber. Dietary fiber can be thought of as a diverse group of polymeric carbohydrate compounds that have in common a resistance to breakdown by mammalian digestive enzymes. Some definitions also include the polyphenolic compound lignin. Dietary fibers may derive from the plant cell wall, such as cellulose, hemicelluloses, pectins, and lignin, or be found intracellularly, such as gums and mucilages. Table 7.1 gives total dietary fiber values for some commonly consumed foods.

Given their diverse origin in plants, it is not surprising that dietary fibers exhibit great differences in their chemical composition and physical characteristics. Until recently, it has been common to categorize dietary fiber based on its solubility in water, i.e., soluble or insoluble fiber. However, it is now widely accepted that this method of categorization by a single chemical property is overly simplistic and does not explain well the range of physiological responses produced by different dietary fibers. It has proven far more useful to define dietary fiber in terms of its physical properties. Of these, two in particular have received the most attention. These are viscosity and susceptibility to fermentation. Although dietary fibers can exhibit a range within each of these properties, e.g., it can be slightly viscous or slightly fermentable, it is common to categorize dietary fibers in a dichotomous fashion, i.e., either highly viscous or not or highly fermentable or not. Table 7.2 indicates the viscosity and fermentability for a number of dietary fibers in such a manner.

There are three universally accepted physiological responses to consumption of dietary fiber. These are lowering of plasma cholesterol concentrations, modification of the glycemic response, and improving large-bowel function. Overwhelming evidence indicates that the reduction of plasma cholesterol and the modification of the glycemic response is associated with consumption of viscous dietary fiber sources.[2] Improving large-bowel function, however, is primarily due to consumption of nonfermentable dietary fibers.[2] In recent years, however, evidence has accumulated pointing to an important role for dietary fiber in body weight regulation. Although the physical property of dietary fiber that may be responsible for this effect and the mechanism by which it occurs is uncertain, this possible new role for dietary fiber is one that may be as important as the physiological responses that are already established.

TABLE 7.1
Dietary Fiber Content of Selected Foods

Food Item	Total Dietary Fiber (g/100 g edible portion)
Cereal grains	
White wheat flour	2.7
Whole wheat flour	12.2
Oat cereal	9.8
Corn meal	4.0
White rice	2.8
Brown rice	3.5
Pearled barley	15.6
Vegetables, raw	
Broccoli	2.6
Carrots	2.8
Cauliflower	2.5
Corn	2.7
Green beans	3.4
Green peas	5.1
Lettuce, iceberg	1.2
Lettuce, romaine	2.1
Onions	1.7
Potatoes	2.4
Spinach	2.2
Tomatoes	1.2
Fruits, raw	
Apples	2.4
Bananas	2.6
Dried plums	7.1
Oranges	2.4
Peaches	1.5
Raisins	3.7
Strawberries	2.0
Legumes, raw	
Black beans	15.2
Chickpeas	17.4
Kidney beans	24.9
Lima beans	19.0
Pinto beans	15.5
Split peas	25.5
White beans	15.2

TABLE 7.2
Viscosity and Susceptibility to Fermentation of Selected
Dietary Fibers

		Viscosity	
		High	**Low**
Fermentability	High	Guar gum β-glucans Glucomannan Pectins	Gum Acacia Oligofructose Inulin
	Low or none	Modified celluloses (e.g. methylcellulose) Psyllium	Cellulose Hemicelluloses

II. EPIDEMIOLOGICAL STUDIES

A. HISTORICAL PERSPECTIVE

Consumption of dietary fiber by ancestral humans was almost certainly vastly greater than that of current western populations. It has been estimated that Paleolithic peoples, who presumably experienced a minimal incidence of obesity, consumed 77–120 g/d,[3] whereas current estimates of fiber intake in the United States range from 16.5 to 17.9 g/d for men and 12.1 to 13.8 g/d for women. Similarly, modern-day subsistence farmers and forager-gatherers who continue to live a traditional lifestyle consume much greater dietary fiber, from 50 to 100 g/d, than those in developed countries.[4] Although these populations have an incidence of obesity far below those in western societies, they of course have many cultural and environmental differences that could account for this difference in incidence. Thus, while this association between dietary fiber consumption and obesity incidence is interesting, it tells us little about whether dietary fiber has a causative role in reducing obesity.

B. LONGITUDINAL STUDIES

A number of epidemiological studies have explored the association between consumption of dietary fiber and body weight. Liu et al.[5] used results from a prospective cohort study of U.S. female nurses, in which food frequency questionnaires were administered at multiple times from 1984 to 1996 to estimate dietary fiber intake. The authors then examined the association between the increase in dietary fiber intake from 1984 and 1994 and body weight gain over the same period. When categorized into quintiles, there was a highly significant trend for an inverse association between the increase in dietary fiber intake and a smaller gain in body weight (Figure 7.1). This smaller body weight gain, however, was much more pronounced in women whose body mass index (BMI) was ≥ 25 compared with women whose BMI was < 25 at the start of the study.

A somewhat similar relationship was found in a longitudinal study of fiber intake and weight gain in a large Mediterranean population.[6] A lower weight gain over the

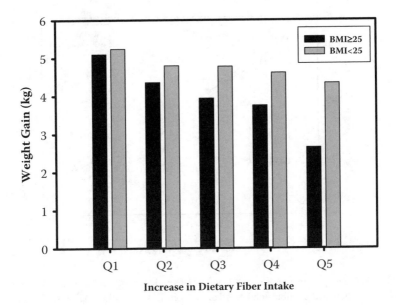

FIGURE 7.1 Weight gain by quintiles (Q) of change in dietary fiber intake from 1984 to 1994, based on BMI in 1984. Adapted from Liu et al., Relation between changes in intakes of dietary fiber and grain products and changes in weight and development of obesity among middle-aged women, *Am. J. Clin. Nutr.,* 78, 920–927, 2003.

previous 5 years was found to be strongly associated with a greater intake of dietary fiber (Figure 7.2), expressed as the change in proportion of subject gaining ≥3 kg. This relationship remained significant after adjustment for a number of potential confounders, such as energy intake, physical activity, snacking, and fat intake. In the Finnish Diabetes Prevention Study, 522 overweight middle-aged men and women were given either standard care (control group) or intensive dietary and exercise counseling and followed for 3 years.[7] Three-day food records were used to determine nutrient consumption. Increasing fiber consumption was strongly associated with greater weight loss and greater reduction in waist circumference.

Changes in waistline due to diet were also examined in the Health Professionals' Follow-Up Study, in which an increase in dietary fiber consumption of 12 g/d was found to be associated with a significant decrease of 0.63 cm in waist circumference.[8] The Coronary Artery Risk Development in Young Adults (CARDIA) Study is of interest because it examined associations between diet and body weight for both blacks and whites.[9] Using a food frequency questionnaire to determine diet history, dietary fiber intake was inversely associated with body weight and waist-to-hip ratios in both black and white men and women. The influence of dietary fiber has also been examined in another large cohort of 2025 men and women, drawn from the Danish Multinational Monitoring of Trends and Determinants in Cardiovascular Disease (MONICA) and a cohort from 1936.[10] Dietary intake was monitored by a 7-day food record. In contrast to the studies described above, no significant correlation

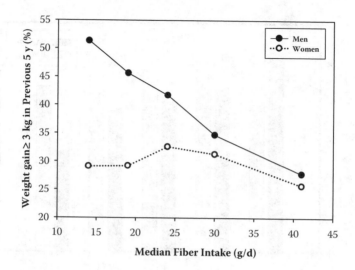

FIGURE 7.2 The proportion of men and women experiencing ≥3 kg weight loss over 5 years as related to their dietary fiber intake. Adapted from Bes-Rasrollo et al. Association of fiber intake and fruit/vegetable consumption with weight gain in a Mediterranean population, *Nutrition*, 22, 504–511, 2006.

was found between dietary fiber intake and change in body weight in men, and only a trend for an inverse correlation in women (p = 0.10), after adjustments for covariates. Clearly, however, a majority of longitudinal studies investigating the relationship between intake of dietary fiber and body weight do find that fiber intake tends to vary inversely with body weight change.

C. Cross Sectional Studies

A number of studies have examined the customary intake of dietary fiber of normal, overweight, and obese subjects. Using hydrostatic weighing to ascertain body composition and 3-day food records and food frequency questionnaires to measure dietary fiber intake, a significantly lower intake of dietary fiber was found in obese men and women than in lean men and women.[11] Total dietary fiber was determined in groups of lean (BMI 20.0–27.0), moderately obese (BMI 27.1–39.9) or severely obese (BMI >39.9) individuals using 3-day food records. After adjusting for potential confounding variables, total dietary fiber, expressed as either g/d or g/1000 kcal, was found to vary inversely with BMI.[12] Similarly, dietary intake was determined in groups of normal weight (BMI <25) and overweight/obese (BMI 25) subjects matched for age and height.[13] Dietary fiber intake was significantly greater in the normal weight group relative to the overweight/obese group (12 ± 5 vs. 9 ± 3 g/1000 kcal, respectively). Further, fiber intake was negatively correlated with percent body fat, determined by dual-energy x-ray absorptiometry (DEXA). In a study of 203 men categorized into three tertiles of body fat based on skinfold measurements, dietary fiber intake, estimated by food frequency questionnaire, was highly significantly inversely correlated with body fat category.[14]

D. SUMMARY

The longitudinal studies and cross sectional studies investigating the relationship between intake of dietary fiber and body weight consistently find that fiber intake is inversely correlated with body weight change. However, these studies must be viewed in the context that the differences in dietary fiber found in them represent differences in consumption of fiber-rich foods, primarily fruits, vegetables, and whole grain cereals. One cannot exclude the possibility that these epidemiological outcomes arise due to other factors besides dietary fiber in these fiber-rich foods. Further, these studies provide little insight as to what physical characteristic, e.g., viscosity, fermentation, etc. of the fiber might be responsible for this association between dietary fiber and body weight reduction.

III. INTERVENTION STUDIES

Two basic approaches have been used to examine the effect of dietary fiber on body weight change experimentally. The majority of studies have administered a purified or semi-purified fiber supplement to subjects, usually in the form of a pill. A few studies have examined the effect of dietary fiber-rich foods on body weight. These latter studies have the advantage of examining the fiber in its native state within the food, but cannot exclude the possibility that food components other than the fiber contribute to or are entirely responsible for any weight loss found.

A. STUDIES USING DIETARY FIBER SUPPLEMENTS

A large number of studies have been conducted on the effect of various types of dietary fiber supplements on body weight. These are summarized in Table 7.3. The majority of studies employed a viscous type of dietary fiber, such as glucomannan

TABLE 7.3
Number of Studies Showing an Increase in Satiety or Reduction in Hunger Relative to a Low-Fiber Control or Placebo Treatment

| | Increased Satiety/Reduced Hunger | | | |
| | Studies ≤ 2 Days | | Studies > 2 Days | |
Fiber Type	Yes	No	Yes	No
Mixed fiber	8[a]	2	5[b]	0
Soluble fiber	8[a]	2	7[a]	1
Insoluble fiber	2	1	5[a]	0

[a] One study showed a statistically nonsignificant increase.
[b] Two studies showed a statistically nonsignificant increase.

Adapted from Howarth, N. C., Saltzman, E., and Roberts, S. B., Dietary fiber and weight regulation, *Nutr. Rev.,* 59, 129–139, 2001 or agar, or a combination of viscous fibers. Widely varying amounts of fiber, duration of study, and use of concurrent weight reduction diets make overall conclusions somewhat challenging. However, in those studies in which the duration of the trial was 1 month or longer, and which used a viscous dietary fiber, all studies except one found a significant reduction in body weight compared with the placebo. In the one exception, the study by Tai et al.,[15] subject compliance with consumption of the fiber supplement was poor. In four of five studies employing a fiber supplement derived from a mix of sources (e.g., cereal and citrus fruit), a significant reduction in body weight occurred. The single study of a wheat fiber supplement found no reduction in body weight. Overall, these intervention trials, when conducted for a reasonable length of time (i.e., 1 month or longer), support the use of dietary fiber supplements as a dietary approach to facilitate body weight loss.

B. STUDIES USING DIETARY FIBER-RICH FOODS

There have been few studies of the effect of fiber-rich foods on body weight. In a study of obese subjects (BMI > 31), individuals consuming a hypocaloric diet high in whole grain cereals while participating in an exercise program lost no more weight than those who consumed a regular hypocaloric diet and also exercised.[16] Fruit and oat intake was examined in a study of overweight women (BMI > 25) consuming a hypocaloric diet.[17] Subjects consumed either 300 g of apple or pear or 60 g of oat cookies for 12 weeks. Those consuming the fruit experienced a significant body weight reduction from baseline, whereas those consuming the oat cookie did not. Since the fruit and oat cookie all supplied approximately the same amount of daily total fiber, this suggests that the fruit fiber was more efficacious in promoting weight loss. The Women's Healthy Eating and Living (WHEL) Study examined the effect in 1010 women of a low--fat, high-vegetable diet intervention on the risk of breast cancer recurrence.[18] Combining results from the intervention and comparison groups, the investigators found that changes in body weight from baseline to 1 year significantly inversely correlated with changes in the energy-adjusted dietary fiber intake. Interestingly, changes in energy intake did not correlate with body weight.

C. SUMMARY

Although the number of investigations is not large, overall the results of intervention studies support a role for dietary fiber in body weight management. However, the limited number of studies precludes the ability to determine what types of dietary fiber may be most efficacious, and provides little guidance about the amount of dietary fiber needed to maximize weight loss.

IV. EFFECTS ON SATIETY AND SATIATION

An important dietary strategy for weight management is to determine what foods or meal patterns will result in a decreased energy intake by inducing quicker satiation (intrameal satiety) and lead to greater satiety (intermeal satiety). Most investigations of the influence of diet on satiation and satiety have focused on macronutrient composition. It is now clear that macronutrients have different effects on satiation and satiety that are independent of their caloric content.[19] Protein appears to have the greatest effect on promoting satiety,[20,21] whereas the relative satiety value of fats and carbohydrates is less clear. In terms of meal patterns, considerable evidence now indicates that the energy density of a meal, defined as the energy content of a given weight of food (kcal/g), has a strong influence on both satiation and satiety.[22] That is, the lower the energy density of the meal or food, the greater the satiety that it produces. Water is the major component of food that impacts the energy density of a food. However, because dietary fiber has a minimal caloric content (approx. 1 kcal/g, due to absorption of colonic fermentation products), it too impacts energy density. Thus, foods high in dietary fiber will tend to be less calorically dense than those with a lower concentration of dietary fiber.

A. EFFECT OF DIETARY FIBER ON SATIETY

Given the importance of satiety in weight management, and the potential for dietary fiber to impact satiety, it is not surprising that a number of studies have examined the role of dietary fiber on satiety and hunger responses. Howarth and colleagues conducted a review of such studies in which healthy nondiabetic subjects were used and that included a control group provided with a meal or diet of equivalent energy and fat content.[23] Their results are summarized in Table 7.3. It is apparent that in both short-term (≤ 2 days) and longer term (> 2 days) trials, the majority of studies found that the presence of dietary fiber in the diet resulted in greater satiety or reduced hunger. There is no discernable difference based on whether the dietary fiber was categorized as of the soluble or insoluble type.

Since the time of the review by Howarth et al. in 2001, a number of other studies of dietary fiber and satiety have been reported. Holt et al. examined the effect of seven different types of bread of equivalent energy on satiety over a 120-minute period.[24] A satiety index score was calculated as the area under the curve of satiety measures of the test breads (based on stone-ground whole-wheat flour or high-gluten wheat flour) divided by the area under the curve for the reference bread (soft white). Although the strongest predictor of the satiety index score was the energy index of the breads, dietary fiber content was also positively associated with the score. Using a similar protocol, but feeding single meals containing different wheat-based or rice-based test meals, a positive correlation was found between the satiety index score and fiber content of the food, but not with other macronutrients.[25] In sausage patties, a substitution of lupin-kernel fiber for fat, but not a substitution of oligofructose, also resulted in a greater satiety score.[26]

Several studies have examined the effect of fiber added to liquid meals. The addition of a pea-fiber/oligofructose fiber mixture to an enteral formula consumed for 14 days increased the sense of fullness and minimal satiety compared with a calorically equivalent fiber-free formula.[27] Finally, consumption of a liquid meal containing either guar gum or a weak- or strong-gelling alginate led to significant increases in the sense of fullness over 2 hours compared with a fiber-free liquid meal.[28]

B. POTENTIAL MECHANISM FOR ENHANCED SATIETY

How dietary fiber increases satiety and reduces hunger is unknown. A number of mechanisms have been postulated with varying degrees of evidence to support them.[23,29] The following is a description of several of the more plausible mechanisms and a discussion of the evidence supporting them.

1. Gastric Distension

Viscous or gel-forming dietary fibers will hydrate in the stomach when mixed with gastric juices, potentially leading to significant gastric distention. It is known that gastric distension will lead to early satiation, an effect mediated by vagus nerve mechanoreceptors, and thus is referred to as a volumetric response.[30] Dietary fiber may delay gastric emptying (discussed below) and thus prolong gastric distension, leading to a prolonged satiating signal. This concept was tested using a synthetic dietary fiber that exists as a liquid at room temperature, but gels at body temperature.[31] This liquid fiber did reduce hunger and increase fullness, and delayed the time to the next meal. Thus, the concept that gelling fibers may increase satiety by increasing gastric distension seems to have some merit. However, there is a synergy between the volumetric signal due to gastric distension and the intestinal nutrient signals of satiety.[30] With a delayed gastric emptying, there may be an attenuation of the intestinal nutrient signal, thus lessening the overall satiety signal. Further, the impact on gastric distension from dietary fiber present in foods may be quite different, and has yet to be determined.

2. Delayed Glucose Absorption

A slower absorption of glucose from a meal, as indicated by a lower postprandial blood glucose concentration over time after consumption of a starch- or sugar-containing meal, is one of the best established physiological effects of viscous dietary fibers. A typical blood glucose curve after ingestion of a viscous fiber is shown in Figure 7.3. This pattern is also typical of the difference between low- and high-glycemic index (GI) foods. The GI is usually defined as the area under the 2-hour postprandial glucose curve after consumption of a test food containing 50 g of carbohydrate, relative to the area under the 2-hour curve for either white bread or glucose.[32] A high-GI food would give a curve similar to the control in Figure 7.3, whereas a low-GI food would appear similar to the viscous fiber. Although dietary fiber is certainly one factor that influences the GI value of a food, a number of other factors are also implicated, included the physical structure of the starch, method of food preparation, protein content, and presence of components such as phytate.[33] Nonetheless, given the similar glucose responses resulting from consumption of viscous fibers and low-GI foods, the effect of low-GI foods on satiety and hunger can provide insight into the likely effect of viscous fibers.

A large number of studies have examined the effect of low-GI foods on satiety or subsequent hunger. As reviewed by Roberts, most short-term (1-meal or 1-day) studies show that they do increase satiety or decrease hunger.[34] However, when only studies were considered in which the intake of energy, macronutrient content, energy density, and palatability were comparable between groups, the results were ambiguous; no clear pattern of low-GI foods promoting satiety or satiation was evident. Several studies have shown that rapid drops in serum glucose precede the onset of hunger or feeding,[35,36] which would be consistent with the idea that the rapid fall in

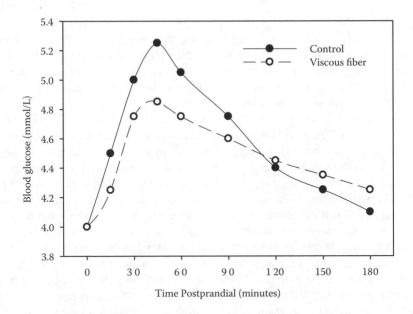

FIGURE 7.3 Typical blood glucose curve after ingestion of a viscous fiber.

serum glucose experienced by those consuming high-GI foods would stimulate hunger. For example, Campfield et al. monitored blood glucose concentrations of healthy adult subjects over time and had them complete ratings of satiety and hunger.[37] In most subjects hunger ratings and requests for a meal were correlated with drops in serum glucose. There was also an association between a rapid drop in serum glucose and desire to eat when the drop in glucose was induced by infusion of insulin. Thus, there is a physiological basis for greater satiety after consumption of viscous fibers that attenuate the decline in serum glucose after a meal.

How viscous dietary fibers attenuate the postprandial blood glucose response has not been determined with certainty. The most cited possibilities include a delayed rate of gastric emptying, delayed starch digestion, or slowed diffusion of glucose within the small intestine. Studies examining the effect of viscous fibers on the rate of glucose absorption within the small intestine have been contradictory, with evidence both for[38] and against[39] a slowing of absorption. Likewise, studies examining the effect of viscous fibers on the rate of gastric emptying have been inconsistent, with both no effect[40] or a delay reported.[39] Since these mechanisms are not mutually exclusive, the effect could be a result of a combination of these effects.

3. Hormonal Effects

The gastrointestinal tract is a major endocrine organ. A number of peptide hormones are released from the stomach, small intestine, and large intestine in response to various stimuli. A number of these hormones appear to play important roles in the regulation of feeding behavior.

a. Cholecystokinin

Cholescystokinin (CCK) is released from the duodenum in response to a meal, primarily in response to fat and protein digestion products, and acts to reduce food intake, although this effect is short-lived.[41] The mechanism of action of CCK in reducing food intake remains uncertain, but may involve an inhibition of gastric emptying or direct activation of vagal afferent fibers.[41]

The effect of dietary fiber on serum CCK has been inconsistent. Pectin feeding to obese subjects caused increased satiety and a delay in gastric emptying, but no change in postprandial serum CCK.[42] Likewise, in a study in which barley pasta enriched with the viscous fiber β-glucan was fed to subjects, no difference in the area under the time curve was found for serum CCK between the control meal containing no viscous fiber and the β-glucan-enriched pasta-containing meals.[43] However, CCK concentrations remained significantly elevated above the baseline value longer in subjects consuming the enriched pasta meals than those consuming the control meal. In another study, the CCK area under the time curve was doubled in subjects who consumed bean flakes, a rich source of dietary fiber, compared with those consuming a low-fiber meal.[44] In a subsequent study, women, but not men, showed a similar increase in the CCK area under the curve when consuming bean flakes in the context of a low-fat meal.[45] However, there was a strong correlation between satiety scores and the plasma CCK response, suggesting that the greater satiety produced by meals containing viscous fiber may be mediated, at least in part, by an enhanced release of CCK.

4. Glucagon-Like Peptide 1

Glucagon-like peptide-1 (7-36) amide (GLP-1) is cleaved from preproglucagon, located in the endocrine L-cells of the distal small intestine, cecum, and colon,[46] and released into the circulation in response to a meal. It is a potent incretin, stimulating the glucose-dependent postprandial release of insulin.[47] Infusion of GLP-1 during a meal into obese humans was shown to decrease the onset of hunger compared with a saline infusion. Subjects also showed decreased stomach emptying and lower postprandial serum glucose,[48] suggesting these responses are the mechanisms by which GLP-1 decreases hunger onset.

A number of studies have examined the effect of dietary fiber consumption on either plasma GLP-1 concentrations after a meal, intestinal tissue GLP-1 protein, or proglucagon mRNA content. Long-term consumption of oligofructose increases circulating GLP-1 in rodents[49,50] and humans.[51] Likewise, feeding a mixture of dietary fibers was found to increase plasma GLP-1 and intestinal proglucagon mRNA in dogs[52] and in rats maintained on a elemental diet.[53]

The characteristic of dietary fiber responsible for the enhanced secretion of GLP-1 in response to a meal appears to be fermentability. Oligofructose, a fiber that increases circulating GLP-1, as described above, is highly fermentable. Rats fed rhubarb stalk fiber, which is highly fermentable, had greater ileal proglucagon mRNA that those fed an equivalent amount of cellulose, a poorly fermented fiber.[54] Yet, rats fed the highly fermentable sugar alcohol lactitol did not have a greater concentration of plasma GLP-1 than the control group,[55] raising some uncertainty regarding the role of fermentation in enhancing GLP-1 secretion. How viscous dietary fibers might effect GLP-1 secretion has yet to be examined.

C. Summary

There is consistent evidence indicating that dietary fiber promotes satiety. However, due to the variety of different fiber types employed, it is difficult to draw conclusions about either the most efficacious type of dietary fiber or the amount needed to provide a significant degree of satiety. There are a number of plausible mechanisms by which dietary fiber may induce satiety, and evidence supporting each of them exists. Given the interrelatedness of some of these mechanisms, for example the effect of CCK and GLP-1 on slowing gastric emptying, it is unlikely that a single mechanism for dietary fiber-induced satiety will be identified.

V. CONCLUSIONS

Consumption of dietary fiber has declined dramatically as humans have adopted what we now refer to as the "western" lifestyle. Concomitant with this adoption of the western lifestyle has been an increase in a constellation of chronic diseases, such as various types of cancer, heart disease, type 2 diabetes, and obesity. The role the decline in dietary fiber consumption has played in the dramatic increases in these chronic diseases remains uncertain and controversial, in spite of considerable study of the relationship. However, sufficient evidence has accumulated to make a compelling case that a high intake of dietary fiber can help normalize body weight. It is likely that at least part of this effect is mediated by an increase in satiety after consumption of high-fiber meals. How dietary fiber promotes weight loss, which types of dietary fiber are most efficacious, and what is the optimal amount of dietary fiber are all questions that future research should be directed toward.

REFERENCES

1. U.S. Obesity Trends 1985–2005. http://www.cdc.gov/nccdphp/dnpa/obesity/trend/maps/index.htm, Accessed November 30, 2005.
2. Gallaher, D. D., Dietary fiber, in *Present Knowledge in Nutrition, 9th ed.*, Bowman, B. A. and Russell, R. M. International Life Sciences Institute, Washington, D.C., 2006, pp. 102–10.
3. Eaton, S. B., Eaton, S. B. 3rd, Konner, M. J., and Shostak, M., An evolutionary perspective enhances understanding of human nutritional requirements, *J. Nutr.,* 126, 1732–1740, 1996.
4. Lee, R., !Kung Bushmen Subsistence: An Input-Output Analysis, in *Environment and Cultural Behavior*, Vayda, AP Natural History Press, New York, 1969, pp. 47–79.
5. Liu, S., Willett, W. C., Manson, J. E., Hu, F. B., Rosner, B., and Colditz, G., Relation between changes in intakes of dietary fiber and grain products and changes in weight and development of obesity among middle-aged women, *Am. J. Clin. Nutr.,* 78, 920–927, 2003.
6. Bes-Rastrollo, M., Martinez-Gonzalez, M. A., Sanchez-Villegas, A., de la Fuente Arrillaga, C., and Martinez, J. A., Association of fiber intake and fruit/vegetable consumption with weight gain in a Mediterranean population, *Nutrition,* 22, 504–511, 2006.

7. Lindstrom, J., Peltonen, M., Eriksson, J. G., Louheranta, A., Fogelholm, M., Uusitupa, M., and Tuomilehto, J., High-fibre, low-fat diet predicts long-term weight loss and decreased type 2 diabetes risk: The Finnish Diabetes Prevention Study, *Diabetologia*, 49, 912–920, 2006.

8. Koh-Banerjee, P., Chu, N. F., Spiegelman, D., Rosner, B., Colditz, G., Willett, W., and Rimm, E., Prospective study of the association of changes in dietary intake, physical activity, alcohol consumption, and smoking with 9-y gain in waist circumference among 16 587 US men, *Am. J. Clin. Nutr.*, 78, 719–927, 2003.

9. Ludwig, D. S., Pereira, M. A., Kroenke, C. H., Hilner, J. E., Van Horn, L., Slattery, M. L., and Jacobs, D. R., Jr., Dietary fiber, weight gain, and cardiovascular disease risk factors in young adults, *JAMA*, 282, 1539–1546, 1999.

10. Iqbal, S. I., Helge, J. W., and Heitmann, B. L., Do energy density and dietary fiber influence subsequent 5-year weight changes in adult men and women?, *Obesity (Silver Spring)*, 14, 106–114, 2006.

11. Miller, W. C., Niederpruem, M. G., Wallace, J. P., and Lindeman, A. K., Dietary fat, sugar, and fiber predict body fat content, *J. Am. Diet. Assoc.*, 94, 612–615, 1994.

12. Alfieri, M. A., Pomerleau, J., Grace, D. M., and Anderson, L., Fiber intake of normal weight, moderately obese and severely obese subjects, *Obes. Res.* 3, 541–547, 1995.

13. Davis, J. N., Hodges, V. A., and Gillham, M. B., Normal-weight adults consume more fiber and fruit than their age- and height-matched overweight/obese counterparts, *J. Am. Diet. Assoc.*, 106, 833–840, 2006.

14. Nelson, L. H. and Tucker, L. A., Diet composition related to body fat in a multivariate study of 203 men, *J. Am. Diet. Assoc.*, 96, 771–777, 1996.

15. Tai, E. S., Fok, A. C., Chu, R., and Tan, C. E., A study to assess the effect of dietary supplementation with soluble fibre (Minolest) on lipid levels in normal subjects with hypercholesterolaemia, *Ann. Acad. Med. Singapore*, 28, 209–213, 1999.

16. Melanson, K. J., Angelopoulos, T. J., Nguyen, V. T., Martini, M., Zukley, L., Lowndes, J., Dube, T. J., Fiutem, J. J., Yount, B. W., and Rippe, J. M., Consumption of whole-grain cereals during weight loss: Effects on dietary quality, dietary fiber, magnesium, vitamin B-6, and obesity, *J. Am. Diet. Assoc.*, 106, 1380–1388; quiz 89–90, 2006.

17. Conceicao de Oliveira, M., Sichieri, R., and Sanchez Moura, A., Weight loss associated with a daily intake of three apples or three pears among overweight women, *Nutrition*, 19, 253–256, 2003.

18. Rock, C. L., Thomson, C., Caan, B. J., Flatt, S. W., Newman, V., Ritenbaugh, C., Marshall, J. R., Hollenbach, K. A., Stefanick, M. L., and Pierce, J. P., Reduction in fat intake is not associated with weight loss in most women after breast cancer diagnosis: Evidence from a randomized controlled trial, *Cancer*, 91, 25–34, 2001.

19. Holt, S. H., Miller, J. C., Petocz, P., and Farmakalidis, E., A satiety index of common foods, *Eur. J. Clin. Nutr.*, 49, 675–690, 1995.

20. Johnstone, A. M., Stubbs, R. J., and Harbron, C. G., Effect of overfeeding macronutrients on day-to-day food intake in man, *Eur. J. Clin. Nutr.*, 50, 418–430, 1996.

21. Marmonier, C., Chapelot, D., and Louis-Sylvestre, J., Effects of macronutrient content and energy density of snacks consumed in a satiety state on the onset of the next meal, *Appetite*, 34, 161–168, 2000.

22. Yao, M. and Roberts, S. B., Dietary energy density and weight regulation, *Nutr. Rev.*, 59, 247–258, 2001.

23. Howarth, N. C., Saltzman, E., and Roberts, S. B., Dietary fiber and weight regulation, *Nutr. Rev.*, 59, 129–139, 2001.

24. Holt, S. H., Brand-Miller, J. C., and Stitt, P. A., The effects of equal-energy portions of different breads on blood glucose levels, feelings of fullness and subsequent food intake, *J. Am. Diet. Assoc.,* 101, 767–73, 2001.

25. Pai, S., Ghugre, P. S., and Udipi, S. A., Satiety from rice-based, wheat-based and rice-pulse combination preparations, *Appetite,* 44, 263–271, 2005.

26. Archer, B. J., Johnson, S. K., Devereux, H. M., and Baxter, A. L., Effect of fat replacement by inulin or lupin-kernel fibre on sausage patty acceptability, post-meal perceptions of satiety and food intake in men, *Br. J. Nutr.,* 91, 591–599, 2004.

27. Whelan, K., Efthymiou, L., Judd, P. A., Preedy, V. R., and Taylor, M. A., Appetite during consumption of enteral formula as a sole source of nutrition: The effect of supplementing pea-fibre and fructo-oligosaccharides, *Br. J. Nutr.,* 96, 350–356, 2006.

28. Hoad, C. L., Rayment, P., Spiller, R. C., Marciani, L., Alonso Bde, C., Traynor, C., Mela, D. J., Peters, H. P., and Gowland, P. A., *In vivo* imaging of intragastric gelation and its effect on satiety in humans, *J. Nutr.,* 134, 2293–3000, 2004.

29. Pereira, M. A. and Ludwig, D. S., Dietary fiber and body-weight regulation. Observations and mechanisms, *Pediatr. Clin. North Am.,* 48, 969–980, 2001.

30. Powley, T. L. and Phillips, R. J., Gastric satiation is volumetric, intestinal satiation is nutritive, *Physiol. Behav.* 82, 69–74, 2004.

31. Tomlin, J., The effect of the gel-forming liquid fibre on feeding behaviour in man, *Br. J. Nutr.,* 74, 427–36, 1995.

32. Wolever, T. M., Jenkins, D. J., Jenkins, A. L., and Josse, R. G., The glycemic index: Methodology and clinical implications, *Am. J. Clin. Nutr.,* 54, 846–854, 1991.

33. Trout, D. L., Behall, K. M., and Osilesi, O., Prediction of glycemic index for starchy foods, *Am. J. Clin. Nutr.,* 58, 873–878, 1993.

34. Roberts, S. B., High-glycemic index foods, hunger, and obesity: Is there a connection?, *Nutr. Rev.,* 58, 163–169, 2000.

35. Louis-Sylvestre, J. and Le Magnen, J., Fall in blood glucose level precedes meal onset in free-feeding rats, *Neurosci. Biobehav. Rev.,* 4 Suppl 1, 13–5, 1980.

36. Smith, F. J. and Campfield, L. A., Meal initiation occurs after experimental induction of transient declines in blood glucose, *Am. J. Physiol.,* 265, R1423–R1429, 1993.

37. Campfield, L. A., Smith, F. J., Rosenbaum, M., and Hirsch, J., Human eating: Evidence for a physiological basis using a modified paradigm, *Neurosci. Biobehav. Rev.* 20, 133–137, 1996.

38. Blackburn, N. A., Redfern, J. S., Jarjis, H., Holgate, A. M., Hanning, I., Scarpello, J. H., Johnson, I. T., and Read, N. W., The mechanism of action of guar gum in improving glucose tolerance in man, *Clin. Sci. (Lond.),* 66, 329–336, 1984.

39. Leclere, C. J., Champ, M., Boillot, J., Guille, G., Lecannu, G., Molis, C., Bornet, F., Krempf, M., Delort-Laval, J., and Galmiche, J. P., Role of viscous guar gums in lowering the glycemic response after a solid meal, *Am. J. Clin. Nutr.,* 59, 914–921, 1994.

40. Bianchi, M. and Capurso, L., Effects of guar gum, ispaghula and microcrystalline cellulose on abdominal symptoms, gastric emptying, orocaecal transit time and gas production in healthy volunteers, *Dig. Liver Dis.,* 34 Suppl 2, S129–S133, 2002.

41. Chaudhri, O., Small, C., and Bloom, S., Gastrointestinal hormones regulating appetite, *Philos. Trans. R. Soc. Lond. B. Biol. Sci.,* 361, 1187–1209, 2006.

42. Di Lorenzo, C., Williams, C. M., Hajnal, F., and Valenzuela, J. E., Pectin delays gastric emptying and increases satiety in obese subjects, *Gastroenterology,* 95, 1211–1215, 1988.

43. Bourdon, I., Yokoyama, W., Davis, P., Hudson, C., Backus, R., Richter, D., Knuckles, B., and Schneeman, B. O., Postprandial lipid, glucose, insulin, and cholecystokinin responses in men fed barley pasta enriched with beta-glucan, *Am. J. Clin. Nutr.*, 69, 55–63, 1999.

44. Bourdon, I., Olson, B., Backus, R., Richter, B. D., Davis, P. A., and Schneeman, B. O., Beans, as a source of dietary fiber, increase cholecystokinin and apolipoprotein b48 response to test meals in men, *J. Nutr.* 131, 1485–1490, 2001.

45. Burton-Freeman, B., Davis, P. A., and Schneeman, B. O., Plasma cholecystokinin is associated with subjective measures of satiety in women, *Am. J. Clin. Nutr.*, 76, 659–67, 2002.

46. Eissele, R., Goke, R., Willemer, S., Harthus, H. P., Vermeer, H., Arnold, R., and Goke, B., Glucagon-like peptide-1 cells in the gastrointestinal tract and pancreas of rat, pig and man, *Eur. J. Clin. Invest.*, 22, 283–291, 1992.

47. Holst, J. J., Orskov, C., Nielsen, O. V., and Schwartz, T. W., Truncated glucagon-like peptide I, an insulin-releasing hormone from the distal gut, *FEBS Lett.*, 211, 169–174, 1987.

48. Naslund, E., Gutniak, M., Skogar, S., Rossner, S., and Hellstrom, P. M., Glucagon-like peptide 1 increases the period of postprandial satiety and slows gastric emptying in obese men, *Am. J. Clin. Nutr.*, 68, 525–530, 1998.

49. Delmee, E., Cani, P. D., Gual, G., Knauf, C., Burcelin, R., Maton, N., and Delzenne, N. M., Relation between colonic proglucagon expression and metabolic response to oligofructose in high fat diet-fed mice, *Life Sci.*, 79, 1007–1013, 2006.

50. Cani, P. D., Neyrinck, A. M., Maton, N., and Delzenne, N. M., Oligofructose promotes satiety in rats fed a high-fat diet: involvement of glucagon-like peptide-1, *Obes. Res.*, 13, 1000–1007, 2005.

51. Piche, T., des Varannes, S. B., Sacher-Huvelin, S., Holst, J. J., Cuber, J. C., and Galmiche, J. P., Colonic fermentation influences lower esophageal sphincter function in gastroesophageal reflux disease, *Gastroenterology*, 124, 894–902, 2003.

52. Massimino, S. P., McBurney, M. I., Field, C. J., Thomson, A. B., Keelan, M., Hayek, M. G., and Sunvold, G. D., Fermentable dietary fiber increases GLP-1 secretion and improves glucose homeostasis despite increased intestinal glucose transport capacity in healthy dogs, *J. Nutr.* 128, 1786–1793, 1998.

53. Reimer, R. A. and McBurney, M. I., Dietary fiber modulates intestinal proglucagon messenger ribonucleic acid and postprandial secretion of glucagon-like peptide-1 and insulin in rats, *Endocrinology*, 137, 3948–3956, 1996.

54. Reimer, R. A., Thomson, A. B., Rajotte, R. V., Basu, T. K., Ooraikul, B., and McBurney, M. I., A physiological level of rhubarb fiber increases proglucagon gene expression and modulates intestinal glucose uptake in rats, *J. Nutr.*, 127, 1923–1928, 1997.

55. Gee, J. M. and Johnson, I. T., Dietary lactitol fermentation increases circulating peptide YY and glucagon-like peptide-1 in rats and humans, *Nutrition*, 21, 1036–1043, 2005.

8 Nutritional Implications of Sex and Age Differences in Energy Metabolism

A.C. Maher and Mark A. Tarnopolsky

CONTENTS

I. INTRODUCTION

It has been assumed for many years that men and women responded similarly to metabolic stress; however, accumulating evidence supports that sex (gender) plays a role in metabolism. Metabolically, women demonstrate higher relative lipid oxidation and lower protein and carbohydrate oxidation at submaximal exercise intensity compared to men.[1-10] Physiologically, men have a greater accumulation of muscle mass and strength following resistance exercise than women.[11,12]

Changes in metabolism are likely genetically regulated either by predetermined expression of genes or by the regulation of gene expression through cell signaling mechanisms, for example, sex hormones.[13,14] Metabolically, the sex hormones appear to have a significant effect on sex- and aging-related differences in substrate utilization. Estrogen appears to favor lipid oxidation as observed when men and male rats are supplemented with 17 β-estradiol.[10,15] In addition, ovariectomized female rodents demonstrated higher carbohydrate oxidation and lower lipid oxidation that is reversed with estrogen supplementation.[16] Interestingly, women have a longer life span and lower mortality rates than men. In terms of muscle mass and strength gains, testosterone has a potent anabolic effect, whereas estrogen has a mild anabolic effect that is important in postmenopausal women, for estrogen replacement therapy may counteract the decline in muscle mass seen at that time.[17] Testosterone supplementation in elderly men to levels of young men increases muscle size and strength.[13]

Recent advances in modern techniques such as proteomics and gene array analysis will likely be useful in helping us understand the molecular basis for sex differences in metabolism, aging, and the influence of sex hormones. The implications of aging and sex differences on substrate metabolism and the impact of this on nutritional recommendations are only just beginning to be elucidated, and specific recommendations for elderly, recreational, and top sport athletes will be an interesting practical area for future research.

II. MUSCLE-RELATED DIFFERENCES BETWEEN SEXES AND WITH AGING

Muscles size and function can be altered by exercise, nutrition, hormones, and aging. All these factors are correlated with muscle metabolism. Before discussing differences in muscle metabolism between sexes and the implications of aging, it is important to review the physiological differences in muscle fiber type between men and women, as well as changes with aging, which might ultimately play a role in metabolism. It is also important to keep in mind that as men and women age there are factors that alter muscle metabolism such as disease, muscle loss, strength and muscle quality reduction, menopause in women, and andropause in men.

Muscle is composed of three types of muscle fibers; Type I, IIA, IIX. In terms of sex differences in fiber type, men have a significantly larger type I fiber area in the biceps brachii, and larger type II fiber area in the vastus lateralis than women.[18,19] Women have a greater type I fiber percent area than men in the vastus lateralis.[19] Similar results were found in rats, where the cross sectional area of type II fibers of the soleus and tibialis were greater in males, and the cross-sectional area of type

I fibers was greater in females; however, there were no significant differences in the percentage of each individual fiber.[20] Metabolically, a higher proportion of type I fibers has been correlated with higher fat oxidation rates. Type I fibers have a greater expression of fatty acid transport protein, FAT/CD36,[21] and women express almost 50% more FAT/CD36 than men.[22]

The myofibril is the contractile component of skeletal muscle and it is likely that age-related losses in muscle strength, mass, and function can be attributed to alterations in myofibrillar protein with age. However, the most consistently reported age-related change in muscle morphology is a reduction in type II fiber size.[23,24] Similarly, older adults have a higher proportion of fibers showing a coexistence of myosin heavy chain type I and IIA, and type IIA and IIX, as compared with young adults,[25] suggesting that fiber-type transitions occur with age. The age-related shift in fiber type affects whole muscle performance, for a greater proportion of type I fibers results in relative fatigue resistance, while a reduced proportion of type II fibers results in a reduction in peak torque.[26] Frontera et al (2002) found that as fiber type shifted toward slow fibers in aging men, there was a reduction in the force per unit muscle mass, maximal force from type I and type IIA single fibers was reduced, type IIA fibers were weaker than type I fibers, and strength in type IIA fibers was not different from type I fibers in older women.[27]

These findings suggest that sex-related differences exist in muscle fiber type and it is important to consider that this may influence metabolism and adaptive responses to exercise. Furthermore, the discrepancy between men and women suggest that age-related sarcopenia may be regulated by different factors for men than for women. The role of estrogen in muscle remains an intriguing potential mechanism underlying the observed sex differences. More research is necessary to decipher these potential sex differences and how they affect aging and muscle metabolism.

Taken together, these observations suggest a general trend toward a decrease in muscle strength through losses in type II fiber size and proportion, and an increase in the proportion of type I fibers with normal human aging. More importantly, these observations suggest that fiber type transitions do occur in the elderly between type I and type II fibers, and that contractile proteins may become less efficient with age. Furthermore, age-related changes of the myofibril appear to be regulated by different factors in men and women.

III. SEX DIFFERENCES IN SUBSTRATE METABOLISM DURING ENDURANCE EXERCISE

The primary source for energy during exercise is fat and carbohydrate; however, protein does contribute a small amount of energy.[28] There are sex differences in energy substrate selection, with women relying primarily on lipid oxidation (62%), with men only utilizing approximately 43% fat.[3,9,28,29] As expected, the greater reliance on lipid oxidation in women during endurance exercise results in a lower proportionate carbohydrate oxidation (Table 7.1).

To compare between two groups of individuals (i.e., sex), several factors known to alter substrate oxidation rate must be controlled for. First, training status and habitual and pre-exercise dietary intake status are important factors when examining exercise and metabolism. One of the best ways to compare between the sexes is to match men and women for training history, and given the higher percent body fat content for females, they should be compared using VO_{2peak} expressed relative to fat-free mass. [30] In addition, with sex comparison studies, the menstrual cycle is known to alter substrate oxidation and must be specified in any study.[31,32] Sex comparison studies should also test men and women at the same time (i.e., during the same experimental period and not with historical data) to control for variation in metabolic charts, different calibrations of CO_2/O_2 gas mixture, and different staff involved in the subject testing.

Irrespective of sex comparisons, key factors that are important to accurately measure whole-body carbohydrate (and lipid) oxidation are to ascertain that subjects are in a steady state and exercising below the anaerobic threshold. For example, the anaerobic threshold in untrained men and women may be as low as 66% of $VO_{2peak,}$ [33] and in the moderate to well trained athlete this may be as high as 80% of $VO_{2peak,}$[3] with no sex difference. Sex comparisons of substrate oxidation rates exceeding the lactate threshold do not yield accurate or valid results.

A. CARBOHYDRATE METABOLISM

1. Sex Differences in Carbohydrate Metabolism

Carbohydrates are a rapidly available source of energy. The Acceptable Macronutrient Distribution Range (AMDR) suggests that 45–65% of the diet should be carbohydrates.[34] Carbohydrates are stored in the muscle and liver in the form of glycogen. Glycogen provides a rapid source of energy to the cells during exercise. For years it was assumed that men and women respond similarly to exercise; however, the majority of cross-sectional studies summarized in a large-scale meta-analysis have found that whole-body carbohydrate oxidation rates are lower for women compared with men during endurance exercise at sub-maximal exercise intensities (Table 7.1).[30] Furthermore, even after 2 or 3 months of exercise training, both men and women show the same sex-related differences in carbohydrate utilization.[1,2,6,35]

The mechanism for the reduction in carbohydrate oxidation in women is unclear, but likely involves an attenuation of predominantly hepatic and possibly muscle glycogen utilization. Recent studies examining glucose kinetics in men and women during exercise and post exercise have demonstrated that the rate of glucose appearance (Ra) and disappearance (Rd) was lower in women then men.[36–38] To elucidate the possible biological factors that may be regulating these differences, upstream substrates have been examined including epinephrine, glucagon, and sex hormones. Interestingly, during exercise, the change in epinephrine concentrations are significantly attenuated in women as compared with men.[4,36,39,40] Studies have found that the adipocytes from women show higher sensitivity to epinephrine as compared with men.[41–43] The latter results imply that there are sex differences in adrenergic receptor density or post-receptor regulation, at least within the adipocytes.

The data regarding a potential role for glucagon in the regulation of exercise metabolism have not been conclusive. Glucagon plays a role in the release of glucose from the liver to maintain blood glucose levels. Horton et al. (2006) observed that the absolute resting value of glucagon was higher in women then men.[36] In contrast,

Tarnopolsky et al. (1990) observed no difference in resting glucagon levels between men and women.[4] Both studies reported that men had a greater reduction in glucagon during exercise, suggesting that glucagon does not affect glucose levels equally based on sex. Further investigation is needed to establish the role of hormonal factors on substrate metabolism in men and women.

Sex hormones such as estrogen and progesterone show a strong correlation with the observed sex-based differences in substrate metabolism. Women in the luteal phase of their menstrual cycle have a significantly lower glucose Ra and glucose Rd.[37,44] Women in the luteal phase also show a reduction in glucose metabolic clearance rates as compared with women in the follicular phase, and women in both follicular and luteal states still had a lower glucose Ra, glucose Rd, and metabolic clearance rates than men.[37] Furthermore, women in the luteal phase of their menstrual cycle had lower proglycogen, macroglycogen, and total glycogen utilization during exercise than women in the follicular phase.[37] Although there are changes in Ra and Rd during different phases of the menstrual cycle, the significance is unknown, as there seems to be no significant change in whole-body substrate metabolism. These data support the possibility that sex hormones regulate some aspects of carbohydrate metabolism between men and women. The specific effects of estrogen supplementation on substrate metabolism will be discussed later.

2. Nutritional Implications of Carbohydrate Loading

The term "carbohydrate loading" is used to describe the dietary strategies used to increase dietary carbohydrate intake in order to maximize muscle (and liver) glycogen storage. Most strategies involve a period of reduced exercise volume and the consumption of a diet that has a higher proportion of energy derived from carbohydrates for a period of 3 to 4 days. This strategy results in an increase in muscle glycogen stores and an improvement in endurance exercise performance in men.[45,46] Muscle glycogen stores are positively correlated with endurance exercise performance at intensities from 60–75% of maximal aerobic power,[47,48] and dietary manipulations lead to a higher carbohydrate intake and can enhance endurance exercise performance in men.[45,46]

Carbohydrate loading was first described in male subjects.[43–46] Interestingly, there appears to be a sex difference in the ability to carbohydrate load. Tarnopolsky et al. (1995) demonstrated that increasing pre-exercise carbohydrates to 75% total energy intake in men and women athletes increased resting muscle glycogen content by 45% in men, which was correlated with a similar increase in performance (43%); whereas the females showed neither an increase in glycogen content nor in exercise performance.[5] These findings have been supported in a study that demonstrated that well trained women athletes showed comparatively modest increases in muscle glycogen and exercise performance following carbohydrate loading.[49] Interestingly, in each of the aforementioned studies there was a lower relative and absolute energy intake by the women, which meant that women consumed fewer carbohydrate on a per kilogram body weight basis (<7 g/kg/d); on the other hand, in studies evaluating carbohydrate loading in men, the corresponding amount of dietary carbohydrate usually amounts to >8 g/kg/d.[5,50,51] In subsequent studies, when women increased their total energy intake by 30% and consumed 75% (>8 g/kg/d) of their energy from carbohydrates there was a significant increase in muscle glycogen content.[52,53] However, the magnitude of the increase in muscle glycogen stores was about 50% that of men on a similar diet.[52,53] Furthermore, there were no differences in the ability of women to carbohydrate load in different stages of their menstrual cycle.[53] From a practical perspective, a female who weighs 60 kg and was consuming 2,500 kcal/d would have to consume 77% of their energy from carbohydrates to attain an intake of >8.0 g/kg/d and nearly 100% would have to come from carbohydrates if her energy intake was ~ 2,000 kcal/d. Increasing energy intake by 33% appears to allow for some ability to carbohydrate load; however, the practical issues of the associated weight gain may attenuate their enthusiasm for such a strategy. Overall, the balance of the data suggests that the ability and practical issues surrounding carbohydrate loading in women may limit the acceptance and efficacy of such a strategy in women. Furthermore, studies have not yet been completed to determine whether any increase in glycogen in women will result in an increase in performance.

The provision of exogenous carbohydrate during endurance exercise can delay the onset of fatigue and promote higher glucose oxidation rates in the latter stages of endurance exercise in men.[54-58] The few studies that have examined the effect of exogenous carbohydrate intake on endurance exercise metabolism and performance in women have found that women who consume a 6%-8% glucose solution have an increase in exercise performance during both the follicular and luteal phases of the menstrual cycle.[32,59] Furthermore, women who oxidized a greater proportion of exogenous carbohydrate had a greater attenuation of endogenous glucose oxidation as compared with men during exercise.[60] A study comparing both men and women showed no sex differences in the metabolic response to exogenous carbohydrate utilization during endurance exercise.[61] These findings suggest that the consumption of exogenous carbohydrates during endurance exercise would be beneficial to exercise performance in both men and women.

The benefits of carbohydrate supplementation in the postexercise recovery period and the impact upon glycogen resynthesis have been examined in men and women. The administration of 1 g/kg carbohydrate or carbohydrate (0.75 g/kg) + protein (0.1 g/kg) + fat (0.02 g/kg), immediately following endurance exercise increased the rate of glycogen resynthesis in men and women similarly.[62] Interestingly, the provision of carbohydrates and protein immediately following endurance exercise during a week of intensified training led to an improvement in nitrogen (protein) retention and an improvement in exercise performance in women.[63] Therefore, in the immediate postexercise period, women and men show similar rates of glycogen resynthesis and women derive performance enhancement from such a strategy during intensified training.

In summary, it appears that women can carbohydrate load if their habitual energy intake results in a relative carbohydrate intake of greater than 8 g/kg/d. With additional energy and an increase in the proportion of carbohydrates, women can increase muscle glycogen content. Men and women show similar responses to exogenous carbohydrate provision during exercise, and both sexes increase performance. Finally, carbohydrate intake immediatelypostexercise increases the rates of glycogen resynthesis in both men and women and can spare protein in women during intensified training.

B. Lipid Metabolism

Fats become proportionately more important as a fuel source with prolonged endurance exercise. One gram of fat yields over twice the energy of carbohydrate.[64,65] The AMDR recommends that 20–35% of an adult's dietary intake should be fat.[34] Fats are predominantly stored as triglycerides in adipocytes; however, fatty acids can also be stored in skeletal muscle as intramyocellular lipids (IMCLs).[66] IMCLs are situated in the sarcoplasma in direct contact with mitochondria, the location of fat oxidation,[67] serving as a direct energy source during exercise. IMCLs are highest in oxidative type I muscle fibers.[68] Trained athletes have a higher IMCL content than sedentary people and IMCL content is lower following prolonged submaximal exercise.[69] Interestingly, one study found that IMCL utilization was apparent in skeletal muscle of women but not men.[70] High dietary fat also increases IMCL content and plays a role in insulin sensitivity in nonathletes.[71]

Similar to the sex differences in carbohydrate metabolism, there are sex differences in whole-body fat oxidation observed by the lower RER in women (Table 8.1). The higher oxidation of lipids in women is observed during endurance-based exercise. Interestingly, women have higher IMCLs than men.[70] The source of the higher lipid use for the women during endurance exercise is likely to be a greater use of IMCL,[70] and to a lesser extent, blood-borne free fatty acids (FFAs).[1,19] High fat diets in men have been shown to increase fat oxidation and whole body lipolysis by increasing the IMCL content, irrespective of changes in plasma FFAs.[72] Using glycerol tracers, several studies have found that women had a higher lipolytic rate than men during endurance exercise.[1,2,73] The higher muscle LPL activity for women may drive FFAs from blood-derived chylomicrons and very low density lipoproteins toward a higher IMCL storage in women with a consequently higher oxidation rate. Trained women runners on a moderate-fat diet restored baseline IMCL content in 22 hours,[74] yet it took trained male cyclists 48 hours to replace IMCL content.[75] Interestingly, a moderate to higher fat diet (35–68% of energy as fat) can restore IMCL content in athletes within 48 hours, but most athletes consume only ~24% of energy as fat, which is not enough to restore IMCL levels within 48 hours.[74–76] It would be of interest to determine if there is a sex difference in the responsiveness to high-fat diets between men and women. One would predict that perhaps women may benefit from a high-fat recovery diet, where as men may not. Further studies need to be done to elucidate the effect of high-fat diets on exercise performance since some studies demonstrate a positive outcome,[77,78] and others no change.[79,80]

In summary, there is strong support that women have higher lipid oxidation during endurance exercise due predominantly to a higher IMCL content and possibly to a more efficient uptake of plasma FFAs than men. Based on the current literature that women demonstrate a preference for fat, metabolism might indicate that sport-related dietary interventions may be different for men and women.

C. Protein Metabolism

Of the 20 different types of amino acids in proteins, nine cannot be synthesized by the body and must be supplied through dietary sources. Protein can serve as an energy source; however, fats and carbohydrates are the preferred energy sources. To allow

TABLE 8.1
Summary of Studies Where Whole Body Substrate Metabolism Was Reported in Men and Women

Reference	Subjects	Exercise	RER (mean)
Costill et al., 1979 [193]	12 F, T 12 M, T	60 min run @ 70% VO_{2max}	F = 0.83 M = 0.84
Froberg and Pederson, 1984 [194]	7 F, T 7 M, T	cycle to exhaustion @80 + 90% VO_{2max}	F = 0.93 M = 0.97
Blatchford, et al., 1985 [195]	6 F, T @ 35% VO_{2max}	90 min walk	F = 0.81 M = 0.85
Tarnopolsky, et al.., 1990 [4]	6 F, T 6 M, T	15.5 km run @ ~65% VO_{2max}	F = 0.876 M = 0.940
Phillips, et al., 1993[3]	6 M, T	90 min cycle @ 65% VO_{2max}	F = 0.820 M = 0.853
Tarnopolsky, et al.., 1995 [5]	8 F, T 7 M, T	60 min cycle @ 75% VO_{2max}	F = 0.892 M = 0.923
Tarnopolsky, et al., 1997 [62]	8 F, T 8 M, T	90 min cycle @ 65% VO_{2max}	F = 0.893 M = 0.918
Horton, et al., 1998[6]	13 F, T + UT 14 M, T + UT	120 min cycle @ 45% VO_{2max}	F = 0.84 M = 0.86
Friedlander, et al., 1998[1]	17 F, UTT 19 M, UTT	60 min cycle @ 45 & 65% VO_{2max}	F = 0.885 M = 0.932
Romijn, et al., 2000 [196]	8 F, T 5 M, T	20–30 min cycle @ 65% VO_{2max}	F = 0.81 M = 0.81
McKenzie, et al., 2000 [35]	6 F, UTT 6 M, UTT	90 min cycle @ 65% VO_{2max}	F = 0.889 M = 0.914
Davis, et al, 2000 [8]	8 F, UT 8 M, UT	90 min cycle @ 50% VO_{2max}	F = 0.92 M = 0.92
Goedecke, et al, 2000 [197]	16 F, T 45 M, T	10 min @ 25, 50, & 75% VO_{2max}	F = 0.90 M = 0.92
Rennie, et al., 2000§	6, F UTT 5, M UTT	90 min cycle @ 60% VO_{2max}	F = 0.893 M = 0.945
Carter, et al., 2001 [2]	8 F, UTT 8 M, UTT	90 min cycle @ 60% VO_{2max}	F = 0.847 M = 0.900
Lamont, et al., 2001 [9]	7 F, UTT 7 M, UTT	60 min cycle @ 50% VO_{2max}	F = 0.808 M = 0.868
Roepstorff, et al., 2002 [38]	7 F, T 7M, T	90 min cycle @ 58% VO_{2max}	F = 0.886 M = 0.905
Melanson, et al., 2002* [198]	8 F,T 8 M,T	400 kcal @ 40 + 70% VO_{2max}	F = 0.87 M = 0.91
Mittendorfer, et al., 2002 [73]	5 F, UT 5 M, UT	90 min cycle @ 50% VO_{2max}	F = 0.87 M = 0.87
Steffensen, et al., 2002 [70]	21 F, T+UT 21 M, T+UT	90 min cycle @ 60% VO_{2max}	F = 0.877 M = 0.893
Riddell, et al., 2003 [60]	7 F, T 7 M, T	90 min cycle @ 60% VO_{2max}	F = 0.93 M = 0.93

(Continued)

TABLE 8.1 (CONTINUED)
Summary of Studies Where Whole Body Substrate Metabolism Was Reported in Men and Women

Reference	Subjects	Exercise	RER (mean)
Lamont, et al., 2003 [82]	4 F, UT 4 M, UT	60 min cycle @ 50% VO_{2max}	F = 0.82 M = 0.83
M'Kaouar, et al., 2004 [199]	6 F, MT 6 M, MT	120 min cycle @ 65% VO_{2max}	F = 93 M = 0.93
Devries, et al., 2005 [37]	13 F, MT 10 M, MT	90 min cycle @ 65% VO_{2max}	F = 0.91 M = 0.94
Zehnder, et al., 2005 [200]	9 F, T 9 M, T	180 min cycle @ 50% VO_{2max}	F = 0.86 M = 0.88
Horton, et al., 2006 [36]	10 F, M T 10 M, MT	90 min cycle@ 57% VO_{2max}	F = 0.865 M = 0.880
Roepstorff, et al., 2006 [201]	9 F M, T 8 M, MT	90 min cycle @ 60% VO_{2max}	F = 0.85 M = 0.89
Wallis, et al., 2006 [61]	8 F, MT 8 M, MT	120 min cycle @ 67% VO_{2max}	F = 0.82 M = 0.85
Mean	n = 249F n = 273 M		F = 0.869 (0.02) M = 0.895 (0.02)[†]

Values are mean (SD). F = females; M = males; T = trained; A = active; U = untrained; UT = longitudinal training study: for longitudinal training studies, the pre/post rides are all collapsed across time for each sex. T + U = trained and untrained in same study. § = master's thesis. * The RER was a combination of those at both exercise intensities. † Significant sex difference (P<0.001, 2 tailed independent t-test).

protein to be used as a source of energy they must be broken down into constituent amino acids, which can be used as fuel in muscle in several ways.[64,65,81] The recommended dietary allowance (RDA) for men and women over the age of 19 is 0.80 g/kg protein. Protein requirements are determined based on the minimum necessary supply of indispensable amino acids and the body's ability to maintain nitrogen balance.[34] Current dietary recommendations do not make allowances for a possible influence of exercise on amino acid and protein requirements.

1. Sex differences in protein utilization

The evidence for whole body carbohydrate oxidation being higher for men as compared with women, during endurance exercise, also predicts that amino acid oxidation would be higher in men. Whole-body experiments using urea excretion demonstrated that overall amino acid oxidation was less for women than for men. Initial studies by our group found that men had higher urinary nitrogen excretion consequent to endurance exercise as compared with women,[4] suggesting that amino acid oxidation was higher during endurance exercise for men tham for women. Further research using ^{13}C-leucine stable isotope methodology in training matched men and women, demonstrating that leucine oxidation was lower for the women as compared with men during endurance exercise.[3,9,35,82,83] Interestingly, one study found that women had a lower rate of leucine, but not lysine oxidation during endurance exercise, as compared with men,[9] showing that the observed sex differences in oxidation may be amino acid specific.

Studies have also examined the effect of menstrual cycle phase on amino acid kinetics. Using ^{13}C-leucine tracers, Lariviere et al. (1994) demonstrated that women had a higher leucine oxidation during the luteal compared with follicular phase,[84] and Lamont et al. (1987) found that that urinary urea nitrogen excretion was higher during the luteal compared with the follicular phase of the menstrual cycle.[85] These findings suggest that sex differences in protein regulation could be related to factors such as estrogen and progesterone levels.

2. Metabolic Regulators as a Mechanism for Sex Differences in Protein Oxidation

There are many possible metabolic regulators including: substrate availability, regulatory enzyme activity, catecholamine responsiveness, and sex steroid hormones. Substrate availability definitely plays a role in metabolic regulation of protein oxidation;[86] however, most well designed sex-comparison studies have ensured that men and women were on controlled diets and received comparable protein based on g/kg. To examine the potential mechanism(s) behind this apparent sex difference in leucine oxidation, McKenzie et al. (2000)[35] measured the active form of branched chain 2-oxo-acid dehydrogenase (BCOAD) in skeletal muscle of six men and six women before and after a 31-day endurance exercise training program. BCOAD is the rate-limiting enzyme for muscle branched-chain amino acid oxidation. They found identical BCOAD total activity levels and the acute exercise-induced percent activation before and after endurance training (although the basal activation was lower in women).[35] The lack of a sex difference in the acute exercise induced BCOAD activation suggested that some of the attenuation of amino acid oxidation in women may be occurring at the hepatic level. This latter finding was also in keeping with an attenuation of hepatic glycogen utilization during exercise for the women.

Sex differences could also be a result of variation in catecholamine responsiveness.[82,87] When the catecholamine receptors (β1– and β2-adrenergic receptors) were blocked pharmacologically with propranalol, men had a further upregulation of leucine oxidation with no observed changes in women.[82,87] In light of these initial studies, further research is needed to determine the metabolic regulation of sex-related differences in amino acid utilization.

3. Athletic Differences in Protein Requirements

There is considerable controversy concerning the optimal dietary protein requirement for endurance athletes. Physical activity is not factored into most dietary protein requirements as exercise-related protein oxidation accounts for only, at most, 6% of total energy requirements.[3,35] Nitrogen-balance studies found that even after a sufficient adaptation period, moderately trained exercising men and women were both in negative nitrogen balance on a diet supplying protein just above the RDA.[3]

Interestingly, the nitrogen balance was more negative for the men (-26 mg/kg/d) versus women (-16 mg/kg/d)[3], indirectly suggesting that any elevation of dietary protein requirements in top sport women athletes will be somewhat less than for men (~ 25% lower).[30] There is also an increase in leucine oxidation during endurance exercise,[3,35] which suggests that dietary protein requirements could be impacted if the exercise duration were sufficiently long or the intensity sufficiently high. The consistent finding of higher exercise induced leucine oxidation in men compared with women[3,9,35,82,83] supports that men may require more protein than women. Finally, the maximal BCOAD activity is greater after endurance exercise training, which suggests that the total capacity to oxidize amino acids is greater in the trained state.[35]

Studies have suggested that optimal protein intake for elite athletes should be in the range of 1.0–1.8 g/kg of body weight.[3,88–91] A recent study examining the level of dietary protein required to achieve positive nitrogen balance in endurance trained males was 1.2 g/kg, and consuming more (3.6 g/kg) protein showed no advantage.[86] In terms of energy requirements, if an athlete is consuming appropriate energy and meeting the AMDR guidelines, he or she will meet these protein requirements, as 1.2 g/kg is approximately 10% of total energy intake. The sports nutritionist counseling an athlete must consider both the percentage as well as the per kilogram requirements, for under some conditions, such as with those on a habitually low energy intake (i.e., amenorrheic women runners, body builders, etc.), 10% of energy may yield a suboptimal protein intake.

In summary, the majority of research supports that elite endurance athletes should consume 1.2–1.8 g/kg protein/d, which is higher than the RDA of 0.80 g/kg, but meets the AMDR, suggesting that the AMDR might be a better measure when trying to determine the appropriate diet for an athlete (assuming that energy intake is adequate). Clearly, more research is needed to determine if and how sex differences in exercise metabolism will impact upon dietary protein requirements and the mechanism(s) behind these findings.

III. EFFECTS OF SEX HORMONES ON SUBSTRATE METABOLISM DURING ENDURANCE EXERCISE

A. ESTROGEN AND SEX DIFFERENCES

Estrogen, the primary sex hormone in women, is well characterized in the regulation of reproduction. Estrogen is also present in lower levels in men and post-menopausal women.[92] Estrogens belong to a group of steroid compounds produced by the enzymatic alteration of androgens, specifically testosterone produces estradiol.[92] Estrogen regulates many physiological functions of the musculoskeletal,[93] gastrointestinal, immune[94], neural,[95] and cardiovascular systems.[96] In ovulating women, estradiol is highest in the later follicular phase of the menstrual cycle, specifically the week prior to ovulation.[92] Estrogen is known to play a role in glucose homeostasis, however, the exact mechanism is unknown. Studies using ovariectomized rodents or via the oral administration of 17β-estradiol to rodents and humans have shown that estrogen has a major influence upon carbohydrate metabolism at the skeletal muscle and hepatic level.[39,97–99] Although several of the earlier studies that examined the effects of 17β-estradiol on substrate metabolism used the hormone at a supra-physiological doses [15,99,100], the same metabolic effects are seen with physiologically relevant doses.[10,16]

Initial studies examining the effects of an ovariectomy on muscle metabolism in female rats resulted in the female rats showing a male-like metabolic pattern with an increase in glycogen utilization and lower lipid utilization in both skeletal muscle and heart.[16,100] These effects could be reverted back to the normal female-like metabolic pattern of increased lipid and lower glycogen utilization by supplementing the rats with 17β-estradiol.[16,100] In rodents, the administration of 17β-estradiol attenuated glycogen degradation in the livers of rats during exercise.[98,99] Results have shown when male or ovariectomized female rats are supplemented with 17β-estrdiol then exercised, there is a sparing of muscle and liver glycogen, and an increase in free fatty acids,[99] leading to an overall improvement in exercise performance. 17β-estradiol also influences lipid storage in mice by increasing intramuscular triglyceride content in both heart and skeletal muscle.[15]

In humans, women demonstrate lower glycogen utilization rates during endurance exercise.[2,7,37] Some studies have found that there does not appear to be a sex difference in basal muscle glycogen content, and women do not show differences in glycogen content at either phase of the menstrual cycle.[35,53,62,101] However, during endurance exercise, women use less muscle glycogen than men,[4] and have a significantly lower proglycogen, macroglycogen, and total glycogen utilization in the luteal versus follicular phase.[37] Interestingly, administration of 17β-estradiol in men reduces the basal level of total muscle glycogen at rest and after exercise.[10] Administration of 17β-estradiol in both men and women attenuated hepatic glucose production during endurance exercise.[39,97] Tarnopolsky et al. (2001)[101] found that administration of 17β-estradiol to men increased their plasma 17-β-estradiol concentration to mid-follicular levels without effecting muscle glycogen breakdown during exercise; however, men given 17β–estradiol had a lower RER, which reflected a reduced reliance upon carbohydrate (CHO) substrate utilization and an increase in lipid metabolism, similar to what was observed in women.[10] Studies have found that glucose rate of appearance and disappearance[1] and glucose metabolic clearance rate[97] were lower for exercising women as compared with men. Interestingly, men given 17β-estradiol had lower proglycogen, total glycogen, hepatic glucose production, and glucose uptake, suggesting whole-body glycogen sparing.[10] These findings imply that 17β-estradiol reduces hepatic glucose production during exercise. At the skeletal muscle level, estrogen also seems to be acting on lipid metabolism. In humans, women show a higher IMCL content and a greater utilization rate during endurance exercise compared to men.[70]

Mechanistically, Ellis et al. (1994)[15] demonstrated that administration of 17β-estradiol increased LPL activity in skeletal muscle and decreased it in adipocytes, suggesting that estrogen might play a role in the preferred storage of lipids in the skeletal muscle for immediate availability in oxidation. Recent studies have shown that women have 160% higher mRNA for LPL than men, but there was no observed sex differences in LPL activity.[22] There are also sex differences in the expression of lipid binding proteins. Fatty acid translocase (FAT/CD36) protein is approximately

50% higher in women compared with men.[22] One study has demonstrated that females have twice the amount of plasma membrane fatty acid transporter (FATP-1) mRNA compared with males;[102] however more research is needed to determine whether this finding translates into functional significance. There appears to be no significant sex differences in carnitine palmitoyl transferase-1 (CPT-1) or β-3-OH-acyl-CoA-dehydrogenase activity in humans; however, 17β-estradiol supplementation in ovariectomized rats demonstrated an increase in the maximal enzyme activities of carnitine palmitoyl transferase-1 (CPT-1) and β-3-OH-acyl-CoA-dehydrogenase.[103]

Estrogen elicits its effects by binding estrogen receptors (ER) α and β, which are known transcription factors for the regulation of genes. ER α and ER β mRNA and protein have been documented in skeletal muscle of humans,[104,105] rats,[106] and mice.[107] A recent study by Wiik et al. (2005)[108] found that ER α and ER β expression was higher in endurance trained men than in moderately active men. However, Lemoine et al. (2002)[106] found that exercising female rats for 7 weeks increased ER α mRNA expression, with no significant change in males. The change in muscle ER expression due to training seems to be muscle-type specific.[109] In rats, ER expression is higher in slow-twitch oxidative muscle than in fast-twitch oxidative-glycolytic and glycolytic muscle.[109] Differences in ER expression in muscle fiber type and increased expression during exercise suggest that ERs are involved in muscle adaptation to exercise, most likely acting at the level of gene regulation.

Murine studies are helping to lead the way in understanding the mechanism and other physiological-related outcomes of the effects of estrogen-based sex differences. Estrogen has been shown to modulate insulin sensitivity in women,[110] possibly by altering insulin-related gene expression.[111,112] The overexpression of GLUT4 in a transgenic murine model resulted in an increase in the percent of glucose disposal through glycolysis in male animals and an increase in that directed toward glycogen storage in female animals.[113] Interestingly, estrogen receptor-α knockout mice exhibit insulin resistance.[114] In a study by Barros et al. (2006)[107] estrogen receptor α was shown to be a positive regulator, and estrogen receptor β a negative regulator, of GLUT-4 expression. More studies are needed to determine the exact signaling pathway for estrogen-related GLUT-4 expression but estrogen has been shown to regulate IP3 signaling,[115] and IP3 is downstream of PI3K, a signaling molecule that has been shown to play a role in GLUT-4 translocation to the sarcoplasm.[116]

A transgenic peripheral peroxisome activating receptor α knockout (PPARα[-/-]) murine model demonstrated that most of the male PPARα[-/-] mice died with severe hypoglycemia when an inhibitor of CPT activity (etomoxir) was given, yet the majority of female mice survived.[117] Furthermore, males administered 17β-estradiol avoided the fatal effects of CPT inhibition.[117] This study demonstrates the interrelatedness of glucose and lipid oxidation and the relationship to 17β-estradiol. Ovariectomized rodent models typically become obese, which can be prevented by administering 17β-estradiol.[118] Further investigation into the molecular mechanism of 17β-estradiol in ovariectomized mice showed that lipogenic genes were downregulated in adipocytes, liver, and skeletal muscle.[119] 17β-estradiol also upregulated the expression of PPAR, and activated AMP-activated protein kinase in mice, suggesting that estrogen promotes the partitioning of FFAs toward oxidation.[119]

In summary, 17β-estradiol appears to be involved in sex-related differences in the use of glucose/glycogen and lipid oxidation during endurance exercise. The exact mechanism by which 17β-estradiol is eliciting these differences is yet to be determined; however, it might have a molecular role in the regulation of genes or protein involved in fatty acid transport and triglyceride hydrolysis (muscle LPL). Although 17β-estradiol offers protection from fatal hypoglycemia in a CPT inhibitor transgenic model of human fatty acid oxidation defects, a significant sex difference in the CPT system and enzymes involved in β-oxidation is apparent only at the mRNA level in human studies. Current gene array analysis techniques will hopefully help elucidate the role of estrogen in metabolic fuel selection.

B. SEX DIFFERENCES DUE TO TESTOSTERONE

The primary sex hormone in men is testosterone. Men have approximately 10 times higher testosterone concentration than women. Testosterone is a steroid-based hormone that promotes secondary sex characteristics in men, including increased muscle mass. Testosterone unequivocally has a stimulatory effect on protein synthesis, resulting in an increase in fat-free mass.[120,121] Similarly, gains in strength and muscle size have been observed with the exogenous administration of testosterone.[122] Research has shown that testosterone administration increased the fractional rate of mixed muscle protein synthesis with no change in fractional protein breakdown rate.[121,123] Furthermore, the protein synthetic stimulation effect was not mediated by an increase in amino acid transport, but rather was due to an increase in the reutilization of intracellular amino acids.[123] Despite these changes in strength and muscle size, reduction or elevation of testosterone in men does not alter substrate metabolism.[124] Braun et al. (2005)[124] observed three levels of testosterone in men, low (~0.8 ng/ml), normal (~5.5 ng/ml), and high (~11 ng/ml), and found no significant difference in carbohydrate oxidation, glucose Rd, plasma glucose, or plasma FFAs. In conclusion, testosterone does not appear to be a candidate in the regulation of sex-observed differences in substrate utilization during endurance exercise.

V. CHANGE IN SUBSTRATE METABOLISM WITH AGING

Aging is accompanied by many physiological changes in metabolism, most of which are poorly understood due to the confounding factors such as poor habitual diet and inactivity. There is an increase in body fat mass and a reduction in fat free mass due to a decrease in protein. There is a reduction in muscle and mitochondrial proteins associated with decreased gene expression.[125] It is still unknown whether reduced physical activity is the sole reason for the observed decreases in muscle mass and strength or whether there is an inevitable effect of age *per se*. Metabolically, muscle mass accounts for ~30% of resting energy expenditure and 40–90% of exercise-related energy expenditure;[126] consequently, it is not surprising that there is a correlation between reduced metabolism and a loss of fat free mass in the elderly. There are also changes in glucose tolerance, increasing the susceptibility for type 2 diabetes,[127] suggesting that one of the contributing factors to reduced metabolism could be insulin signaling or abundance, given that insulin controls the flux of metabolic substrates. Aging can impair insulin secretion or response,[128] and the increase in IMCL content in skeletal muscle from older adults[129,130] will also lead to insulin resistance.[131] Interestingly, both endurance and resistance exercise can counteract some of these effects, suggesting that some of these changes are due to muscular inactivity's causing reduced metabolic capabilities.

A. CARBOHYDRATE METABOLISM WITH AGING

As discussed in section 3 of this chapter, carbohydrates and lipids are the primary fuel sources during exercise, but vary in percent utilization depending on sex. Interestingly, fat and carbohydrate utilization also differ between the young and the elderly. It is well documented that metabolism is lower with aging; however, exercise can alter metabolism in the elderly. During moderate-intensity endurance exercise, mean carbohydrate oxidation was higher in elderly men and women at the same absolute exercise intensity as compared with young men and women, but significantly lower at similar relative intensities.[132,133] During high-intensity endurance exercise (15% above ventilatory threshold) in older men, carbohydrate oxidation was significantly higher; whereas young men increased fat oxidation with no changes in carbohydrate oxidation.[133,134] Interestingly, 16 weeks of moderate endurance exercise training in elderly men and women decreases the rate of carbohydrate oxidation and lowered glucose Ra.[135] These findings confirm the differences in carbohydrate oxidation with aging, and that exercise can alter carbohydrate oxidation differently in young and old.

Mechanistically, aging has been shown to reduce insulin-mediated glucose disposal even in glucose-tolerant elderly subjects.[128] Also, glycogen storage in the liver is usually higher with aging, which could be due to an increase in insulin resistance; however, glycogen storage is lower in skeletal muscle.[136] Aerobic exercise can aid in maintaining normal glucose homeostasis and alter insulin sensitivity.[137–140] Similarly, resistance exercise has been shown to improve whole-body glucose disposal in elderly subjects, but has little effect on insulin sensitivity.[141] Exercise increases the ability of skeletal muscle from older adults to extract glucose, and exercise in combination with insulin stimulation has an additive effect on whole-body glucose uptake and clearance.[138] When comparing endurance trained young and elderly subjects there is still a significantly lower insulin sensitivity in the elderly population; however, the difference is significantly less than in sedentary elderly subjects compared with sedentary young subjects.[134,140] The improvement in insulin sensitivity seems to be less sustainable in older people, consequently, the long-term benefits are only observed with regular long-term exercise.[139,142] Rasmussen et al. (2006) [143] demonstrated that in older subjects, skeletal muscle protein synthesis was resistant to insulin supplementation, and this may contribute to sarcopenia. Interestingly, aerobic exercise in older adults increases muscle mitochondrial enzyme activity (citrate synthase, cytochrome c oxidase)[139,144–146] and genes involved in mitochondrial biogenesis (PGC-1α, NRF-1, TFAM),[139] which could aid in the oxidation of carbohydrates and lipids.

In summary, aerobic exercise can improve insulin sensitivity and mitochondrial function in the aging population. Changes in glucose tolerance and insulin sensitivity in elderly populations can also be affected by diet. High dietary carbohydrates

(63–85% total calories) can improve insulin sensitivity compared to low-carbohydrate (30% total calories) diets,[147–149] although, by caloric displacement, diets that are too high in carbohydrates can compromise the consumption of adequate amounts of fats and protein. Although diet alone can improve changes in insulin sensitivity, it seems more practical to recommend regular endurance or resistance exercise to counteract changes in muscle metabolism, such as mitochondrial function. It has been demonstrated that a high-carbohydrate diet (63% total calories) in combination with aerobic exercise training is likely the best prescription for elderly patients, as the two in combination improve insulin sensitivity and promote healthy weight loss.[149]

B. Lipid Metabolism

Aging increases fat mass in humans and the distribution of stored fats is different for men and women as they age. Specifically, women have a higher percent subcutaneous and intrahepatocelluar lipid compartments and lower visceral adipose tissue compared with men.[136,150] Interestingly, there are no significant differences in IMCL content between men and women as they age;[136] however, the total amount increases with age,[150] which may impair insulin signaling, as there is a significant correlation between increased IMCL content and insulin resistance.[151,152] Studies correlating basal fat oxidation to fat mass showed no correlation; however there was a positive correlation with fat-free mass.[153] Plasma FFA concentrations are the simplest approach to study the turnover of fats, as they indirectly represent lipolysis, de-novo synthesis, and oxidation; however, FFA levels in the elderly have been shown to increase, decrease, and remain the same.[154–156] Results likely vary based on insulin, as insulin effects FFA concentrations.[154]

Aerobic exercise studies examining fat metabolism in young versus elderly have demonstrated that elderly men and women have a lower mean fat oxidation rate at the same absolute or relative exercise intensity as young men and women.[132] FFA Ra is significantly lower (~35%) in elderly men and women at relative exercise intensities similar to young men and women.[132] Sixteen weeks of moderate endurance exercise training in elderly men and women increases the rate of fat oxidation, but does not significantly change glycerol Ra, FFA Ra, or FFA Rd.[135] These results suggest that exercise training in elderly men and women increases fat oxidation through alterations in skeletal muscle fatty acid metabolism.[135]

The mechanisms contributing to alterations in fat accumulation and distribution are under investigation. As discussed above, the mechanisms in fat oxidation are likely similar to that of carbohydrate and involve changes in gene regulation of transporters and mitochondrial function. Again, aerobic exercise in the elderly increases muscle mitochondrial enzyme activity of citrate synthase and cytochrome c oxidase,[139,144–146] and genes involved in mitochondrial biogenesis like PGC-1α, NRF-1 and TFAM,[139] which are involved in the final pathway of the oxidation of lipids.

C. Protein Metabolism

Aging is associated with sarcopenia and whether it is due to a slow process of muscle protein catabolism or other factors such as a reduced ability to process and build muscle requires further investigation. Approximately 50% of the proteins in the human body are located in the skeletal muscle, which constitutes approximately 15% of an adult's body weight.[157] With aging, muscle size decreases, as does strength and muscle quality (the force per unit area). These changes can be attenuated to varying degrees with endurance exercise, resistance exercise, or protein supplementation.

Whole-body protein turnover is significantly lower in older adults.[139,158,159] Several studies have shown a lower fractional synthetic rate of mixed muscle protein in older as compared with younger men and women.[144,158,160–162] Short et al. (2004)[144] demonstrated that, at the whole-body level, protein breakdown, protein synthesis, and leucine oxidation declined at a rate of ~4–5% per decade, irrespective of sex. The rate of myofibrillar protein synthesis and MHC are also reduced in older as compared with younger adults.[163] These reduction are associated with a reduction in functional strength.[158] Furthermore, mitochondrial protein synthesis is also reduced in older as compared with younger adults.[164] The mechanism(s) behind the reduction in protein is associated with a lower abundance of mRNA species involved in electron transport chain and myofibrillar gene expression.[125,165]

These changes can be alleviated by an acute bout of resistance exercise, leading to the stimulation of myofibrillar proteins and mixed muscle protein synthesis rates [11,144,166–168], most likely mediated by translational or post-translational mechanisms.[168,169] The benefits of resistance exercise are further supported by studies that have found no difference in protein breakdown between younger and older adults.[160,167] Similarly, 4 months of aerobic exercise can increase mixed muscle protein synthesis, but does not seem to alter whole body protein turnover.[144]

From a nutritional standpoint, traditional nutritional supplements *per se* have been ineffective at improving muscle mass in the elderly;[170] however, ingestion or infusion of essential amino acids does stimulate muscle protein synthesis in the elderly,[171,172] although the extent of stimulation of protein synthesis by amino acids is lower in older adults.[172] A combination of protein or essential amino acids and exercise training further enhances muscle protein synthesis in older adults[173] and improves muscle strength by more than 125%.[174] In younger adults, the consumption of proteins, essential amino acids, with and without carbohydrate in the immediate postexercise period increases the rate of muscle protein synthesis and improves net balance.[175] A recent study found that protein synthesis rates between young and old were similar following activity of daily living exercise with the ingestion of leucine and protein.[176] From a practical perspective, one study found that the consumption of a protein/carbohydrate and fat snack immediately following acute exercise resulted in an enhancement of the muscle mass gains following a period of resistance exercise training.[177] Finally, it does not appear that the source of protein is important in the enhancement of strength and muscle mass gains following resistance exercise, for a meat-based diet and a lacto-ovo vegetarian diet were comparable.[178]

In general, the mechanism behind muscle protein loss and aging needs further investigation. There could be a genetic component as there is a decrease in the expression of skeletal muscle mRNA encoding for proteins involved in protein turnover and energy metabolism in aged compared with young humans and animals. These age-related changes can be reduced by exercise in combination with protein supplementation. The timing of protein administration appears to be important, with strength gains being enhanced if the nutrition is consumed shortly after exercise.

D. BENEFITS OF EXERCISE AND HORMONE REPLACEMENT THERAPY IN THE ELDERLY

Aging is associated with changes in body composition such as increase in body fat mass, decrease in protein mass, and decrease in contractile and mitochondrial-related proteins.[126] Research has attempted to determine if age-associated changes in muscle function are a cause or effect of aging. Evidence is accumulating to suggest that progressive resistance exercise is a useful non-pharmacological treatment for age-related losses in muscle mass, quality, and function. Long-term habitual exercise can result in similar dynamic strength, maximum voluntary isometric strength, cross-sectional area, specific tension, power, and proportion of myosin heavy chain iso-forms in older men compared with young men.[126,179] Mitochondrial function has been reported to decline with age; however, Brierly et al. (1996)[180] demonstrated that oxidative metabolism was poorly correlated with chronological age and strongly correlated with markers of physical activity, and subsequently found that mitochondrial respiratory chain function was not significantly different between young and elderly athletes.[181] Exercise alone increases aerobic capacity, muscle protein synthesis, and mitochondrial enzyme activity in older men and women.[144] This data suggests that an active lifestyle is able to preserve muscle function during aging to levels similar to those of sedentary young adults.

There are specific sex differences in the process of aging. In men, the process of aging is usually gradual and levels of testosterone slowly decrease such that half of men aged 50–70 years are hypogonadal.[158] In men, both acute and chronic resistance exercise alone increases free testosterone, although the effect is attenuated in younger compared with older men.[182,183] Testosterone replacement in elderly men to levels similar to that of young males increased muscle size and strength.[13] A recent study examining the combined effects of testosterone and exercise in untrained frail elderly men concluded there was no synergistic effects of the combination.[184] These findings are similar to a study that compared hypogonadal men with HIV-related muscle wasting and found that both resistance exercise and testosterone administration and the combination of both resulted in similar increases in muscle strength and mass.[122] This is contrary to the interactive effects of testosterone and exercise in young healthy males where fat-free mass, muscle size and strength were greater in the testosterone plus resistance exercise group as compared with a non-exercising group receiving testosterone.[120] These studies suggest that there are age-related differences in the response to hormonal intervention in men.

Women undergo menopause at approximately 50 years of age. Menopause is the cessation of menses and reduction of estrogen production. It is associated with increased adiposity and greater risk of metabolic disease.[185–187] Estrogen supplementation in menopausal and postmenopausal women can attenuate gains in adipose tissue, improve insulin sensitivity, and reduce the likeliness to develop type 2 diabetes.[188–190] Furthermore, estrogen replacement therapy in post-menopausal women can counteract the decline in muscle mass.[17] Although estrogen replacement therapy for postmenopausal females might have a synergistic effect in combination with resistance training, current research suggests there is no significant effect of the combination in comparison with exercise alone.[191] There is also a growing interest in testosterone therapy in postmenopausal women as women experience a 28% decrease in testosterone as they age,[192] and the anabolic effects of testosterone, particularly in combination with exercise could improve overall health and longevity of women as they age.

Currently, the interactive effect between hormone replacement therapy and resistance exercise is only beginning to be explored. In terms of muscle mass and strength gains, testosterone has a potent anabolic effect, whereas estrogen has a mild anabolic effects in younger adults however in elderly people the benefits of hormone replacement therapy with (and even without) resistance exercise need further investigation. These results suggest that, over a lifetime, regular exercise alone may have the best protective effect on muscle strength, function, and oxidative capacity.

VI. SUMMARY

There are sex differences in metabolic fuel selection during endurance exercise. Specifically, females oxidize more lipids and less carbohydrate than men. The mechanism behind these findings is ultimately differences in gene regulation, but the mechanism by which this genetic regulation is occurring needs further investigation, although the sex hormone estrogen is a potential candidate. The implications of sex differences on nutritional recommendations need further investigation but remain a promising area, especially for athletes.

There are also differences in substrate metabolism with aging, and whether sex-related differences are maintained remains to be determined; however, menopause plays an important role in changes in substrate metabolism in women. Evidence is overwhelming that the best way to counteract the effects of sarcopenia is with exercise, although protein or amino acid supplementation either alone or in combination with exercise also seems to be beneficial for the elderly. Research into the genetic regulation of substrate pathway differences is in its infancy but will ultimately unfold the conundrum of sex and age-related differences in metabolism.

REFERENCES

1. Friedlander, A.L., Casazza, G.A., Horning, M.A., Huie, M.J., Piacentini, M.F., Trimmer, J.K., Brooks, G.A. Training-induced alterations of carbohydrate metabolism in women: Women respond differently from men. *J. Appl. Physiol.* 85, 1175–1186, 1998.
2. Carter, S.L., Rennie, C., Tarnopolsky, M.A. Substrate utilization during endurance exercise in men and women after endurance training. *Am. J. Physiol. Endocrinol. Metab.* 280, E898–907, 2001.
3. Phillips, S.M., Atkinson, S.A., Tarnopolsky, M.A., MacDougall, J.D. Gender differences in leucine kinetics and nitrogen balance in endurance athletes. *J.App. Physiol.* 75, 2134–2141, 1993.
4. Tarnopolsky, L.J., MacDougall, J.D., Atkinson, S.A., Tarnopolsky, M.A., Sutton, J.R. Gender differences in substrate for endurance exercise. *J.Appl. Physiol.* 68, 302–308, 1990.
5. Tarnopolsky, M.A., Atkinson, S.A., Phillips, S.M., MacDougall, J.D. Carbohydrate loading and metabolism during exercise in men and women. *J. Appl. Physiol.* 78, 1360–1368, 1995.

6. Horton, T.J., Pagliassotti, M.J., Hobbs, K., Hill, J.O. Fuel metabolism in men and women during and after long-duration exercise. *J. Appl. Physiol.* 85, 1823–1832, 1998.

7. Ruby, B.C., Coggan, A.R., Zderic, T.W. Gender differences in glucose kinetics and substrate oxidation during exercise near the lactate threshold. *J. Appl. Physiol.* 92, 1125–1132, 2002.

8. Davis, S.N., Galassetti, P., Wasserman, D.H., Tate, D. Effects of gender on neuroendocrine and metabolic counterregulatory responses to exercise in normal man. *J. Clin. Endocrinol. Metab.* 85, 224–230, 2000.

9. Lamont, L.S., McCullough, A.J., Kalhan, S.C. Gender differences in leucine, but not lysine, kinetics. *J. Appl. Physiol.* 91, 357–362, 2001.

10. Devries, M.C., Hamadeh, M.J., Graham, T.E., Tarnopolsky, M.A. 17β-estradiol supplementation decreases glucose rate of appearance and disappearance with no effect on glycogen utilization during moderate intensity exercise in men. *J. Clin. Endocrinol. Metab.* 90, 6218–6225, 2005.

11. Yarasheski, K.E., Pak-Loduca, J., Hasten, D.L., Obert, K.A., Brown, M.B., Sinacore, D.R. Resistance exercise training increases mixed muscle protein synthesis rate in frail women and men ≥ = 76 yr old. *Am. J. Physiol.* 277, E118–125, 1999.

12. Tarnopolsky, M.A., Parise, G., Yardley, N.J., Ballantyne, C.S., Olatinji, S., Phillips, S.M. Creatine-dextrose and protein-dextrose induce similar strength gains during training. *Med. Sci. Sports. Exerc.* 33, 2044–2052, 2001.

13. Ferrando, A.A., Sheffield–Moore, M., Yeckel, C.W., Gilkison, C., Jiang, J., Achacosa, A., Lieberman, S.A., Tipton, K., Wolfe, R.R., Urban, R.J. Testosterone administration to older men improves muscle function: Molecular and physiological mechanisms. *Am. J. Physiol. Endocrinol. Metab.* 282, E601–607, 2002.

14. Wolfe, R., Ferrando, A., Sheffield-Moore, M., Urban, R. Testosterone and muscle protein metabolism. *Mayo. Clin. Proc.* 75 Suppl, S55–59; discussion S59–60, 2000.

15. Ellis, G.S., Lanza-Jacoby, S., Gow, A., Kendrick, Z.V. Effects of estradiol on lipoprotein lipase activity and lipid availability in exercised male rats. *J. Appl. Physiol.* 77, 209–215, 1994.

16. Kendrick, Z.V., Steffen, C.A., Rumsey, W.L., Goldberg, D.I. Effect of estradiol on tissue glycogen metabolism in exercised oophorectomized rats. *J. Appl. Physiol.* 63, 492–496, 1987.

17. Dionne, I.J., Kinaman, K.A., Poehlman, E.T. Sarcopenia and muscle function during menopause and hormone-replacement therapy. *J. Nutr. Health. Aging.* 4, 156–161, 2000.

18. Miller, A.E., MacDougall, J.D., Tarnopolsky, M.A., Sale, D.G. Gender differences in strength and muscle fiber characteristics. *Eur. J. Appl. Physiol. Occup. Physiol.* 66, 254–262, 1993.

19. Carter, S.L., Rennie, C.D., Hamilton, S.J., Tarnopolsky, M.A. Changes in skeletal muscle in males and females following endurance training. *Can. J. Physiol. Pharmacol.* 79, 386–392, 2001.

20. Fox, J., Garber, P., Hoffman, M., Johnson, D., Schaefer, P., Vien, J., Zeaton, C., Thompson, L.V. Morphological characteristics of skeletal muscles in relation to gender. *Aging Clin. Exp. Res.* 15, 264–269, 2003.

21. Vistisen, B., Roepstorff, K., Roepstorff, C., Bonen, A., van Deurs, B., Kiens, B. Sarcolemmal FAT/CD36 in human skeletal muscle colocalizes with caveolin-3 and is more abundant in type 1 than in type 2 fibers. *J. Lipid Res.* 45, 603–609, 2004.

22. Kiens, B., Roepstorff, C., Glatz, J.F., Bonen, A., Schjerling, P., Knudsen, J., Nielsen, J.N. Lipid binding proteins and lipoprotein lipase activity in human skeletal muscle: Influence of physical activity and gender. *J. Appl. Physiol.* 2004.

23. Lexell, J., Henriksson-Larsen, K., Winblad, B., Sjostrom, M. Distribution of different fiber types in human skeletal muscles: Effects of aging studied in whole muscle cross sections. *Muscle Nerve.* 6, 588–595, 1983.

24. Coggan, A.R., Spina, R.J., King, D.S., Rogers, M.A., Brown, M., Nemeth, P.M., Holloszy, J.O. Histochemical and enzymatic comparison of the gastrocnemius muscle of young and elderly men and women. *J. Gerontol.* 47, B71–76, 1992.

25. Klitgaard, H., Mantoni, M., Schiaffino, S., Ausoni, S., Gorza, L., Laurent-Winter, C., Schnohr, P., Saltin, B. Function, morphology and protein expression of ageing skeletal muscle: A cross-sectional study of elderly men with different training backgrounds. *Acta. Physiol. Scand.* 140, 41–54, 1990.

26. Cupido, C.M., Hicks, A.L., Martin, J. Neuromuscular fatigue during repetitive stimulation in elderly and young adults. *Eur. J. Appl. Physiol. Occup. Physiol.* 65, 567–572, 1992.

27. Frontera, W.R., Suh, D., Krivickas, L.S., Hughes, V.A., Goldstein, R., Roubenoff, R. Skeletal muscle fiber quality in older men and women. *Am. J. Physiol. Cell Physiol.* 279, C611–618, 2000.

28. Lamont, L.S. Gender differences in amino acid use during endurance exercise. *Nutr. Rev.* 63, 419–422, 2005.

29. Tarnopolsky, M.A. Gender differences in substrate metabolism during endurance exercise. *Can. J. Appl. Physiol.* 25, 312–327, 2000.

30. Tarnopolsky, M.A., Saris, W.H. Evaluation of gender differences in physiology: an introduction. *Curr. Opin. Clin. Nutr. Metab. Care.* 4, 489–492, 2001.

31. Nicklas, B.J., Hackney, A.C., Sharp, R.L. The menstrual cycle and exercise: performance, muscle glycogen, and substrate responses. *Int. J. Sports Med.* 10, 264–269, 1989.

32. Campbell, S.E., Angus, D.J., Febbraio, M.A. Glucose kinetics and exercise performance during phases of the menstrual cycle: Effect of glucose ingestion. *Am. J. Physiol. Endocrinol. Metab.* 281, E817–825, 2001.

33. Pritzlaff-Roy, C.J., Widemen, L., Weltman, J.Y., Abbott, R., Gutgesell, M., Hartman, M.L., Veldhuis, J.D., Weltman, A. Gender governs the relationship between exercise intensity and growth hormone release in young adults. *J. Appl. Physiol.* 92, 2053–2060, 2002.

34. Zello, G.A. Dietary Reference Intakes for the macronutrients and energy: Considerations for physical activity. *Appl. Physiol. Nutr. Metab.* 31, 74–79, 2006.

35. McKenzie, S., Phillips, S.M., Carter, S.L., Lowther, S., Gibala, M.J., Tarnopolsky, M.A. Endurance exercise training attenuates leucine oxidation and BCOAD activation during exercise in humans. *Am. J. Physiol. Endocrinol. Metab.* 278, E580–587, 2000.

36. Horton, T.J., Grunwald, G.K., Lavely, J., Donahoo, W.T. Glucose kinetics differ between women and men, during and after exercise. *J. Appl. Physiol.* 100, 1883–1894, 2006.

37. Devries, M.C., Hamadeh, M.J., Phillips, S.M., Tarnopolsky, M.A. Menstrual Cycle Phase and Sex Influence Muscle Glycogen Utilization and Glucose Turnover During Moderate Intensity Endurance Exercise. *Am. J. Physiol. Regul. Integr. Comp. Physiol.* 2006.

38. Roepstorff, C., Steffensen, C.H., Madsen, M., Stallknecht, B., Kanstrup, I.L., Richter, E.A., Kiens, B. Gender differences in substrate utilization during submaximal exercise in endurance-trained subjects. *Am. J. Physiol. Endocrinol. Metab.* 282, E435–447, 2002.

39. Ruby, B.C., Robergs, R.A., Waters, D.L., Burge, M., Mermier, C., Stolarczyk, L. Effects of estradiol on substrate turnover during exercise in amenorrheic females. *Med. Sci. Sports Exerc.* 29, 1160–1169, 1997.

40. Brooks, S., Nevill, M.E., Meleagros, L., Lakomy, H.K., Hall, G.M., Bloom, S.R., Williams, C. The hormonal responses to repetitive brief maximal exercise in humans. *Eur. J. Appl. Physiol. Occup. Physiol.* 60, 144–148, 1990.

41. Jensen, M.D., Cryer, P.E., Johnson, C.M., Murray, M.J. Effects of epinephrine on regional free fatty acid and energy metabolism in men and women. *Am. J. Physiol.* 270, E259–264, 1996.

42. Monjo, M., Rodriguez, A.M., Palou, A., Roca, P. Direct effects of testosterone, 17 beta–estradiol, and progesterone on adrenergic regulation in cultured brown adipocytes: potential mechanism for gender-dependent thermogenesis. *Endocrinology.* 144, 4923–4930, 2003.

43. Ramis, J.M., Salinas, R., Garcia-Sanz, J.M., Moreiro, J., Proenza, A.M., Llado, I. Depot- and gender-related differences in the lipolytic pathway of adipose tissue from severely obese patients. *Cell Physiol. Biochem.* 17, 173–180, 2006.

44. Zderic, T.W., Coggan, A.R., Ruby, B.C. Glucose kinetics and substrate oxidation during exercise in the follicular and luteal phases. *J. Appl. Physiol.* 90, 447–453, 2001.

45. Bergstrom, J., Hermansen, L., Hultman, E., Saltin, B. Diet, muscle glycogen and physical performance. *Acta. Physiol. Scand.* 71, 140–150, 1967.

46. Costill, D.L., Sherman, W.M., Fink, W.J., Maresh, C., Witten, M., Miller, J.M. The role of dietary carbohydrates in muscle glycogen resynthesis after strenuous running. *Am. J. Clin. Nutr.* 34, 1831–1836, 1981.

47. Hultman, E. Studies on muscle metabolism of glycogen and active phosphate in man with special reference to exercise and diet. *Scand. J. Clin. Lab. Invest. Suppl.* 94, 1–63, 1967.

48. Bergstrom, J., Hultman, E. A study of the glycogen metabolism during exercise in man. *Scand. J. Clin. Lab. Invest.* 19, 218–228, 1967.

49. Walker, J.L., Heigenhauser, G.J., Hultman, E., Spriet, L.L. Dietary carbohydrate, muscle glycogen content, and endurance performance in well-trained women. *J. Appl. Physiol.* 88, 2151–2158, 2000.

50. Sherman, W.M., Costill, D.L., Fink, W.J., Miller, J.M. Effect of exercise-diet manipulation on muscle glycogen and its subsequent utilization during performance. *Int. J. Sports Med.* 2, 114–118, 1981.

51. Karlsson, J., Saltin, B. Diet, muscle glycogen, and endurance performance. *J. Appl. Physiol.* 31, 203–206, 1971.

52. Tarnopolsky, M.A., Zawada, C., Richmond, L.B., Carter, S., Shearer, J., Graham, T., Phillips, S.M. Gender differences in carbohydrate loading are related to energy intake. *J. Appl. Physiol.* 91, 225–230, 2001.

53. James, A.P., Lorraine, M., Cullen, D., Goodman, C., Dawson, B., Palmer, T.N., Fournier, P.A. Muscle glycogen supercompensation: Absence of a gender-related difference. *Eur. J. Appl. Physiol.* 85, 533–538, 2001.

54. Febbraio, M.A., Chiu, A., Angus, D.J., Arkinstall, M.J., Hawley, J.A. Effects of carbohydrate ingestion before and during exercise on glucose kinetics and performance. *J. Appl. Physiol.* 89, 2220–2226, 2000.

55. Coggan, A.R., Swanson, S.C. Nutritional manipulations before and during endurance exercise: effects on performance. *Med. Sci. Sports Exerc.* 24, S331–335, 1992.

56. Coggan, A.R., Coyle, E.F. Metabolism and performance following carbohydrate ingestion late in exercise. *Med. Sci. Sports Exerc.* 21, 59–65, 1989.

57. Coggan, A.R., Coyle, E.F. Carbohydrate ingestion during prolonged exercise: effects on metabolism and performance. *Exerc. Sport Sci. Rev.* 19, 1–40, 1991.

58. Burelle, Y., Peronnet, F., Charpentier, S., Lavoie, C., Hillaire-Marcel, C., Massicotte, D. Oxidation of an oral [13C]glucose load at rest and prolonged exercise in trained and sedentary subjects. *J. Appl. Physiol.* 86, 52–60, 1999.

59. Bailey, S.P., Zacher, C.M., Mittleman, K.D. Effect of menstrual cycle phase on carbohydrate supplementation during prolonged exercise to fatigue. *J. Appl. Physiol.* 88, 690–697, 2000.

60. Riddell, M.C., Partington, S.L., Stupka, N., Armstrong, D., Rennie, C., Tarnopolsky, M.A. Substrate utilization during exercise performed with and without glucose ingestion in female and male endurance trained athletes. *Int. J. Sport Nutr. Exerc. Metab.* 13, 407–421, 2003.

61. Wallis, G.A., Dawson, R., Achten, J., Webber, J., Jeukendrup, A.E. Metabolic response to carbohydrate ingestion during exercise in males and females. *Am. J. Physiol. Endocrinol. Metab.* 290, E708–715, 2006.

62. Tarnopolsky, M.A., Bosman, M., Macdonald, J.R., Vandeputte, D., Martin, J., Roy, B.D. Postexercise protein-carbohydrate and carbohydrate supplements increase muscle glycogen in men and women. *J. Appl. Physiol.* 83, 1877–1883, 1997.

63. Roy, B.D., Luttmer, K., Bosman, M.J., Tarnopolsky, M.A. The influence of postexercise macronutrient intake on energy balance and protein metabolism in active females participating in endurance training. *Int. J. Sport Nutr. Exerc. Metab.* 12, 172–188, 2002.

64. Stanley, W.C., Connett, R.J. Regulation of muscle carbohydrate metabolism during exercise. *FASEB J.* 5, 2155–2159, 1991.

65. Powers, S.K., Howley, E.T., *Exercise Physiology*, 3rd edition, McGraw-Hill, Boston, Massachusetts, 1996.

66. Morgan, T.E., Short, F.A., Cobb, L.A. Effect of long-term exercise on skeletal muscle lipid composition. *Am. J. Physiol.* 216, 82–86, 1969.

67. Hoppeler, H. Exercise-induced ultrastructural changes in skeletal muscle. *Int. J. Sports Med.* 7, 187–204, 1986.

68. Hwang, J.H., Pan, J.W., Heydari, S., Hetherington, H.P., Stein, D.T. Regional differences in intramyocellular lipids in humans observed by *in vivo* 1H-MR spectroscopic imaging. *J. Appl. Physiol.* 90, 1267–1274, 2001.

69. Staron, R.S., Hikida, R.S., Murray, T.F., Hagerman, F.C., Hagerman, M.T. Lipid depletion and repletion in skeletal muscle following a marathon. *J. Neurol. Sci.* 94, 29–40, 1989.

70. Steffensen, C.H., Roepstorff, C., Madsen, M., Kiens, B. Myocellular triacylglycerol breakdown in females but not in males during exercise. *Am.J. Physiol. Endocrinol. Metab.* 282, E634–642, 2002.

71. Goodpaster, B.H., He, J., Watkins, S., Kelley, D.E. Skeletal muscle lipid content and insulin resistance: Evidence for a paradox in endurance-trained athletes. *J. Clin. Endocrinol. Metab.* 86, 5755–5761, 2001.

72. Zderic, T.W., Davidson, C.J., Schenk, S., Byerley, L.O., Coyle, E.F. High-fat diet elevates resting intramuscular triglyceride concentration and whole body lipolysis during exercise. *Am. J. Physiol. Endocrinol. Metab.* 286, E217–225, 2004.

73. Mittendorfer, B., Horowitz, J.F., Klein, S. Effect of gender on lipid kinetics during endurance exercise of moderate intensity in untrained subjects. *Am. J. Physiol. Endocrinol. Metab.* 283, E58–65, 2002.

74. Larson-Meyer, D.E., Newcomer, B.R., Hunter, G.R. Influence of endurance running and recovery diet on intramyocellular lipid content in women: A 1H NMR study. *Am. J. Physiol. Endocrinol. Metab.* 282, E95–E106, 2002.

75. van Loon, L.J., Schrauwen-Hinderling, V.B., Koopman, R., Wagenmakers, A.J., Hesselink, M.K., Schaart, G., Kooi, M.E., Saris, W.H. Influence of prolonged endurance cycling and recovery diet on intramuscular triglyceride content in trained males. *Am. J. Physiol. Endocrinol. Metab.* 285, E804–811, 2003.

76. Starling, R.D., Trappe, T.A., Parcell, A.C., Kerr, C.G., Fink, W.J., Costill, D.L. Effects of diet on muscle triglyceride and endurance performance. *J. Appl. Physiol.* 82, 1185–1189, 1997.

77. Lambert, E.V., Speechly, D.P., Dennis, S.C., Noakes, T.D. Enhanced endurance in trained cyclists during moderate intensity exercise following two weeks adaptation to a high fat diet. *Eur. J. Appl. Physiol. Occup. Physiol.* 69, 287–293, 1994.

78. Rowlands, D.S., Hopkins, W.G. Effects of high-fat and high-carbohydrate diets on metabolism and performance in cycling. *Metabolism.* 51, 678–690, 2002.

79. Phinney, S.D., Bistrian, B.R., Evans, W.J., Gervino, E., Blackburn, G.L. The human metabolic response to chronic ketosis without caloric restriction: Preservation of submaximal exercise capability with reduced carbohydrate oxidation. *Metabolism.* 32, 769–776, 1983.

80. Goedecke, J.H., Christie, C., Wilson, G., Dennis, S.C., Noakes, T.D., Hopkins, W.G., Lambert, E.V. Metabolic adaptations to a high-fat diet in endurance cyclists. *Metabolism.* 48, 1509–1517, 1999.

81. MacLean, D.A., Spriet, L.L., Hultman, E., Graham, T.E. Plasma and muscle amino acid and ammonia responses during prolonged exercise in humans. *J. Appl. Physiol.* 70, 2095–2103, 1991.

82. Lamont, L.S., McCullough, A.J., Kalhan, S.C. Gender differences in the regulation of amino acid metabolism. *J. Appl. Physiol.* 95, 1259–1265, 2003.

83. Kobayashi, R., Shimomura, Y., Murakami, T., Nakai, N., Fujitsuka, N., Otsuka, M., Arakawa, N., Popov, K.M., Harris, R.A. Gender difference in regulation of branched-chain amino acid catabolism. *Biochem. J.* 327 (2), 449–453, 1997.

84. Lariviere, F., Moussalli, R., Garrel, D.R. Increased leucine flux and leucine oxidation during the luteal phase of the menstrual cycle in women. *Am. J. Physiol.* 267, E422–428, 1994.

85. Lamont, L.S., Lemon, P.W., Bruot, B.C. Menstrual cycle and exercise effects on protein catabolism. *Med. Sci. Sports Exerc.* 19, 106–110, 1987.

86. Gaine, P.C., Pikosky, M.A., Martin, W.F., Bolster, D.R., Maresh, C.M., Rodriguez, N.R. Level of dietary protein impacts whole body protein turnover in trained males at rest. *Metabolism.* 55, 501–507, 2006.

87. Lamont, L.S., McCullough, A.J., Kalhan, S.C. Beta-adrenergic blockade heightens the exercise-induced increase in leucine oxidation. *Am. J. Physiol.* 268, E910–916, 1995.

88. Friedman, J.E., Lemon, P.W. Effect of chronic endurance exercise on retention of dietary protein. *Int. J. Sports Med.* 10, 118–123, 1989.

89. Meredith, C.N., Zackin, M.J., Frontera, W.R., Evans, W.J. Dietary protein requirements and body protein metabolism in endurance-trained men. *J. Appl. Physiol.* 66, 2850–2856, 1989.

90. Lemon, P.W., Dolny, D.G., Yarasheski, K.E. Moderate physical activity can increase dietary protein needs. *Can. J. Appl. Physiol.* 22, 494–503, 1997.

91. Tarnopolsky, M. Protein requirements for endurance athletes. *Nutrition.* 20, 662–668, 2004.

92. Simpson, E.R. Sources of estrogen and their importance. *J. Steroid Biochem. Mol. Biol.* 86, 225–230, 2003.

93. Srivastava, S., Toraldo, G., Weitzmann, M.N., Cenci, S., Ross, F.P., Pacifici, R. Estrogen decreases osteoclast formation by down-regulating receptor activator of NF-kappa B ligand (RANKL)-induced JNK activation. *J. Biol. Chem.* 276, 8836–8840, 2001.

94. Wilder, R.L. Hormones, pregnancy, and autoimmune diseases. *Ann.N. Y. Acad. Sci.* 840, 45–50, 1998.

95. McEwen, B.S., Alves, S.E. Estrogen actions in the central nervous system. *Endocr. Rev.* 20, 279–307, 1999.

96. Mendelsohn, M.E., Karas, R.H. The protective effects of estrogen on the cardiovascular system. *N. Engl. J. Med.* 340, 1801–1811, 1999.

97. Carter, S., McKenzie, S., Mourtzakis, M., Mahoney, D.J., Tarnopolsky, M.A. Short-term 17β-estradiol decreases glucose R(a) but not whole body metabolism during endurance exercise. *J. Appl. Physiol.* 90, 139–146, 2001.

98. Rooney, T.P., Kendrick, Z.V., Carlson, J., Ellis, G.S., Matakevich, B., Lorusso, S.M., McCall, J.A. Effect of estradiol on the temporal pattern of exercise-induced tissue glycogen depletion in male rats. *J. Appl. Physiol.* 75, 1502–1506, 1993.

99. Kendrick, Z.V., Ellis, G.S. Effect of estradiol on tissue glycogen metabolism and lipid availability in exercised male rats. *J. Appl. Physiol.* 71, 1694–1699, 1991.

100. Hatta, H., Atomi, Y., Shinohara, S., Yamamoto, Y., Yamada, S. The effects of ovarian hormones on glucose and fatty acid oxidation during exercise in female ovariectomized rats. *Horm. Metab. Res.* 20, 609–611, 1988.

101. Tarnopolsky, M.A., Roy, B.D., MacDonald, J.R., McKenzie, S., Martin, J., Ettinger, S. Short-term 17-β-estradiol administration does not affect metabolism in young males. *Int. J. Sports Med.* 22, 175–180, 2001.

102. Binnert, C., Koistinen, H.A., Martin, G., Andreelli, F., Ebeling, P., Koivisto, V.A., Laville, M., Auwerx, J., Vidal, H. Fatty acid transport protein-1 mRNA expression in skeletal muscle and in adipose tissue in humans. *Am. J. Physiol. Endocrinol. Metab.* 279, E1072–1079, 2000.

103. Campbell, S.E., Febbraio, M.A. Effect of ovarian hormones on mitochondrial enzyme activity in the fat oxidation pathway of skeletal muscle. *Am. J. Physiol. Endocrinol. Metab.* 281, E803–808, 2001.

104. Wiik, A., Glenmark, B., Ekman, M., Esbjornsson-Liljedahl, M., Johansson, O., Bodin, K., Enmark, E., Jansson, E. Oestrogen receptor beta is expressed in adult human skeletal muscle both at the mRNA and protein level. *Acta. Physiol. Scand.* 179, 381–387, 2003.

105. Lemoine, S., Granier, P., Tiffoche, C., Rannou-Bekono, F., Thieulant, M.L., Delamarche, P. Estrogen receptor alpha mRNA in human skeletal muscles. *Med. Sci. Sports Exerc.* 35, 439–443, 2003.

106. Lemoine, S., Granier, P., Tiffoche, C., Berthon, P.M., Rannou-Bekono, F., Thieulant, M.L., Carre, F., Delamarche, P. Effect of endurance training on oestrogen receptor alpha transcripts in rat skeletal muscle. *Acta. Physiol. Scand.* 174, 283–289, 2002.

107. Barros, R.P., Machado, U.F., Warner, M., Gustafsson, J.A. Muscle GLUT4 regulation by estrogen receptors ERbeta and ERalpha. *Proc. Natl. Acad. Sci. U. S. A.* 103, 1605–1608, 2006.

108. Wiik, A., Gustafsson, T., Esbjornsson, M., Johansson, O., Ekman, M., Sundberg, C.J., Jansson, E. Expression of oestrogen receptor alpha and beta is higher in skeletal muscle of highly endurance-trained than of moderately active men. *Acta. Physiol. Scand.* 184, 105–112, 2005.

109. Lemoine, S., Granier, P., Tiffoche, C., Berthon, P.M., Thieulant, M.L., Carre, F., Delamarche, P. Effect of endurance training on oestrogen receptor alpha expression in different rat skeletal muscle type. *Acta. Physiol. Scand.* 175, 211–217, 2002.

110. Godsland, I.F. Oestrogens and insulin secretion. *Diabetologia.* 48, 2213–2220, 2005.

111. Morimoto, S., Cerbon, M.A., Alvarez-Alvarez, A., Romero-Navarro, G., Diaz-Sanchez, V. Insulin gene expression pattern in rat pancreas during the estrous cycle. *Life Sci.* 68, 2979–2985, 2001.

112. von Wolff, M., Ursel, S., Hahn, U., Steldinger, R., Strowitzki, T. Glucose transporter proteins (GLUT) in human endometrium: Expression, regulation, and function throughout the menstrual cycle and in early pregnancy. *J. Clin. Endocrinol. Metab.* 88, 3885–3892, 2003.

113. Tsao, T.S., Li, J., Chang, K.S., Stenbit, A.E., Galuska, D., Anderson, J.E., Zierath, J.R., McCarter, R.J., Charron, M.J. Metabolic adaptations in skeletal muscle overexpressing GLUT4: Effects on muscle and physical activity. *FASEB J.* 15, 958–969, 2001.

114. Heine, P.A., Taylor, J.A., Iwamoto, G.A., Lubahn, D.B., Cooke, P.S. Increased adipose tissue in male and female estrogen receptor-alpha knockout mice. *Proc. Natl. Acad. Sci. U. S. A.* 97, 12729–12734, 2000.

115. Simoncini, T., Hafezi-Moghadam, A., Brazil, D.P., Ley, K., Chin, W.W., Liao, J.K. Interaction of oestrogen receptor with the regulatory subunit of phosphatidylinositol-3-OH kinase. *Nature.* 407, 538–541, 2000.

116. Jessen, N., Goodyear, L.J. Contraction signaling to glucose transport in skeletal muscle. *J. Appl. Physiol.* 99, 330–337, 2005.

117. Djouadi, F., Weinheimer, C.J., Saffitz, J.E., Pitchford, C., Bastin, J., Gonzalez, F.J., Kelly, D.P. A gender-related defect in lipid metabolism and glucose homeostasis in peroxisome proliferator-activated receptor alpha-deficient mice. *J. Clin. Invest.* 102, 1083–1091, 1998.

118. Richard, D. Effects of ovarian hormones on energy balance and brown adipose tissue thermogenesis. *Am. J. Physiol.* 250, R245–249, 1986.

119. D'Eon, T.M., Souza, S.C., Aronovitz, M., Obin, M.S., Fried, S.K., Greenberg, A.S. Estrogen regulation of adiposity and fuel partitioning. Evidence of genomic and non-genomic regulation of lipogenic and oxidative pathways. *J. Biol. Chem.* 280, 35983–35991, 2005.

120. Bhasin, S., Storer, T.W., Berman, N., Callegari, C., Clevenger, B., Phillips, J., Bunnell, T.J., Tricker, R., Shirazi, A., Casaburi, R. The effects of supraphysiologic doses of testosterone on muscle size and strength in normal men. *N. Engl. J. Med.* 335, 1–7, 1996.

121. Griggs, R.C., Kingston, W., Jozefowicz, R.F., Herr, B.E., Forbes, G., Halliday, D. Effect of testosterone on muscle mass and muscle protein synthesis. *J. Appl. Physiol.* 66, 498–503, 1989.

122. Bhasin, S., Storer, T.W., Javanbakht, M., Berman, N., Yarasheski, K.E., Phillips, J., Dike, M., Sinha-Hikim, I., Shen, R., Hays, R.D., Beall, G. Testosterone replacement and resistance exercise in HIV-infected men with weight loss and low testosterone levels. *JAMA.* 283, 763–770, 2000.

123. Ferrando, A.A., Tipton, K.D., Doyle, D., Phillips, S.M., Cortiella, J., Wolfe, R.R. Testosterone injection stimulates net protein synthesis but not tissue amino acid transport. *Am. J. Physiol.* 275, E864–871, 1998.

124. Braun, B., Gerson, L., Hagobian, T., Grow, D., Chipkin, S.R. No effect of short-term testosterone manipulation on exercise substrate metabolism in men. *J. Appl. Physiol.* 99, 1930–1937, 2005.

125. Welle, S., Bhatt, K., Thornton, C.A. High-abundance mRNAs in human muscle: comparison between young and old. *J. Appl. Physiol.* 89, 297–304, 2000.

126. Karakelides, H., Sreekumaran Nair, K. Sarcopenia of aging and its metabolic impact. *Curr. Top Dev. Biol.* 68, 123–148, 2005.

127. Davidson, M.B. The effect of aging on carbohydrate metabolism: A review of the English literature and a practical approach to the diagnosis of diabetes mellitus in the elderly. *Metabolism.* 28, 688–705, 1979.

128. Tessari, P. Role of insulin in age-related changes in macronutrient metabolism. *Eur. J. Clin. Nutr.* 54 Suppl 3, S126–130, 2000.
129. Wolfe, R.R., Klein, S., Carraro, F., Weber, J.M. Role of triglyceride-fatty acid cycle in controlling fat metabolism in humans during and after exercise. *Am. J. Physiol.* 258, E382–389, 1990.
130. Sinha, R., Dufour, S., Petersen, K.F., LeBon, V., Enoksson, S., Ma, Y.Z., Savoye, M., Rothman, D.L., Shulman, G.I., Caprio, S. Assessment of skeletal muscle triglyceride content by (1)H nuclear magnetic resonance spectroscopy in lean and obese adolescents: relationships to insulin sensitivity, total body fat, and central adiposity. *Diabetes.* 51, 1022–1027, 2002.
131. Petersen, K.F., Befroy, D., Dufour, S., Dziura, J., Ariyan, C., Rothman, D.L., DiPietro, L., Cline, G.W., Shulman, G.I. Mitochondrial dysfunction in the elderly: possible role in insulin resistance. *Science.* 300, 1140–1142, 2003.
132. Sial, S., Coggan, A.R., Carroll, R., Goodwin, J., Klein, S. Fat and carbohydrate metabolism during exercise in elderly and young subjects. *Am. J. Physiol.* 271, E983–989, 1996.
133. Manetta, J., Brun, J.F., Perez-Martin, A., Callis, A., Prefaut, C., Mercier, J. Fuel oxidation during exercise in middle-aged men: Role of training and glucose disposal. *Med. Sci. Sports Exerc.* 34, 423–429, 2002.
134. Manetta, J., Brun, J.F., Prefaut, C., Mercier, J. Substrate oxidation during exercise at moderate and hard intensity in middle-aged and young athletes vs sedentary men. *Metabolism.* 54, 1411–1419, 2005.
135. Sial, S., Coggan, A.R., Hickner, R.C., Klein, S. Training-induced alterations in fat and carbohydrate metabolism during exercise in elderly subjects. *Am. J. Physiol.* 274, E785–790, 1998.
136. Machann, J., Thamer, C., Schnoedt, B., Stefan, N., Stumvoll, M., Haring, H.U., Claussen, C.D., Fritsche, A., Schick, F. Age and gender related effects on adipose tissue compartments of subjects with increased risk for type 2 diabetes: A whole body MRI/MRS study. *Magma.* 18, 128–137, 2005.
137. Dela, F., Mikines, K.J., Larsen, J.J., Galbo, H. Training-induced enhancement of insulin action in human skeletal muscle: The influence of aging. *J. Gerontol. A Biol. Sci. Med. Sci.* 51, B247–252, 1996.
138. Dela, F., Mikines, K.J., Larsen, J.J., Galbo, H. Glucose clearance in aged trained skeletal muscle during maximal insulin with superimposed exercise. *J. Appl. Physiol.* 87, 2059–2067, 1999.
139. Short, K.R., Vittone, J.L., Bigelow, M.L., Proctor, D.N., Rizza, R.A., Coenen-Schimke, J.M., Nair, K.S. Impact of aerobic exercise training on age-related changes in insulin sensitivity and muscle oxidative capacity. *Diabetes.* 52, 1888–1896, 2003.
140. Clevenger, C.M., Parker Jones, P., Tanaka, H., Seals, D.R., DeSouza, C.A. Decline in insulin action with age in endurance-trained humans. *J. Appl. Physiol.* 93, 2105–2111, 2002.
141. Ferrara, C.M., Goldberg, A.P., Ortmeyer, H.K., Ryan, A.S. Effects of aerobic and resistive exercise training on glucose disposal and skeletal muscle metabolism in older men. *J. Gerontol. A Biol. Sci. Med. Sci.* 61, 480–487, 2006.
142. Seals, D.R., Hagberg, J.M., Hurley, B.F., Ehsani, A.A., Holloszy, J.O. Effects of endurance training on glucose tolerance and plasma lipid levels in older men and women. *JAMA.* 252, 645–649, 1984.
143. Rasmussen, B.B., Fujita, S., Wolfe, R.R., Mittendorfer, B., Roy, M., Rowe, V.L., Volpi, E. Insulin resistance of muscle protein metabolism in aging. *FASEB J.* 20, 768–769, 2006.

144. Short, K.R., Vittone, J.L., Bigelow, M.L., Proctor, D.N., Nair, K.S. Age and aerobic exercise training effects on whole body and muscle protein metabolism. *Am. J. Physiol. Endocrinol. Metab.* 286, E92–101, 2004.

145. Coggan, A.R., Abduljalil, A.M., Swanson, S.C., Earle, M.S., Farris, J.W., Mendenhall, L.A., Robitaille, P.M. Muscle metabolism during exercise in young and older untrained and endurance-trained men. *J. Appl. Physiol.* 75, 2125–2133, 1993.

146. Spina, R.J., Chi, M.M., Hopkins, M.G., Nemeth, P.M., Lowry, O.H., Holloszy, J.O. Mitochondrial enzymes increase in muscle in response to 7–10 days of cycle exercise. *J. Appl. Physiol.* 80, 2250–2254, 1996.

147. Chen, M., Bergman, R.N., Porte, D., Jr. Insulin resistance and beta-cell dysfunction in aging: The importance of dietary carbohydrate. *J. Clin. Endocrinol. Metab.* 67, 951–957, 1988.

148. Fukagawa, N.K., Anderson, J.W., Hageman, G., Young, V.R., Minaker, K.L. High-carbohydrate, high-fiber diets increase peripheral insulin sensitivity in healthy young and old adults. *Am. J. Clin. Nutr.* 52, 524–528, 1990.

149. Hays, N.P., Starling, R.D., Sullivan, D.H., Fluckey, J.D., Coker, R.H., Williams, R.H., Evans, W.J. Effects of an ad libitum, high carbohydrate diet and aerobic exercise training on insulin action and muscle metabolism in older men and women. *J. Gerontol. A Biol. Sci. Med. Sci.* 61, 299–304, 2006.

150. Cree, M.G., Newcomer, B.R., Katsanos, C.S., Sheffield-Moore, M., Chinkes, D., Aarsland, A., Urban, R., Wolfe, R.R. Intramuscular and liver triglycerides are increased in the elderly. *J. Clin. Endocrinol. Metab.* 89, 3864–3871, 2004.

151. Krssak, M., Falk Petersen, K., Dresner, A., DiPietro, L., Vogel, S.M., Rothman, D.L., Roden, M., Shulman, G.I. Intramyocellular lipid concentrations are correlated with insulin sensitivity in humans: a 1H NMR spectroscopy study. *Diabetologia.* 42, 113–116, 1999.

152. Levin, K., Daa Schroeder, H., Alford, F.P., Beck-Nielsen, H. Morphometric documentation of abnormal intramyocellular fat storage and reduced glycogen in obese patients with Type II diabetes. *Diabetologia.* 44, 824–833, 2001.

153. Calles-Escandon, J., Arciero, P.J., Gardner, A.W., Bauman, C., Poehlman, E.T. Basal fat oxidation decreases with aging in women. *J. Appl. Physiol.* 78, 266–271, 1995.

154. Bonadonna, R.C., Groop, L.C., Simonson, D.C., DeFronzo, R.A. Free fatty acid and glucose metabolism in human aging: Evidence for operation of the Randle cycle. *Am. J. Physiol.* 266, E501–509, 1994.

155. Sandberg, H., Yoshimine, N., Maeda, S., Symons, D., Zavodnick, J. Effects of an oral glucose load on serum immunoreactive insulin, free fatty acid, growth hormone and blood sugar levels in young and elderly subjects. *J. Am. Geriatr Soc.* 21, 433–439, 1973.

156. Fraze, E., Chiou, Y.A., Chen, Y.D., Reaven, G.M. Age-related changes in postprandial plasma glucose, insulin, and free fatty acid concentrations in nondiabetic individuals. *J. Am. Geriatr. Soc.* 35, 224–228, 1987.

157. Tessari, P. Changes in protein, carbohydrate, and fat metabolism with aging: possible role of insulin. *Nutr. Rev.* 58, 11–19, 2000.

158. Balagopal, P., Rooyackers, O.E., Adey, D.B., Ades, P.A., Nair, K.S. Effects of aging on *in vivo* synthesis of skeletal muscle myosin heavy-chain and sarcoplasmic protein in humans. *Am. J. Physiol.* 273, E790–800, 1997.

159. Rooyackers, O.E., Balagopal, P., Nair, K.S. Measurement of synthesis rates of specific muscle proteins using needle biopsy samples. *Muscle Nerve Suppl.* 5, S93–96, 1997.

160. Yarasheski, K.E., Zachwieja, J.J., Bier, D.M. Acute effects of resistance exercise on muscle protein synthesis rate in young and elderly men and women. *Am. J. Physiol.* 265, E210–214, 1993.

161. Welle, S., Thornton, C., Jozefowicz, R., Statt, M. Myofibrillar protein synthesis in young and old men. *Am. J. Physiol.* 264, E693–698, 1993.
162. Welle, S., Totterman, S., Thornton, C. Effect of age on muscle hypertrophy induced by resistance training. *J. Gerontol. A Biol. Sci. Med. Sci.* 51, M270–275, 1996.
163. Short, K.R., Vittone, J.L., Bigelow, M.L., Proctor, D.N., Coenen-Schimke, J.M., Rys, P., Nair, K.S. Changes in myosin heavy chain mRNA and protein expression in human skeletal muscle with age and endurance exercise training. *J. Appl. Physiol.* 99, 95–102, 2005.
164. Rooyackers, O.E., Adey, D.B., Ades, P.A., Nair, K.S. Effect of age on *in vivo* rates of mitochondrial protein synthesis in human skeletal muscle. *Proc. Natl. Acad. Sci. U S A.* 93, 15364–15369, 1996.
165. Lee, C.K., Klopp, R.G., Weindruch, R., Prolla, T.A. Gene expression profile of aging and its retardation by caloric restriction. *Science.* 285, 1390–1393, 1999.
166. Hasten, D.L., Pak-Loduca, J., Obert, K.A., Yarasheski, K.E. Resistance exercise acutely increases MHC and mixed muscle protein synthesis rates in 78–84 and 23–32 yr olds. *Am. J. Physiol. Endocrinol. Metab.* 278, E620–626, 2000.
167. Welle, S., Thornton, C., Statt, M. Myofibrillar protein synthesis in young and old human subjects after three months of resistance training. *Am. J. Physiol.* 268, E422–427, 1995.
168. Balagopal, P., Schimke, J.C., Ades, P., Adey, D., Nair, K.S. Age effect on transcript levels and synthesis rate of muscle MHC and response to resistance exercise. *Am. J. Physiol. Endocrinol. Metab.* 280, E203–208, 2001.
169. Welle, S., Bhatt, K., Thornton, C.A. Stimulation of myofibrillar synthesis by exercise is mediated by more efficient translation of mRNA. *J. Appl. Physiol.* 86, 1220–1225, 1999.
170. Wolfe, R.R. Optimal nutrition, exercise, and hormonal therapy promote muscle anabolism in the elderly. *J. Am. Coll. Surg.* 202, 176–180, 2006.
171. Volpi, E., Ferrando, A.A., Yeckel, C.W., Tipton, K.D., Wolfe, R.R. Exogenous amino acids stimulate net muscle protein synthesis in the elderly. *J. Clin. Invest.* 101, 2000–2007, 1998.
172. Katsanos, C.S., Kobayashi, H., Sheffield-Moore, M., Aarsland, A., Wolfe, R.R. Aging is associated with diminished accretion of muscle proteins after the ingestion of a small bolus of essential amino acids. *Am. J. Clin. Nutr.* 82, 1065–1073, 2005.
173. Biolo, G., Tipton, K.D., Klein, S., Wolfe, R.R. An abundant supply of amino acids enhances the metabolic effect of exercise on muscle protein. *Am. J. Physiol.* 273, E122–129, 1997.
174. Fiatarone, M.A., O'Neill, E.F., Ryan, N.D., Clements, K.M., Solares, G.R., Nelson, M.E., Roberts, S.B., Kehayias, J.J., Lipsitz, L.A., Evans, W.J. Exercise training and nutritional supplementation for physical frailty in very elderly people. *N. Engl. J. Med.* 330, 1769–1775, 1994.
175. Tipton, K.D., Elliott, T.A., Cree, M.G., Aarsland, A.A., Sanford, A.P., Wolfe, R.R. Stimulation of net muscle protein synthesis by whey protein ingestion before and after exercise. *Am. J. Physiol. Endocrinol. Metab.* 2006.
176. Koopman, R., Verdijk, L., Manders, R.J., Gijsen, A.P., Gorselink, M., Pijpers, E., Wagenmakers, A.J., van Loon, L.J. Co-ingestion of protein and leucine stimulates muscle protein synthesis rates to the same extent in young and elderly lean men. *Am. J. Clin. Nutr.* 84, 623–632, 2006.
177. Esmarck, B., Andersen, J.L., Olsen, S., Richter, E.A., Mizuno, M., Kjaer, M. Timing of postexercise protein intake is important for muscle hypertrophy with resistance training in elderly humans. *J. Physiol.* 535, 301–311, 2001.

178. Haub, M.D., Wells, A.M., Tarnopolsky, M.A., Campbell, W.W. Effect of protein source on resistive-training-induced changes in body composition and muscle size in older men. *Am. J. Clin. Nutr.* 76, 511–517, 2002.

179. Saris, W.H., Tarnopolsky, M.A. Biological ageing: A physiological perspective. *Curr. Opin. Clin. Nutr. Metab. Care.* 3, 469–472, 2000.

180. Brierley, E.J., Johnson, M.A., James, O.F., Turnbull, D.M. Effects of physical activity and age on mitochondrial function. *QJM.* 89, 251–258, 1996.

181. Brierley, E.J., Johnson, M.A., James, O.F., Turnbull, D.M. Mitochondrial involvement in the ageing process. Facts and controversies. *Mol. Cell. Biochem.* 174, 325–328, 1997.

182. Kraemer, W.J., Hakkinen, K., Newton, R.U., Nindl, B.C., Volek, J.S., McCormick, M., Gotshalk, L.A., Gordon, S.E., Fleck, S.J., Campbell, W.W., Putukian, M., Evans, W.J. Effects of heavy-resistance training on hormonal response patterns in younger vs. older men. *J. Appl. Physiol.* 87, 982–992, 1999.

183. Kraemer, W.J., Staron, R.S., Hagerman, F.C., Hikida, R.S., Fry, A.C., Gordon, S.E., Nindl, B.C., Gothshalk, L.A., Volek, J.S., Marx, J.O., Newton, R.U., Hakkinen, K. The effects of short-term resistance training on endocrine function in men and women. *Eur. J. Appl. Physiol. Occup. Physiol.* 78, 69–76, 1998.

184. Sullivan, D.H., Roberson, P.K., Johnson, L.E., Bishara, O., Evans, W.J., Smith, E.S., Price, J.A. Effects of muscle strength training and testosterone in frail elderly males. *Med. Sci. Sports Exerc.* 37, 1664–1672, 2005.

185. Tchernof, A., Desmeules, A., Richard, C., Laberge, P., Daris, M., Mailloux, J., Rheaume, C., Dupont, P. Ovarian hormone status and abdominal visceral adipose tissue metabolism. *J. Clin. Endocrinol. Metab.* 89, 3425–3430, 2004.

186. Toth, M.J., Tchernof, A., Sites, C.K., Poehlman, E.T. Effect of menopausal status on body composition and abdominal fat distribution. *Int. J. Obes. Relat. Metab. Disord.* 24, 226–231, 2000.

187. Carr, M.C. The emergence of the metabolic syndrome with menopause. *J. Clin. Endocrinol. Metab.* 88, 2404–2411, 2003.

188. Margolis, K.L., Bonds, D.E., Rodabough, R.J., Tinker, L., Phillips, L.S., Allen, C., Bassford, T., Burke, G., Torrens, J., Howard, B.V. Effect of oestrogen plus progestin on the incidence of diabetes in postmenopausal women: Results from the Women's Health Initiative Hormone Trial. *Diabetologia.* 47, 1175–1187, 2004.

189. Kritz-Silverstein, D., Barrett-Connor, E. Long-term postmenopausal hormone use, obesity, and fat distribution in older women. *JAMA.* 275, 46–49, 1996.

190. Sayegh, R.A., Kelly, L., Wurtman, J., Deitch, A., Chelmow, D. Impact of hormone replacement therapy on the body mass and fat compositions of menopausal women: A cross-sectional study. *Menopause.* 6, 312–315, 1999.

191. Brooke-Wavell, K., Prelevic, G.M., Bakridan, C., Ginsburg, J. Effects of physical activity and menopausal hormone replacement therapy on postural stability in post-menopausal women—a cross-sectional study. *Maturitas.* 37, 167–172, 2001.

192. Khosla, S., Melton, L.J., 3rd, Atkinson, E.J., O'Fallon, W.M., Klee, G.G., Riggs, B.L. Relationship of serum sex steroid levels and bone turnover markers with bone mineral density in men and women: A key role for bioavailable estrogen. *J. Clin. Endocrinol. Metab.* 83, 2266–2274, 1998.

193. Costill, D.L., Fink, W.J., Getchell, L.H., Ivy, J.L., Witzmann, F.A. Lipid metabolism in skeletal muscle of endurance-trained males and females. *J. Appl. Physiol.* 47, 787–791, 1979.

194. Froberg, K., Pedersen, P.K. Sex differences in endurance capacity and metabolic response to prolonged, heavy exercise. *Eur. J. Appl. Physiol. Occup. Physiol.* 52, 446–450, 1984.

195. Blatchford, F.K., Knowlton, R.G., Schneider, D.A. Plasma FFA responses to prolonged walking in untrained men and women. *Eur. J. Appl. Physiol. Occup. Physiol.* 53, 343–347, 1985.

196. Romijn, J.A., Coyle, E.F., Sidossis, L.S., Rosenblatt, J., Wolfe, R.R. Substrate metabolism during different exercise intensities in endurance-trained women. *J. Appl. Physiol.* 88, 1707–1714, 2000.

197. Goedecke, J.H., St Clair Gibson, A., Grobler, L., Collins, M., Noakes, T.D., Lambert, E.V. Determinants of the variability in respiratory exchange ratio at rest and during exercise in trained athletes. *Am. J. Physiol. Endocrinol. Metab.* 279, E1325–1334, 2000.

198. Melanson, E.L., Sharp, T.A., Seagle, H.M., Horton, T.J., Donahoo, W.T., Grunwald, G.K., Hamilton, J.T., Hill, J.O. Effect of exercise intensity on 24-h energy expenditure and nutrient oxidation. *J. Appl. Physiol.* 92, 1045–1052, 2002.

199. M'Kaouar, H., Peronnet, F., Massicotte, D., Lavoie, C. Gender difference in the metabolic response to prolonged exercise with [13C]glucose ingestion. *Eur. J. Appl. Physiol.* 92, 462–469, 2004.

200. Zehnder, M., Ith, M., Kreis, R., Saris, W., Boutellier, U., Boesch, C. Gender-specific usage of intramyocellular lipids and glycogen during exercise. *Med. Sci. Sports. Exerc.* 37, 1517–1524, 2005.

201. Roepstorff, C., Thiele, M., Hillig, T., Pilegaard, H., Richter, E.A., Wojtaszewski, J.F., Kiens, B. Higher skeletal muscle {alpha}2AMPK activation and lower energy charge and fat oxidation in men than in women during submaximal exercise. *J. Physiol.* 2006.

9 Body Weight Regulation and Energy Needs

Melinda M. Manore and Janice L. Thompson

CONTENTS

I. INTRODUCTION

For many athletes, either weight loss or weight gain may be a goal depending on their sport. For sports such as basketball, American football, and weight-lifting, weight gain is often a goal, with a focus on gaining muscle mass. Conversely, for other sports such as wrestling, distance running, gymnastics, diving, and dance, a low body weight is considered a necessity for ensuring successful performance. For those sports where performance is judged based on some aesthetic component (e.g., dance, diving, and gymnastics), the pressure is even greater to be thin. In addition to performance pressures, athletes are also susceptible to the societal pressures to be thin or to have a particular body shape and size. This is especially true among many female athletes where the drive for thinness can become obsessive, leading to disordered eating behaviors and potential detrimental health consequences.[1]

When is it appropriate for an athlete to lose weight? There are situations in which weight loss in an athlete may be warranted. Some athletes may gain body fat in the off-season, and their performance is enhanced when they lose the excess body fat. However, there are also many circumstances in which the athlete or coaching staff may have unrealistic goals and expectations regarding body weight and performance. If weight loss is necessary, what is the safest way to encourage healthy weight loss in an athlete? If weight gain is warranted, how can muscle mass gains be optimized without resorting to unproven supplements or ergogenic aids? This chapter will address these questions. First, a review of energy balance, fuel oxidation, and the relationship of these factors to weight loss and gain is given. Second, we review the safe weight loss strategies athletes can use. We then discuss the pathogenic weight loss strategies athletes should not use and their associated health concerns. Finally, we review the recommendations for safe weight gain, with a focus on gaining muscle mass. In the athlete, both weight loss and weight gain need to be approached with care, prudence, and realistic expectations for all involved in the process.

II. MANIPULATION OF ENERGY BALANCE TO INDUCE WEIGHT LOSS OR WEIGHT GAIN

Weight loss or gain requires an imbalance between energy intake and energy expenditure. For weight loss, energy intake will be intentionally reduced below the level of energy expenditure or energy intake can remain stable, while energy expenditure is increased. For weight gain, the reverse is true. Energy intake needs to be increased above energy expenditure, while also incorporating both resistance-training (RT) and aerobic exercise into the weight gain plan. While manipulating energy balance appears simple, a number of factors affect an individual's ability to either lose or gain weight. These factors include changes in the components of the energy balance equation and the manipulation of fuel oxidation through alterations in the macronutrient composition of the diet. In addition, a number of other factors unique to each individual need to be considered, such as genetic make-up, lifestyle, environmental conditions, social and behavioral circumstances, stage of growth, and diet and exercise habits.[2]

A. ENERGY BALANCE EQUATION

The energy balance equation comprises energy intake and energy expenditure, and states that body weight is maintained if energy intake equals energy expenditure:

$$\text{Energy balance occurs when: } E_{in} = E_{out}$$

Where E_{in} = Energy in (kJ/d or kcal/d) and E_{out} = Energy expended (kJ/d or kcal/d)

The oxidation rates of the macronutrients must also balance and are discussed later in this chapter.

Each side of the energy balance equation must be assessed. The three components of total daily energy expenditure (TDEE) are resting metabolic rate (RMR), thermic effect of food (TEF), and the thermic effect of activity (TEA). RMR represents the energy expended to support all resting metabolic functions (e.g., maintaining body temperature, ventilation, cellular electrical activity). The TEF represents the energy expended as a result of digestion, absorption, transport, and storage of foods consumed. The TEA includes a number of factors associated with movement: (1) programmed physical activity, (2) activities of daily living, which would include all movement/activities done above resting level, including very low level activities such as sitting and standing, and (3) spontaneous physical activity and/or fidgeting, which includes small movements such as changing your position in a chair, tapping your foot, shivering, and maintaining your posture.

Levine[3] has suggested that the activities of daily living (e.g., everything we do that is not sleeping, eating, or sport/exercise activities) be classified as non-exercise activity thermogenesis (NEAT). He has hypothesized that NEAT may help explain why some people are obese and others are not and why some people can maintain their body weight, while others gain weight.[4,5,] He and colleagues[5] compared the NEAT in 10 mildly obese and 10 lean sedentary individuals and found that obese individuals were seated 2 h/d longer than lean individuals, who were standing or walking 2.5 h/d more than obese individuals. This difference in NEAT accounted for a difference of 350 ± 65 kcal/d (5,6). Thus, this component of TDEE needs to be considered when looking at athletes' daily activities. Are the athletes extremely sedentary during the day, except when they are training for their sport? If they are, they may be expending less energy than might be estimated or anticipated for someone considered to be physically active. This was demonstrated by Thompson et al., when they compared the energy expenditures of two groups of highly trained male triathletes matched for age, fat free mass (FFM) and weight. These researchers found that those triathletes who appeared to have low energy intakes compared with energy expenditures (energy intakes that were 1535 ± 524 kcal < estimated energy expenditures), yet reported being weight stable, had significantly lower spontaneous physical activity levels than those athletes whose energy intake more closely matched their energy expenditure. Data were collected in a metabolic chamber where all meals and activity were controlled. Thus, the athletes originally estimated to have inadequate energy intake were actually in energy balance.

For most sedentary individuals, RMR accounts for 60–75% of TDEE, with the TEF and TEA accounting for 6–10% and 15–34% of TDEE, respectively.[8] Of course, athletes will have a higher level of TEA because of their high level of programmed physical activity. Increasing TDEE to result in weight loss can be accomplished by manipulating one or more of these three components, as discussed below. The reverse is also true for weight gain. Increasing total energy intake above TDEE can result in weight gain.

B. MANIPULATION OF THE COMPONENTS OF THE ENERGY BALANCE EQUATION

Although it has long been claimed that exercise increases RMR, its effects are equivocal. Since RMR is dependent primarily on level of muscle and organ tissue, the impact of exercise and becoming more fit on RMR will depend on whether there is a change in FFM and total body weight. Although some cross-sectional studies comparing athletes with untrained subjects have found athletes to have significantly higher RMR values,[9,10] others have found no difference in RMR among untrained and trained individuals.[11,12] These studies have compared RMR values using kcal/kg FFM, thus controlling for the differences in FFM between trained and untrained controls. Results of more recent training studies show that most individuals do not experience an increase in RMR with training, when data are expressed as kcal/kg FFM.[13,14]

It is important to remember that results from a particular study may depend on how the data are expressed and collected. For example, Byrne and Wilmore[13] compared the effect of RT or RT plus walking on RMR in sedentary, moderately obese (37.5% body fat) women over a 20-wk training program. They found a significant increase in RMR in the RT-only group and a significant decrease in RMR in the RT-plus-walking group, when RMR was expressed as either ml O_2/min or total kcal/d, but no differences when RMR was expressed as kcal/kg FFM/day. In fact, RMR expressed as kcal/kg FFM decreased in both groups, but was only significantly lower in the RT-plus-walking group. In this study, FFM increased by 1.9 kg in both groups due to the training programs, with similar increases in total body weight, but no change in fat mass or relative body fat. Thus, based on increases in body weight alone, we would expect RMR to increase. It is likely that many factors affect one's metabolic response to exercise, including genetics; the type, intensity, and duration of exercise training; the timing of RMR measurement in relationship to the last exercise bout; and how the data are collected and expressed. In summary, the research data are not clear on whether exercise increases RMR; however, we do know that significant increases in FFM can increase RMR. Thus, the impact of any training program on RMR will depend on how body weight and composition change and to what degree.

RMR is known to have a genetic component, with approximately 40% of the variability in RMR explained by genetics in twins and pairs of parents and children after adjusting for the influences of age, gender and FFM.[15] The type of training employed could have an impact on changing the RMR. The strongest predictor of RMR is FFM, with approximately 80% of the variance in RMR accounted for by FFM.[8] As indicated above, it would seem that increasing one's FFM through RT would increase FFM, and in turn, increase RMR.[13] Interestingly, Bosselaers et al.[16] found that body builders had significantly higher absolute 24-h energy expenditure than inactive controls, but this difference disappeared when adjustments were made for differences in FFM among the two groups. However, exercise has been found to prevent some of the decline in RMR that occurs with energy restriction and dieting,[17] but appears to be protective only when energy restriction is not severe.[18]

Exercise intensity and duration can also have an impact on RMR and TDEE. Fat is the predominant fuel source during endurance-type exercise of low to moderate intensity. As exercise intensity increases above 60–70% of VO_{2max}, carbohydrate contributes proportionately more energy than fat. In addition, most individuals can perform low- to moderate-intensity exercise for a longer duration than high-intensity exercise, resulting in greater energy expenditure over time. These findings led to the recommendation that weight loss is best achieved by performing moderate-intensity endurance-type exercise for 45–60 min duration.

However, a study by Tremblay et al.[19] challenged these assumptions. They found that individuals participating in high-intensity bicycling training were shown to have a greater reduction in skinfold thickness than individuals who performed moderate-intensity continuous bicycling training. The high-intensity training reduced body fat more despite the fact that the energy cost of the high-intensity training was less than half of moderate-intensity training. The authors concluded that high-intensity training may have significantly increased loss of body fat by affecting an increase in β-oxidation enzyme activity. This study has led to important changes in how we make weight loss recommendations to athletes. Today, all athletes incorporate high-intensity workouts, including RT training programs, into their overall training programs for their sports. We know that high-intensity workouts build strength and FFM and expend more energy per minute than slower, more aerobic-type exercises. Thus, including all types of exercise into a weight-loss program along with moderate energy restriction will allow athletes to continue to perform at high intensities while experiencing desirable body fat changes.

In addition to its potential impact on RMR, exercise can also increase TDEE through an increase in energy expenditure above RMR during a brief period following the exercise bout. This increase in energy expenditure is referred to as excess postexercise oxygen consumption (EPOC). It has been well documented in the exercise literature that exercise (both endurance and RT) increases EPOC.[20] However, the degree of EPOC that occurs with exercise varies dramatically (4–21%) depending on the type, intensity, and duration of exercise that occurs.[21] For example, Bahr et al.[22] found that 80 min of exercise at 70% VO_{2max} significantly increased EPOC by 15% at 12-h postexercise, while EPOC was only 5.1% at 12-h postexercise when the exercise lasted only 20 min. When three bouts of exercise at 108% VO_{2max} for 2 min were performed, EPOC lasted 4 h following exercise.[23]

RT (90–100 min) has also been found to increase EPOC. Melby et al.[24] and Osterberg and Melby[25] found EPOC was elevated 5–10% and 4% above RMR when measured the morning following RT in both men and women, respectively. It is generally agreed that exercise can increase EPOC for a period of time after exercise, but exercise needs to be of either long duration or high intensity to increase EPOC to any significant extent. If exercise is intense enough or long enough to increase EPOC, then we would expect an overall increase in TDEE. However, moderate levels of physical activity for approximately 30 min (40–70% VO_{2max}) do not significantly increase EPOC for any significant length of time and RMR returns to baseline with ~30–50 min.[21,26]

The TEF is influenced by the composition of the diet (% of energy from fat, carbohydrate, protein, and alcohol). The thermogenic effects of a nutrient depend on the energy costs of digesting, transporting, and metabolizing that nutrient for energy (ATP) or storing the energy as fat. The thermic effect of carbohydrate (or glucose), fat, and protein are 6–8%, 2–3% and 25–40%, respectively, of the total energy consumed.[27,28] This means that very little energy is needed to metabolize and store fat, while processing and storing protein and carbohydrate are less energy efficient. The magnitude of TEF is also dependent upon the total daily energy intake. TEF typically accounts for 6–10% of the energy intake, but can vary from 4–15% depending on the individual.[29] Using a typical individual with a daily energy intake of 2500 kcal/d, the TEF would be 150–250 kcal/d. To affect an increase in TEF, one would need to increase energy intake, which could result in positive balance and weight gain, or alter the nutrient composition of the diet.

The third component of TDEE is the TEA, which accounts for energy expended above RMR and TEF. Because the TEA is the most variable of the components of energy expenditure, it is the one most easily manipulated to result in weight loss. Increasing this component in some athletes is not practical, as they may already be exercising a great deal. In fact, it is common for many endurance athletes to expend 1000–2000 kcal/d while engaging in sport-related activities. Thompson et al.[7] found that the RMR of a group of elite male endurance athletes accounted for only 38–47% of TDEE (as opposed to 60–75% in most sedentary individuals) due to their high levels of exercise training. Thus, the present physical activity level of the athlete must be assessed before recommendations regarding changing the other components of TEA can be made.

III. DIET COMPOSITION AND FUEL UTILIZATION

The ability of an individual to lose or gain body weight and change body composition is influenced not only by alterations in energy intake and TDEE, but also by the oxidation rates of the macronutrients consumed. For weight and body composition to be maintained over time, energy intake must equal energy expenditure and substrates consumed must equal their oxidation rates. Therefore, macronutrient balance occurs when:

$$Protein_{in} = Protein_{oxidation}$$
$$CHO_{in} = CHO_{oxidation}$$
$$Fat_{in} = Fat_{oxidation}$$
$$Alcohol_{in} = Alcohol_{oxidation}$$

where $Protein_{in}$ is the amount of protein intake (g/d) and $Protein_{oxidation}$ is the amount of protein oxidized (g/d). These same notations apply to CHO, fat, and alcohol.

It is now known that under normal physiological conditions, carbohydrate, protein, and alcohol are not readily converted to triglycerides or stored as adipose tissue.[30-33] This is due to an increase in oxidation rates in response to increased intakes of carbohydrate, protein, and alcohol. When carbohydrates are consumed, glycogen storage and glucose oxidation are increased, while fat oxidation is decreased.[31,34] Under normal feeding conditions, glucose that is not stored is utilized for energy,[34] with little *de novo* lipogenesis occurring from excess carbohydrate intake.[31,32] As with carbohydrate, increased protein intake is also accompanied by an increase in protein oxidation, and any excess amino acids are deaminated and the carbon skeletons can be used to meet energy demands.[34] Because alcohol cannot be converted to body fat, alcohol is considered a priority fuel that is oxidized above protein and carbohydrat.[35] Alcohol consumption suppresses fat oxidation and can indirectly contribute to body fat storage by providing alternative sources of fuel for oxidation, while the fat in the meal is stored as body fat. Thus, when discussing weight loss with an athlete, the amount of alcohol consumed in the diet cannot be ignored. High alcohol consumption can be a major reason that athletes do not reach their weight loss goals.

The effect of inadequate energy or carbohydrate intake has a unique impact on protein balance and is a key concern for athletes attempting to lose weight. Inadequate intakes of carbohydrate or energy will result in a negative protein balance.

Thus, a higher protein/kcal ratio is required to maintain protein balance when energy or carbohydrate intake is insufficient. To prevent loss of FFM, it is important that both carbohydrate and protein are eaten in adequate quantities to maximize protein sparing in the athlete attempting to lose body fat.

Fat balance differs from protein and carbohydrate balance in that the oxidation of fat does not immediately increase proportionately with increased fat intake.[34] The failure to oxidize dietary fat in response to increased fat intake results in the excess energy consumed as dietary fat being converted to fat for storage in the adipose tissue. The varied responses of carbohydrate, protein, alcohol, and fat oxidation to changes in intake emphasize the importance of nutrient composition when designing weight-loss programs for athletes.

A. High-Carbohydrate, Low-Fat Diets

According to the energy balance equation, weight loss will occur when energy intake is lower than energy expenditure. However, the composition of the diet plays an important role in the composition of the weight lost and in providing the energy necessary for exercise training. A common recommendation for weight loss is the consumption of a high-carbohydrate, low-fat diet. The previous discussion of fuel oxidation sheds light on how this type of diet can result in the loss of body fat. The consumption of excess energy results in fat storage due to the efficiency of storing dietary fat over other fuels, as it is the fuel least likely to be oxidized in proportion to its intake. Since excess carbohydrate is not readily stored as body fat, a high-carbohydrate, lower-fat diet will less likely result in body-fat accumulation.

The macronutrient dietary recommendations made to most athletes fall within those recommend by the Institute of Medicine (IOM), Food and Nutrition Board, for the general public. The IOM established the acceptable macronutrient distribution ranges (AMDRs)[36] for adults; these ranges are 45–65% of energy from carbohydrate and 20–35% of energy from fat, with the remainder coming from protein. These recommendations assume that individuals are meeting their protein requirements, which have been set at 0.8 g/kg.[36] Protein requirements of athletes are discussed elsewhere in this text, but the requirements are typically higher than in sedentary individuals.[37]

Because athletes need carbohydrate for energy during exercise and must replace their glycogen stores after exercise is over, we typically recommend higher carbohydrate diets to athletes, with the exact percentage dependent on the athlete's sport. Thus, for an endurance athlete a high-carbohydrate, low-fat diet would provide approximately 60–65% of energy from carbohydrate and approximately 20–25% of energy from fat, with 10–20% of total energy from protein. Weight loss has been accomplished with this type of diet even when dieters are given *ad libitum* access to food, as long as low-fat meat, milk and dairy products are used along with unprocessed carbohydrates (whole grains/cereals, whole fruits, vegetables). The weight loss that accompanies *ad libitum* food intake may be beneficial to athletes who are maintaining heavy training schedules while trying to lose body fat. Two primary mechanisms have been identified to explain weight loss despite *ad libitum* food intake on high-carbohydrate diets that primarily comprise whole grains/cereals, fruits, and vegetables, plus low-fat protein sources. These hypothesized mechanisms are listed below:

- Significantly less energy (kcal/g of food) is consumed with a high-carbohydrate diet comprising unprocessed carbohydrates, due to its higher fiber and lower fat content[38-40]
- Sense of fullness and less hunger when consuming a high-carbohydrate unprocessed diet, due to the increased bulk of the foods eaten[38,41,42]
- Suppression of appetite and decreased energy consumed in the subsequent meal when consuming low-energy-dense foods (kcal/g or volume of food) such as broth-based soups and salads before a meal.[43]

The high-carbohydrate, low-fat diets that benefit athletes should contain an abundance of unprocessed carbohydrate foods such as legumes and beans, whole grains/cereals, whole fruits, vegetables, and low-fat meat and dairy products. It is very easy to consume a high-carbohydrate, low-fat diet by eating a diet high in simple carbohydrates, such as soda, cookies, candy, high-sugar cereals, processed grains (crackers, pasta, white bread) and beverages high in added sugars, such as some fruit, coffee, tea and energy drinks. While these types of foods provide glucose, they supply few other nutrients (such as vitamins, minerals, and fiber), and they can also lead to excess energy intake. While the excess simple carbohydrates will not likely be stored as fat, any dietary fat included in the meal that is not utilized for energy will be stored in the adipose tissue, and body fat and weight gain can result.

B. LOW-CARBOHYDRATE, HIGH-PROTEIN DIETS

Low-carbohydrate, high-protein weight loss plans are in abundance. While packaged under a variety of names and marketing strategies, this type of diet typically comprises foods containing at least 30% or more of the energy from protein, less than 45% of total energy from carbohydrate, and the balance of energy derived from fat. Although the Atkins diet[44] falls in and out of favor with dieters, this type of low-carbohydrate diet (less than 20g/day) has never been recommended for athletes because the carbohydrate level is too low to support exercise, maintain blood glucose levels, and replace muscle glycogen. The recommended dietary allowance (RDA) for carbohydrate is 130 g/d, which is the average minimum amount of glucose utilized by the brain.[36] This level of carbohydrate is higher than that recommended by the Atkins diet,[44] but is too low for athletes. There are two mechanisms proposed to support the use of the high protein-type diets for athletes:

1. The thermic effect of protein is high, which means that more energy is expended in the absorption, digestion and metabolism of protein. Higher protein diets are more satiating, which may make it easier to adhere to the dietary plan.
2. Reducing dietary carbohydrate will prevent the excessive production of insulin (or insulin "surges") that result from eating a high carbohydrate meal; lower levels of insulin leads to reduced fat storage and improved glucose regulation.

Research examining whether low-carbohydrate, high-protein/fat diets result in greater weight loss than energy-equivalent low-fat, high-carbohydrate diets (e.g., conventional diet) shows that, initially, people lose weight faster on the low-carbohydrate, high-protein/fat diets, but after 12 months total weight loss is similar.[45] The major disadvantage of applying a low-carbohydrate diet plan to the lifestyle of an athlete is that this type of diet will result in glycogen depletion, leaving the athlete with limited or no capability of performing high-intensity activities. Another disadvantage of a low-carbohydrate diet plan is that body weight decreases more rapidly due to the increased diuresis, or loss of body water, that accompanies the oxidation of stored carbohydrate. While the weight-loss goals are achieved, these diets leave one feeling lethargic, short-tempered, dehydrated, and unable to perform much physical activity. Carbohydrate is the most critical fuel for athletic performance, and consuming inadequate amounts of carbohydrate will hinder the athlete's cognitive ability and the ability to train and perform optimally, and could lead to fluid and electrolyte imbalances that can be harmful.

Claims regarding the risks of consuming a high-carbohydrate diet include concerns about the regulation of glucose and insulin metabolism and the storage of excess carbohydrate as body fat. As insulin signals the cells to store glucose and fat, and dietary carbohydrate results in the secretion of insulin, dietary carbohydrate is claimed to be dangerous if consumed in large proportions, and is blamed for insulin insensitivity, mood swings, and increased body fat. It is important to understand that much of the research published on glucose/insulin regulation, weight loss, and responses to various diets include obese subjects and individuals with type 2 diabetes or other glucose regulation problems. These individuals are not the metabolic peers of highly trained athletes. Athletes have improved glucose tolerance and insulin sensitivity compared with their healthy sedentary counterparts,[46] and respond quite differently to the dietary regimens imposed upon sedentary obese and individuals with diabetes. For example, Niakaris et al.[46] gave healthy lean male sprint runners, endurance runners, and sedentary controls a 75-g oral glucose-tolerance test. They found that the basal plasma insulin and the insulinemic responses to glucose were significantly higher in controls than the athletes ($p < 0.05$, $p < 0.02$, respectively). There were no differences for these variables between endurance and sprint runners. In addition, both groups of athletes were more insulin-sensitive than controls, regardless of the measure of insulin sensitivity used ($p < 0.05$). These results show that exercise training improves the ability of the body to metabolize glucose.

Recommendations for carbohydrate intake to ensure glycogen repletion will vary depending on the size of the individual, his or her gender, and the type of sport in which the athlete is participating. Of course, some sports rely much more heavily on glycogen stores (e.g., long-distance endurance sports) than sports that are shorter in duration or are intermittent in nature (e.g., gymnastics, wrestling, volleyball). In general, 7–10 g of carbohydrate/kg body weight will be adequate to normalize carbohydrate stores in 24-h after exercise.[47] In smaller individuals, such as women and children, this recommendation may be too high and carbohydrate intakes between 5–6 g/kg body weight may be adequate. These goals are achievable if one monitors total energy needs and reduces excess dietary fat from the diet, while assuring that adequate amounts of dietary unprocessed carbohydrates consumed.

IV. OPTIMAL BODY WEIGHT AND COMPOSITION FOR EXERCISE PERFORMANCE

While body weight can affect performance in sports requiring moving the body horizontally or vertically through space, the composition of the body, or amount of body fat, appears to be a more significant predictor of performance than body weight. Examples of sports where lower body fat is advantageous include distance running, diving, gymnastics, wrestling, and figure skating. Some sports also have judges who rate performance, such as gymnastics and body building. In these sports, a lean physique is generally required for successful performance. There are many instances where fat mass, in adequate amounts, is advantageous. Examples include contact sports, where the application and absorption of force and momentum are critical components, in addition to long-distance swimming, where fat mass assists with maintaining buoyancy and body temperature.

While all athletes need to be fit and prepared for competition, not all individuals should be classified into the same body-weight category. Unfortunately, many abuses of weight standards occur, and extreme dieting behaviors can lead to poor performance, illness, disordered eating behaviors, menstrual dysfunction in female athletes, and in extreme cases, even death.[48–50] How can healthy and responsible weight recommendations be made for athletes? In reality, weight standards for groups of athletes are not appropriate and should not be applied if at all possible. There are some sports, such as gymnastics, where physical appearance is critical to performance and closely linked with the maintenance of a relatively low body weight. Thus, it is important to assist these athletes with combining a competitive body weight with healthy eating practices.

The most effective strategy for assessing appropriate weight loss is to measure the body composition of the athlete, and if body fat levels are higher than is considered optimal, weight loss can be responsibly guided by reducing body fat and maintaining FFM. A detailed description of the procedure to assist an athlete with healthy and responsible weight loss is provided in section V of this chapter. Assessment of body composition is helpful in determining both the levels of body fat and FFM. Body composition is not error-free, however, and the results should be applied appropriately. Even when the best assessment methods are used (e.g., hydrostatic weighing and bone density assessment or DXA), the error associated with estimating body fat ranges from 1–3%.[51] Using other methods increases this range of error. Using skinfold or bioelectrical impedence measures very carefully, and applying the correct prediction equations will at best result in a prediction error of 3% body fat.[51] This means that if percentage body fat is measured at 16%, actual percentage body fat may be as low as 13% or as high as 19%. Because many individuals who assess body composition in athletes are not adequately trained, the prediction error could be even greater.

As with body weight standards, many abuses of values are derived using measures of body composition. The following is an example of inappropriate use of skinfold measures in an athlete: A female distance runner has her body composition assessed using skinfold calipers. Her body fat is calculated to be 15%. The team standard for body fat is 14%, and this athlete is instructed to lose approximately

10 pounds (4.5 kg) in an attempt to reduce her body fat to desirable levels. As just reviewed, even under the best circumstances of measurement this athlete's body fat may be as low as 12% or as high as 18%. Thus, this athlete may already have a percentage body fat within desirable ranges, and weight loss is not necessary. In addition, the goal for weight loss is based on an arbitrary decision, and is not based on the athlete's existing body fat stores.

It has been suggested[51] that the minimal levels of body fat that are compatible with health are 12% for women and 5% for men. The scenario just presented is common, especially among collegiate athletic teams. In this type of situation, it is important not only to have realistic and healthy percentage body-fat goals, but to measure body composition using another, preferably more accurate method to get a clearer picture of whether this athlete has a percentage body fat that falls within desirable ranges.

Unfortunately, there are numerous situations in which starting line-ups, scholarship status, and punitive exercise measures are determined solely based upon an athlete's percentage body fat. Athletes can also be devastated by the results of these tests, and may be driven to extreme measures to reach a goal that may or may not be realistic. It is critical that the athlete, coach, and family of the athlete are aware of the limitations of body composition assessments in order to gain a realistic attitude toward ways to improve performance, and avoid focusing on reducing body weight and body fat entirely as factors to enhance performance.

If weight loss is indicated, it is important to maintain as much FFM as possible. This can be accomplished by setting realistic body-weight and body-fat goals based upon the existing FFM. The new goal weight can be calculated using the following formula:[52]

$$\text{Goal Weight} = \frac{\text{Fat-free mass (FFM)}}{1 - \text{desired \% body fat}}$$

For example, a male basketball player has been measured at 230 pounds (104.5 kg), 17% body fat and has a FFM of 191 pounds (85.4 kg). The goal for this player is to reduce body fat to a range of 10–13%. Applying the range of desired percentage body fat values, this athlete's goal weight range is 212–220 pounds (96–100 kg). This calculation assumes that the athlete will lose predominantly fat mass and maintain FFM. If we apply this equation to the scenario with the female athlete discussed previously (assuming she weighs 115 pounds or 52.3 kg), we find that to reduce her percentage body fat from 15% to 13%, she would need to lose only 2 to 3 pounds (1–1.4 kg), not the 10 pounds (4.5 kg) recommended.

V. WEIGHT LOSS STRATEGIES

While there are a variety of healthy plans an athlete can follow for weight loss, there also is an abundance of strategies available that can be harmful and potentially deadly for the athlete. A review of both safe and pathogenic weight-loss strategies is provided in this section.

A. SAFE WEIGHT LOSS STRATEGIES

Successful and safe weight loss is dependent upon many factors. As training and performance are dependent upon sound nutrition, designing a program that addresses individual habits, food preferences, health needs, and training schedules will help ensure that the athlete will meet weight loss and performance goals. Table 9.1 outlines the steps to follow when designing a weight-loss plan for an athlete. While the athlete can use this information to design a weight-loss program, it is most beneficial to seek assistance from a registered dietitian (RD) who is trained in sports nutrition. Many universities have full- and part-time RDs who can assist athletes with meeting their weight loss goals, and there are also RDs working in the community who specialize in sports nutrition. If possible, weight loss should be accomplished during the off-season, as losing weight during the season can negatively impact training and performance. The ideal rate of weight loss is 1–2 pounds per week (0.5–1kg), as faster weight loss can lead to loss of FFM. Measuring the body composition, current dietary intake, and typical activity level of an athlete are necessary to determine the energy and macronutrient needs of the athletes. As discussed earlier, prescribing a diet high in unprocessed carbohydrates (whole grains/cereals, fruits and vegetables) will ensure adequate carbohydrate for training and glycogen repletion and help control hunger. It is always a good idea for an athlete to take a general multi-vitamin/mineral supplement when dieting, especially if energy intake is less than 2000 kcal/d.

B. PATHOGENIC STRATEGIES AND HEALTH CONCERNS

Pathogenic weight loss strategies include any weight loss behaviors or actions that are potentially harmful to the athlete. These strategies include restrained eating, chronic dieting, bingeing and purging, skipping meals, fasting, excessive exercise, laxative or diet pill abuse, and dehydration. Although participating in these behaviors can lead to weight loss, numerous health problems can result, so athletes need to be educated about the risks of these types of behaviors. Some of the most common health concerns that can result from practicing pathogenic weight-loss strategies are nutritional deficiencies, eating disorders, and severe dehydration. Each of these concerns can have a negative impact on the health and performance of athlete. While many athletes and coaches may view these problems as acute (short term) and having no long-term impact on health, the following evidence suggests that these dietary practices can seriously threaten the long-term health of the athlete. Below we have "bulleted" some of the adverse health effects associated with various weight-loss practices:

- **Nutritional deficiencies**. In order to lose weight, athletes frequently restrict food intake by skipping meals, eliminating food groups, fasting, or eating only one to three foods a day. Anytime athletes regularly restrict energy intake to <1500 kcal/d for females and <1800 kcal/d for men, they are at increased risk for poor nutrient intakes. This level of energy intake is too low to meet the macro- and micronutrients needs of the body and fuel the body for exercise, especially if physical activity is high. Severe energy restriction is especially a problem for female athletes, since they

TABLE 9.1
Steps To Follow When Designing a Weight Loss Plan for an Athlete*

- Assess body composition using the most accurate method(s) available. Calculate a reasonable goal weight range for the athlete using the following equation:

$$\text{Goal weight} = \frac{\text{fat-free mass (FFM)}}{1 - \text{desired \% body fat}}$$

- Assess current dietary intake using weighed diet records.* Information should be considered regarding dietary habits, including the time and places where food is consumed. Determine situations that may trigger the athlete to overeat.
- Determine the athlete's current activity level using activity records or published questionnaires. Analyze the athlete's activity patterns. Are they optimal for inducing weight loss? If not, determine any adjustments that need to be made in daily activity patterns to increase TDEE.
- Estimate energy balance by subtracting energy expenditure from energy intake. Energy restriction should equal about 300–500 kcal/d less than the current energy needed to maintain body weight. Remember, it is common for individuals to under-report energy intake[65] and over-report physical activity levels. If the energy intake of the athlete appears to be low, use either the energy-expenditure estimate from the activity records or the midpoint value between reported energy intake and energy expenditure as the energy-intake goal for weight loss.
- The diet plan should be designed around the recommended macronutrient intakes of athletes while taking into account the athlete's individual needs based on sport, food preferences, and costs. Diets should be high in unprocessed carbohydrate, such as beans and legumes, whole grain cereals and breads, fruits, vegetables, and low-fat meats and dairy.
- All athletes on a reduced-energy diet plan should take a multivitamin/mineral supplement. Women may also need to take an additional calcium supplement, with vitamin D added. Iron supplementation can benefit those at risk for iron depletion and deficiency anemia. Before taking iron supplements, iron status should be assessed, current dietary sources determined and excess iron losses identified. Iron supplementation should be done under the direction of a health professional.
- Encourage regular fluid intake. Athletes need to consume enough fluid to replace losses that occur with training and normal metabolism.
- Encourage athletes to eat small meals and snacks throughout the day to reduce feelings of hunger. Select foods that have low energy density (kcal/g) such as salads, whole fruits, broth-based soups, and vegetables.
- Encourage the athlete to maintain healthy dietary practices. Stress the importance of maintaining training and performance while achieving gradual weight loss of 1–2 pounds (0.5–1 kg) per week.
- Athletes should limit or avoid consuming alcoholic beverages and other forms of high-sugar, low-nutrient-dense beverages. Alcohol decreases fat oxidation and increases fat storage while increasing appetite.[66]

* For details on using diet and activity records to estimate energy balance refer to Thompson and Manore.[21]

---

typically need less energy than male athletes due to their smaller body size. In addition, even female athletes who are not dieting frequently have energy and nutrient intakes that are below recommended levels.[53,4] Carbohydrate, iron, calcium, B-vitamins (B_6. B_{12}, folate), vitamin D, magnesium, iron, and zinc are nutrients particularly affected by energy restriction among athletes. All of these nutrients are critical for optimal health and performance. Chronically low-energy and -nutrient intakes can lead to glycogen depletion, decreased oxygen-carrying capacity, increased incidence of bone fractures, and higher injury rates due to fatigue and impaired cell growth and repair. With these concerns in mind, athletes reducing body weight will benefit from taking a complete multivitamin/mineral supplement, and female athletes may also need to take supplemental calcium and vitamin D.

- **Disordered eating.** For some athletes, chronically dieting to maintain a low body weight can be the first step toward developing a clinical eating disorder such as bulimia nervosa or anorexia nervosa, or eating disorders not otherwise specified (EDNOS).[1,48,55] See Beals[1] for a complete review of disordered eating issues in athletes. The rates of eating disorders and disordered eating among athletes participating in aesthetic, thin-build and weight-dependent sports (e.g., gymnastics, dance, distance running, and figure skating) are significantly higher than in sports where weight is not such an issue.[48] Persistent dietary restriction can lead to binge-and-purge eating. Bingeing includes consuming large quantities of food at one time, followed by purging using practices such as self-induced vomiting, laxatives, diuretics, and excessive exercise. Bingeing and purging are extremely dangerous practices that can lead to clinical eating disorders, tooth decay, poor performance, dehydration, and even death due to fluid and electrolyte imbalances.[1] Excessive exercise is one form of purging, and is commonly used by athletes to attempt to prevent storage of any excess energy that may be consumed. Our personal experiences have shown that many college females keep a meticulous count of energy (kcals) consumed over the day and use exercise as a means to punish self-proclaimed "bad" eating behaviors. Athletes should not deprive themselves of favorite foods or use excessive exercise as a punitive measure.

  One negative health consequence related to disordered eating and eating disorders, such as anorexia nervosa, is menstrual dysfunction in female athletes. Menstrual dysfunction, which includes amenorrhea, oligomenorrhea, and subclinical ovulatory disturbances, also occurs in many female athletes who do not have an eating disorder but may be under eating for their sport. Physical and psychological stress, low energy intakes, and intense training have been implicated in contributing to menstrual disturbances in female athletes.[50,53,56,57] The athlete's hormonal status and energy stores, and the severity of energy restriction interact to play a significant role in the onset of menstrual dysfunction.[58] The potential health problems associated with menstrual dysfunction are currently being examined by a number of investigators and include decreased bone mineral density, impaired reproductive function, and increased risk for cardiovascular disease.

- **Dehydration and laxative abuse**. Participation in weight-class sports, such as wrestling, boxing, crew, and horse racing (jockeys), can push athletes to lose weight rapidly to qualify for a lower weight category or meet a designated weight. Weight-class athletes frequently participate in rapid weight loss practices such as fasting, dehydrating, and bingeing and purging.[49] Dehydration is a practice commonly used for rapid weight loss in athletes needing to "make weight." Wrestlers are among certain groups of athletes who dehydrate themselves by exercising intensely in hot environments while wearing vapor-impermeable suits. They may also combine this activity with fluid restriction, the use of diuretics and laxatives, and vomiting.[49] This practice is extremely dangerous and the National Collegiate Athletic Association (NCAA) has restricted weight loss for wrestlers to no more than 1.5% of body weight per week.[59,60] Despite these attempts to prevent the use of dehydration to achieve rapid weight loss, these practices are still used by high school and collegiate-level wrestlers. In extreme cases, death can result.

The deaths of three collegiate wrestlers emphasize the risk of using dehydration to achieve rapid weight loss.[61] All three wrestlers used similar rapid weight loss strategies over 3–12 h, including restricted food and fluid intake and excessive exercise in hot environments while wearing vapor-impermeable suits. Preliminary reports suggest that death resulted from hyperthermia, which was induced by the use of pathogenic strategies. A recent survey of 43 college wrestling teams found that the most weight lost during the season was 5.3 ± 2.8 kg or 6.9% ± 4.7%, while the most weight during the week was 2.9 ± 1.3 kg or 4.3% ± 2.3%.[49] The three wrestlers who died lost an average of 30 pounds (13.6 kg) or 15% of total pre-season weight.[61] It is obvious from these findings that practicing dehydration during periods of extreme weight loss can be fatal. Thus, strategies for maintaining regular fluid intake should be an integral part of a safe weight loss plan.

VI. WEIGHT GAIN STRATEGIES

At first glance, it would seem that weight gain in an athlete should be easy — it would be a natural result of simply eating more food (kilocalories) each day. However, the reality is not that simple for athletes who are trying to gain weight. As with weight loss, a number of factors (lifestyle, genetics, environment, social interaction, stage of growth, and exercise training program) must be considered if successful weight gain (e.g., gains in strength and FFM) are to occur. Since neither weight loss nor weight gain is easy, a number of supplements have been developed "promising" to help athletes achieve their weight goals. Of course, if these products worked, there would not be so many athletes unsuccessful at reaching their weight goals. When these products do work, they usually contain banned substances (e.g., ephedra for weight loss; anabolic steroids for weight gain) that can get athletes eliminated from their sports.[62] Below is a discussion of techniques for assuring that weight gain is composed primarily of FFM, follows sound training and dietary guidelines, and is done within a reasonable time frame. It is important to recognize that the energy recommendations made for someone who wants to gain weight will be different from the individual who wants to maintain current body weight but change body composition. For weight gain, energy intake must exceed energy expenditure, placing the athlete in positive energy balance.

A. GAINING MUSCLE MASS

For most athletes, weight gain really means increases in muscle mass and strength. To assure that the weight gained is muscle mass and not fat, the athlete must participate in a well-designed RT program, continue to participate in the training program of their individual sport, and consume an energy-dense diet that puts them into positive energy balance. The athlete still needs to allow time for rest and recovery, since overtraining will not allow for the synthesis of new muscle tissue. Working with a strength coach will help assure that the RT program is realistic and will help athletes achieve their goals. Athletes also need to work with a sports dietitian to assure that weight gain goals are realistic (1–2 pounds/wk; 0.25–0.50 kg/wk) within the time frame set. If weight gain is too rapid, the result may be a gain in fat mass and not muscle mass. Gains in muscle mass are best done in the off-season, when the demands of athletes' individual training programs for their sport will be less intense. This allows them to focus on their diets and their RT programs, while also allowing adequate time for rest.

As with weight loss, to gain weight the energy balance equation must be considered. Energy intake must be higher than energy expenditure and careful attention needs to be paid to the composition of the diet. The dietary recommendations for increases in body weight, with a focus on muscle mass, are listed below.[63] This topic is discussed in more detail by Tarnopolosky.[37]

Estimate total energy expenditure and increase total energy intake by 300–500 kcal/d above estimated energy expenditure, while maintaining a healthy composition to the diet (~55–65% of energy from carbohydrate; ~20–25% of energy from fat; ~10–20% of energy from protein). The actual macronutrient composition of the diet will depend on the individual athlete, since some athletes eat so many kcal/d that even a diet that contains 50% of the energy from carbohydrate is adequate to replace muscle glycogen.[21,64]

Increase meal and snack frequency, which should naturally increase energy intake. If the athlete is already consuming a number of meals and snack, using meal-replacement drinks or high-carbohydrate glycogen-replacement drinks between meals or immediately after exercise is an easy way to increase energy intake without contributing to feeling too full.

Increase protein intake to approximately 1.6 g/kg body weight. This level of protein intake will provide the additional protein needed for new tissue synthesis and will increase the percentage of energy from protein while decreasing the energy from carbohydrate and fat. A dietary protein intake that represents about 15% of energy from protein, in an energy-sufficient or -positive diet, should be adequate to cover the requirements of most athletes, including both strength and endurance athletes.[37] Thus, most athletes do not need to add protein powders or shakes to their diet in order to achieve their protein needs unless this is a dietary preference for them.

Timing of meals and snacks around exercise training will assure that the athlete has numerous opportunities to increase energy intake, goes to practice well fueled, and provides the nutrients required for building muscle and replacing glycogen once exercise is over. A post-training snack that provides both carbohydrate and high-quality protein (7–10g) may help optimize the body's ability to synthesize protein while minimizing protein catabolism.[37]

Monitor amount and type of fat intake. Although weight gain is the objective, fat gain is not. Athletes still need to select healthy fats (olive and canola oil, fatty fish, nuts, lower-fat meat and dairy) and reduce intakes of saturated and trans fatty acids.

VII. CONCLUSIONS AND RECOMMENDATIONS

It is apparent that a plethora of weight loss strategies is available for use by athletes. The key to successful weight loss includes providing a diet plan that allows for maintenance of exercise training, health, and performance. Pathogenic weight-loss strategies, while used frequently by some athletes, should be avoided at all times. For the athlete who wants to gain weight, the struggle can be just as challenging as weight loss is for the athlete who wants to lose weight. For them, the keys to success depend on a good RT program, a diet plan that allows for positive energy balance while containing nutrient-rich foods, and adequate time to achieve the weight-gain goal. Working with a sports dietitian will make this process easier and reduce the risk of using unhealthy weight gain strategies.

REFERENCES

1. Beals, K. A., *Disordered Eating Among Athletes*. Human Kinetics, Champaign, IL, 2004.
2. O'Conner, H, and Caterson, I.,Weight loss and the athlete. In Burke L., Deakin V., Eds. *Clinical Sports Nutrition, 3rd Edition.* McGraw-Hill: Boston, 2006, pp. 135–173.
3. Levine, J.A., Non-exercise activity thermogenesis (NEAT). *Nutrition Reviews*, 62, S82–S97, 2004.
4. Levine, J.A., Eberhardt, N.L., and Jensen, M.D., Role of non-exercise activity thermogenesis in resistance to fat gain in humans. *Science,* 283, 212–214, 1999.
5. Levine, J.A., Lanningham-Foster, L.M., McCrady, S.K., Krizan, A.C., Olson, L.R., Kane, P.H., Jensen, M.D., and Clark, M.M., Interindividual variation in posture allocation: Possible role in human obesity. *Science*, 307, 584–589, 2005.
6. Ravussin, E., A NEAT way to control weight? *Science*, 307, 530–531, 2005.
7. Thompson, J.L., Manore, M.M., Skinner, J.S., Ravussin, E., and Spraul, M. Daily energy expenditure in male endurance athletes with differing energy intakes. *Med. Sci. Sports Exerc.,* 27,347–354, 1995.
8. Ravussin, E. and Bogardus, C., Relationship of genetics, age and physical fitness to daily energy expenditure and fuel utilization. *Am. J. Clin. Nutr.*; 49,968–75, 1989.
9. Bullough, R. C., Gillette, C. A., Harris, M. A., and Melby, C. L. Interaction of acute changes in exercise energy expenditure and energy intake on resting metabolic rate. *Am. J. Clin. Nutr.*, 61, 473–481, 1995.
10. Poehlman, E. T., McAuliffe, T .L., VanHouten, D. R., and Danforth, E., Influence of age and endurance training on metabolic rate and hormones in healthy men. *Am. J. Physiol.*, 259, E66–E72, 1990.

11. Broeder, C. E., Burrhus, K. A., Svanevik, L. A., and Wilmore, J. H., The effects of aerobic fitness on resting metabolic rate. *Am. J. Clin. Nutr.*, 55, 795–801, 1992.

12. Horton, T. J. and Geissler, C. A., Effect of habitual exercise on daily energy expenditure and metabolic rate during standardized activity. *Am. J. Clin. Nutr.*; 59,13–19, 1994.

13. Byrne, H. K. and Wilmore, J. H., The effects of a 20-week exercise training program on resting metabolic rate in previously sedentary, moderately obese women. *Int. J. Sport Nutr. Exerc. Metab.*, 11,15–31, 2001.

14. Keytel, L. R., Lambert, M. I., Johnson, J., Noakes, T. D., and Lambert, E. V., Free living energy expenditure in post menopausal women before and after training. *Int. J. Sport Nutr. Exerc. Metab.*, 22, 226–237, 2001.

15. Bouchard, C., Tremblay, A., Nadeau, A., Despres, J. P., Theriault, G., Boulay, M. R., Lortie, G., Leblanc, C., and Fournier, G., Genetic effect in resting and exercise metabolic rates. *Metabolism*, 38, 364–370, 1989.

16. Bosselaers, I., Buemann, B., Victor, O. J., and Astrup, A., Twenty-four-hour energy expenditure and substrate utilization in body builders. *Am. J. Clin. Nutr.*, 59,10–12, 1994.

17. Thompson, J. L., Manore, M. M., and Thomas, J., Effect of diet and diet-plus-exercise on resting metabolic rate: A meta analysis. *Int. J. Sport Nutr.*, 6: 41–61, 1996.

18. Donnelly, J. E., Jacobsen, D. L., Jakacic, J. M., and Whatley, J. E. Very low calorie diet with concurrent versus delayed and sequential exercise. *Int. J. Obesity*, 18, 469–475, 1994.

19. Tremblay, A., Simoneau, J., and Bouchard, C., Impact of exercise intensity on body fatness and skeletal muscle metabolism. *Metabolism*. 43, 814–818, 1994.

20. Poehlman, E. T. and Melby, C. Resistance training and energy balance. *Int. J. Sport Nutr.* 8, 143–159, 1998.

21. Manore, M.M. and Thompson, J.L., *Sport Nutrition for Health and Performance*. Human Kinetics Publishers, Champaign, IL, 2000, ch. 5.

22. Bahr, R., Ingnes, I., Vaage, O., Sejersted, O.,M., Newsholme, E. A., Effect of duration of exercise on excess post-exercise O$_2$ consumption. *J. Appl. Physiol.*, 62, 485–490, 1987.

23. Bahr, R., Gronnerod, O., Sejersted, O.M., Effect of supramaximal exercise on excess postexercise O$_2$ consumption. *Med. Sci. Sport Exer.*, 24, 66–71, 1992.

24. Melby, C., Scholl, C., Edwards, G., and Bullough, R., Effect of acute resistance exercise on postexercise energy expenditure and resting metabolic rate. *J. Appl. Physiol.*, 75(4), 1847–1853, 1993.

25. Osterberg ,K. L., and Melby, C. L., Effect of acute resistance exercise on postexercise oxygen consumption and resting metabolic rate in young women. *Int. J. Sport Nutr. Exerc. Metab.* 10, 71–81, 2000.

26. Smith, J. and McNaughton, L., The effects of intensity of exercise on excess post-exercise oxygen consumption and energy expenditure in moderately trained men and women. *Eur. J. Appl. Physiol.*, 67, 420–425, 1993.

27. Flatt, J. P., The biochemistry of energy expenditure. In: Bray, G., ed. *Recent Advances in Obesity Research II*. London: John Libbey, 1978, pp. 211–228

28. Jequier, E., Regulation of thermogenesis and nutrient metabolism in the human: Relevance for obesity. In: Bjorntorp, P., Brodoff, B. N., eds. *Obesity*. Philadelphia: Lippincott, 1992, pp. 130–135.

29. Hollis, J. H., Mattes, R. D. Are all calories created equal? Emerging issues in weight management. *Curr. Diabetes Reports*, 5, 374–378, 2005.

30. Swinburn, B. and Ravussin, E., Energy balance or fat balance? *Am. J. Clin. Nutr.*, 57(suppl), 766S–71S, 1993.

31. Flatt, J. P., Macronutrient composition and food selection. *Obesity Res.,* 9, 256S–262S, 2001.

32. Saris, W. H. M., Sugars, energy metabolism and body weight control. *Am. J. Clin. Nutr.,* 78(suppl):850S–857S, 2003.

33. Saris, W. H. M. and Tarnopolsky, M.A., Controlling food intake and energy balance: Which macronutrient should we select? *Curr. Opinion Clin. Nutr. Metab. Care,* 6, 609–613, 2003.

34. Thomas, C. D., Peters, J. C., Reed, W. G., Abumrad, N. N., Sun, M., and Hill. J. O., Nutrient balance and energy expenditure during ad libitum feeding of high-fat and high-carbohydrate diets in humans. *Am. J. Clin. Nutr.,* 55, 934–942, 1992.

35. Suter, P.M., Is alcohol consumption a risk factor for weight gain and obesity? *Critical Rev. Clin. Lab. Sci.,* 43, 197–227, 2005.

36. Institute of Medicine (IOM), Food and Nutrition Board. *Dietary Reference Intakes for Energy, Carbohydrate, Fiber, Fat, Fatty Acids, Cholesterol, Protein, and Amino Acids.* Washington DC: National Academy Press, 2005.

37. Tarnopolosky, M., Protein and amino acids needs for training and bulking up. In: Burke, L., Deakin, V., eds. *Clinical Sports Nutrition, 3rd Edition.* McGraw-Hill: Boston, 2006, pp.73–98.

38. Duncan, K. H., Bacon, J. A., and Weinsier, R. L., The effects of a high and low energy dense diets on satiety, energy intake and eating time of obese and non-obese subjects. *Am. J. Clin. Nutr.,* 37, 763–767, 1983.

39. Lissner, L., Levitsky, D. A., Strupp, B. J., Kalkwarf, H. J., and Roe, D. A. Dietary fat and the regulation of energy intake in human subjects. *Am. J. Clin. Nutr.,* 46, 886–886, 1987.

40. Tremblay, A., Plourde, G., Depres, J. P., and Bouchard, C., Impact of dietary fat content and fat oxidation on energy intake in humans. *Am. J. Clin. Nutr.,* 49, 799–895, 1989.

41. Ledikwe, E. J., Blanck, H. M., Kettle K. L., Serdula, M. K., Seymour, J. D., Tohill, B. C., and Rolls, B. J. Dietary energy density is associated with energy intake and weight status in US adults. *Am. J. Clin. Nutr.,* 84, 1362–1268, 2006.

42. Rolls, B. J., Drewnowski, A., and Ledikwe, J. H., Changing the energy density of the diet as a strategy for weight management. *J. Am. Diet. Assoc.,* 105, S98–103, 2005.

43. Rolls, B. J., Roe, L. S., and Meengs, J. S., Salad and satiety: energy density and portion size of a first-course salad affect energy intake at lunch. *J. Am. Diet. Assoc.,* 104, 1570–1576, 2004.

44. Atkins, R.C., *Atkins for Life.* St. Martin's Press, New York, 2003.

45. Foster, G. D., Wyatt, H, R., Hill, J. O., McGuckin, B. G., Brill, C., Mohammed, B. S., Szapary, P. O., Rader, D. J., Edman, J. S., and Klein, S. A randomized trial of a low-carbohydrate diet for obesity. *N.Engl J.Med.,* 348, 2082–2090, 2003.

46. Niakaris, K., Magkos, F., Geladas, N., Sidossis, L. S., Insulina sensitivity derived from oral glucosa tolerante testing in athletes: disagreement between available indicies. *J. Sports Sci.,* 23, 1065–1073, 2005.

47. Burke, L. Preparation for competition. In: Burke, L. and Deakin, V., Eds. *Clinical Sports Nutrition, 3rd Edition.* McGraw-Hill: Boston, 2006, pp. 335–384.

48. Beals, K. A., Manore, M. M., Disordered eating and menstrual dysfunction in female collegiate athletes. *Int. J. Sport Nutr. Exerc. Metab.,* 12, 281–293, 2002.

49. Oppliger, R. A., Steen, S. A. N., Scott, J. R., Weight loss practices of college wrestlers. *Int. J. Sport Nutr. Exerc. Metab.* 13, 29–46, 2003.

50. Otis, C. L., Drinkwater, B., Johnson, M., Loucks, A., and Wilmore, J., The female athlete triad. *Med. Sci. Sports Exerc.,* 29, i–ix, 1997.

51. Lohman, T. G., *Advances in Body Composition Assessment*, Human Kinetics, Champaign, IL, 1992, p. 7.
52. Wilmore, J. H., Body weight standards and athletic performances, In: *Eating, Body Weight and Performance in Athletes. Disorders of Modern Society*. Brownell, K. D., Rodin, J., and Wilmore, J. H., Eds., Lea and Febiger, Philadelphia, 1992, 315–329.
53. Manore, M. M., Nutritional recommendations and athletic menstrual dysfunction. *Int. Sport Med. J.*, 5, 45–55, 2004.
54. Manore, M. M. and Woolf, K., Nutritional concerns of the female athlete. In: *Ensuring the Health of Active and Athletic Girls and Women*. Ransdell, L. and Petlichkoff, L. eds., Waldorf, MD: National Association for Girls and Women in Sport, American Alliance for Health, Physical Education, Recreation and Dance, 2005, pp. 167–203.
55. Beals, K.A. and Manore, M.M.. Behavioral, psychological, and physical characteristics of female athletes with subclinical eating disorders. *Int. J. Sport Nutr. Exerc. Metab.*, 10,128–143, 2000.
56. Dueck, C.A., Manore, M.M., and Matt, K.S., Role of energy balance in athletic menstrual dysfunction. *Int. J. Sport Nutr.*, 6, 90–116, 1996.
57. Manore, M.M., Running on empty: Health consequences of chronic dieting in active women. *ACMS's Hlth. Fitness J.*, 2, 24–31, 1998.
58. Loucks, A. B., Energy balance and body composition in sports and exercise. *J. Sports Sci.*, 22, 1–14, 2004.
59. National Collegiate Athletic Association (NCAA), NCAA Sports Medicine Handbook 2005–06, http://www.ncaa.org. Accessed October, 2006.
60. National Collegiate Athletic Association (NCAA), NCAA 2007 Wrestling Rules and Interpretations. http://www.ncaa.org. Accessed October, 2006.
61. Division of Nutrition and Physical Activity, Hyperthermia and dehydration-related deaths associated with intentional rapid weight loss in three collegiate wrestlers — North Carolina, Wisconsin, and Michigan. *Morbidity Mortality Wkly.*, 47, 105, 1998.
62. Maughan, R. J. Contamination of dietary supplements and positive drug test in sport. *J Sports Sci.*, 23, 883–889, 2004.
63. Slater, G., Practical Tips — Bulking up. In: Burke, L. and Deakin, V., Eds. *Clinical Sports Nutrition, 3rd Edition*. McGraw-Hill Publ: Boston, 2006, pp. 99–103.
64. Manore, M. M., and Thompson, J. L., Energy requirements of the athlete: Assessment and evidence of energy efficiency. In: Burke, L. and Deakin, V., Eds. *Clinical Sports Nutrition, 3rd Edition*. McGraw-Hill: Boston, MA, 2006, pp. 113–134.
65. Trabulis, J. and Schoeller, D. A., Evaluation of dietary assessment instruments against doubly labeled water, a biomarker of habitual energy intake. *Am. J. Physiol. Endocrinol. Metab.*, 281, E891–E899, 2001.
66. Yoemans, M. R., Caton, S., and Hetherington, M. M., Alcohol and food intake. *Curr. Opin. Clin. Nutr. Metab. Care*, 6, 639–644, 2003.

Index